PEDIATRIC
MANUAL MEDICINE

For my patients

who challenge me daily to learn more,
work harder and be a better physician.

For Elsevier

Publisher: *Sarena Wolfaard*
Development Editors: *Claire Wilson, Barbara Simmons*
Project Manager: *Emma Riley*
Designer: *Charles Gray*
Illustration Manager: *Merlyn Harvey*
Illustrator: *Joanna Cameron*

PEDIATRIC MANUAL MEDICINE

AN OSTEOPATHIC APPROACH

Jane E Carreiro DO

Osteopathic Physician, Associate Professor and Chair
Department of Osteopathic Manipulative Medicine
University of New England College of Osteopathic Medicine
Biddeford, Maine, USA

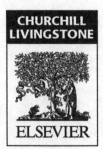

Edinburgh London New York Oxford Philadelphia St Louis Sydney Toronto 2009

CHURCHILL
LIVINGSTONE
ELSEVIER

First published 2009

ISBN: 978-0-443-10308-7

British Library Cataloguing in Publication Data
A catalogue record for this book is available from the British Library

Library of Congress Cataloging in Publication Data
A catalog record for this book is available from the Library of Congress

Notice
Neither the Publisher nor the Author assumes any responsibility for any loss or injury and/or damage to persons or property arising out of or related to any use of the material contained in this book. It is the responsibility of the treating practitioner, relying on independent expertise and knowledge of the patient, to determine the best treatment and method of application for the patient.

The Publisher

ELSEVIER your source for books, journals and multimedia in the health sciences
www.elsevierhealth.com

Working together to grow libraries in developing countries

www.elsevier.com | www.bookaid.org | www.sabre.org

ELSEVIER   BOOK AID International   Sabre Foundation

The Publisher's policy is to use **paper manufactured from sustainable forests**

Printed in China

Contents

This text attempts to provide guidance for the use of manipulative techniques in children. It focuses on common pediatric conditions affecting the neuromusculoskeletal system, but other conditions are discussed as well. The book is organized by body region rather than pathophysiological process. Each chapter consists of discussions of common clinical conditions, their presentation (Clinical Notes) and treatment (Treatment Notes), including descriptions of specific manipulative techniques that may be useful in management. Appropriate techniques are presented and adapted for different age groups: newborn, infant, toddler, child and athlete (the models resented being called adolescents).

The text is written from the perspective of the osteopathic structure–function models. These models, described in the chapter on basic principles, provide the framework for the discussion of each condition's pathophysiology, presentation, resulting compensatory responses and treatment philosophy. The medical and surgical information is current as of the completion of writing, but it is strongly recommended that the reader seek out the most recent publications in the appropriate journals.

Anatomical dissections, diagrams and radiographs have been included to aid in understanding many of the musculoskeletal relationships described. However, manipulation is like surgery: you cannot learn it from reading a book. This text assumes that the reader is well grounded in the principles and skills of manual medicine and manipulation. This text is not meant to be used as an introduction to the manipulative disciplines, but as an aid in applying these skills to help bring some relief to the younger members of our communities.

Our children are our future.

JE Carreiro
2008

Unless otherwise indicated, all photographs have been used with the permission of the Willard & Carreiro Collection.

Acknowledgements

Somehow, when I started this project I thought this would be very easy… Take some pictures, write some text, then Bob's your uncle (as the Brits say) and it would be done. Somehow I forgot that 2-year-olds will not sit still and let you re-shoot the same photograph. They don't want to take their clothes off and sit on a vinyl table for hours. Newborns grow REALLY fast and stop looking like newborns, and it takes a long time before another one arrives. Teenagers have hormones (that summarizes it nicely). So this project was not as easy as I thought it would be. In fact, the part I thought would be most time consuming – the dissections – were actually the easy part (cadavers are always there when you need them). Having said all that, this text owes its existence to a few very helpful, cooperative, reliable, hard-working, generous and extremely nice people: Nicholas Carreiro, Brayden Rattigan, Kendra Emery, Hunter Ferrill, Michael Willard, and Lauren Jane Willard. Their patience, help and wonderful smiles made the job a real pleasure, as did the man often behind the camera, my colleague, partner and friend Frank Willard PhD.

In addition, I owe a tremendous debt to Lynette Bassett DO, Heather Ferrill DO, and Noelle Sheretts-Ratigan DO. Their support in this project was instrumental to its completion. Jude Viola (soon to be DO) provided the most conscientious, thorough and complete help with editing, as well as her Zimstrer cookies, which kept me going.

I would like to thank my colleagues in the Osteopathic Manipulative Medicine department at the University of New England: Stephanie Waecker DO, Ron Mosiello DO, Bill Papura DO, Steve Goldbas DO, Doris Newman DO, John Pelletier DO, Mary Spang and Nancy Goulet, who have encouraged and supported this work. Others who have contributed to this process through discussion and analysis include Dr Kerstim Schmidt, Herr Dr Mathias Reidel, Herr Dr Bernhard Ewen, Herr Dr Johannes Mayer, Herr Dr Theo Rudolf , Karen Steele DO, Lisa Milder DO, and especially Hugh Ettlinger DO. Many thanks to Sarena Wolfaard, Claire Wilson, Barbara Simmons and the staff at Elsevier for their help and support with this project.

I am grateful for the support of the University of New England. The intellectual curiosity, enthusiasm and commitment of the students at the University's College of Osteopathic Medicine continue to be an inspiration for me, as are the dedication, passion, skill and contentiousness of the OPP/Anatomy Fellows with whom I have the exquisite pleasure to work.

Finally, I am grateful to all the individuals in this text who so selflessly gave of themselves so that we could learn from their sacrifice.

Chapter One

Basic principles

OVERVIEW

The body's inherent capacity for healing provides the cornerstone for the osteopathic approach to diagnosis and treatment of musculoskeletal conditions. Rather than limit palpatory diagnosis to the biomechanics of joints, the osteopathic concept expands the view of musculoskeletal dysfunction to include the impaired or altered function of all related components of the skeletal, visceral, arthrodial and myofascial structures and their vascular, lymphatic and neural elements. Musculoskeletal conditions need to be addressed from several perspectives, of which normalization of joint biomechanics is but one. Promoting lymphatic and venous drainage from an area may accelerate the removal of the byproducts of inflammation and cell death, and thus normalize tissue pH. Facilitating arterial flow increases oxygen and nutrient delivery to tissues undergoing repair. Compensatory tissue stresses and restrictions that develop subsequent to an injury or dysfunction alter biomechanics and potentially increase muscle workload. Nociception and pain can influence autonomic function at the spinal, brainstem and cortical levels. Tissue irritation can generate reflexive changes in smooth and striated muscle tone. Altered joint biomechanics may influence compressive loads on the joint, the function of related myofascial tissues, vascular and lymphatic flow, and overall homeostasis. This perspective is summarized in the osteopathic models of structure and function.

The structure–function models can be used to interpret clinical information, including biomechanical dysfunction, and to formulate plans for treatment. There are several models. The Biomechanical Model views the body as an integration of somatic components that relate as a posture and balance mechanism. Stresses or imbalances within this mechanism have the potential to affect dynamic function, increase energy expenditure, alter proprioception, change joint structure, impede neurovascular function and alter tissue metabolism. Working within this model, clinical management, including osteopathic manipulative techniques, focuses on restoring posture and balance relationships and enhancing the efficient use of the musculoskeletal components.

The second model, the Neurological Model, considers the interactions between spinal facilitation, proprioceptive function, the autonomic nervous system, and primary afferent nociceptors. The model expands to include the influence of these systems on the neuroendocrine immune network. The interrelatedness of the musculoskeletal and visceral systems through the autonomic nervous system is particularly important in this model, within which clinical interventions, including manipulative treatment, are used to reduce mechanical stresses, balance neural inputs and decrease afferent nociceptive drive.

The third model is called the Respiratory/Circulatory Model. It concerns itself with the maintenance of extra- and intracellular environments through the unimpeded delivery of oxygen and nutrients and the removal of cellular waste products. Any tissue stress interfering with the flow or circulation of any body fluid can affect tissue health. Within this model osteopathic manipulation and other clinical interventions are used to address the dysfunction or impedance of respiratory mechanics and the circulation and the flow of body fluids.

The fourth model is the Bioenergetic Model. This recognizes that the body seeks to maintain a balance between energy production, distribution and expenditure, thereby aiding its ability to adapt to various stressors. From the perspective of this model patient care, including manipulation, focuses on clinical findings such as somatic dysfunction, which have the potential to dysregulate the production, distribution or expenditure of energy.

The final model is the Biopsychosocial Model, which acknowledges the various reactions and psychological stresses with which the patient must contend. Health and the ability to heal may be affected by cultural, environmental, socioeconomic, physiological and psychological factors. Somatic dysfunction may be exacerbated or maintained as a response to environmental, socioeconomic, cultural or psychological conditions, and in turn may contribute to the patient's overall level of physiological stress.

The manual treatment techniques chosen should be based on the pathophysiology of the problem, the body's response, and the 'tissue feel.' In the concept of osteopathy 'tissue feel' includes texture, tone, tension, and movement characteristics. Depending on their structure and function, tissues respond differently to pathophysiological processes. Terminology has been created to describe or categorize the primary tissue types or phenomena noted with palpation. The most common terms include 'osseous' or 'articular,' referring to joints and bones; 'membranous' referring to ligaments; 'fascial' or 'myofascial,' which includes muscles, fascia, peritoneum and myometrium; 'fluid,' referring to intravascular and extravascular fluids; and 'potency,' referring to inherent energy.

The pathophysiology of neuromusculoskeletal conditions in children encompasses a wide variety of processes, each of which will elicit a different response from different tissues of the body. The osteopathic models of structure–function relationships can be used to understand the response of the body and determine the best way to facilitate healing. Therapeutically, the models are used in combination. For example, a condition having an inflammatory component, such as a tendinitis, could be viewed using the Respiratory/Circulatory Model to promote lymphatic drainage and arterial delivery, the Biomechanical Model to normalize tissue stresses around the joint, and the Neurological Model to reduce afferent drive. As a result, techniques addressing biomechanical dysfunction, fluid drainage and pain management might be employed. The specific techniques are chosen based on the tissue feel or phenomena that are most affected. Inflammatory diseases are immunologically mediated and primarily affect connective tissue. The elements of the immune system travel through the intravascular and extravascular fluids. Very often in patients with these disease processes abnormal tissue texture quality is palpable in the membranous, fascial and fluid phenomena. Techniques that address these phenomena and meet the goals of the structure–function models would be most appropriate for treatment. For example, the treatment of rheumatoid arthritis would encompass techniques that facilitate flow in the arterial and the low-pressure circulatory (lymphatic and venous drainage) systems to assist in maintaining a healthy environment for the tissue, and techniques that address nociception and the neuroendocrine immune system.

SOME KEY DIFFERENCES TO REMEMBER WHEN TREATING CHILDREN

Joint mechanics are influenced by the level of ossification present. The anatomical and functional barriers of any given joint are not present early in the ossification process. This may increase the joint's vulnerability to direct techniques and the vulnerability of joint surfaces to compressive forces. Ossification centers vary in the timing of their development (Table 1.1). Some first appear early in infancy but are not completed until young adulthood. Others begin much later and close in late puberty, which increases their susceptibility to shearing and tensile forces during a time of life associated with escalated physical activity. Areas of bone growth are at risk for localized ischemia and inflammation, both of which increase the threat of degenerative changes later in life.

Table 1.1 Age of onset and completion of ossification for selected areas

Bone area	Onset of ossification	Closure of ossification
Iliac crest	11–14 years	20 years
Anterior inferior iliac spine	13–15 years	16–18 years
Ischial tuberosity	13–15 years	16–18 years
Acetabulum	Birth	14–16 years
Femoral head	4 months	16–18 years
Greater trochanter	4–6 years	16–17 years
Lesser trochanter	11–12 years	15–16 years
Femoral condyles	Birth	16–18 years
Tibial plateau	Birth	16–20 years
Fibula head	3–4 years	16–20 years
Distal tibia	6 months	17–18 years
Clavicle, proximal end	17 years	20 years
Acromial process	14–15 years	18–20 years
Coracoid process	14–15 years	18–20 years
Humeral head	1st year	18–20 years
Distal humerus	Various centers 12 months to 10 years	14–17 years
Ulnar trochanter	8–10 years	14–17 years
Radial head	3–6 years	14–17 years
Ribs and sternum	1st year	25 years

The relationships that are maintained between the articular surfaces of any given joint are governed by the proprioceptive input from the surrounding ligaments, tendons and muscles. In adults there are well-defined body maps influencing the relationship of joint surfaces and the resting lengths of agonist and antagonist muscle groups. Movement patterns are also well established. These body maps serve to reinforce normal relationships after trauma or injury. Arguably, they must also play a role in the correction of biomechanical dysfunction using manual therapies. In many techniques, manual therapies rely on inherent somatosensory and motor mapping for the therapeutic process to succeed. Various terminologies may be used, depending on the manual approach, but no approach claims to create these functional maps or processes. Rather, manual therapy is applied to remove obstructions and impediments to normal function. In adults, one of the reasons there is a resolution of

biomechanical strains and a normalization of biomechanical relationships after manual therapy, be it osteopathy, chiropractic, or massage, etc., is because somatic maps exist that can reinforce those normal relationships. In children these maps are immature, and in some cases poorly established. As a result, tissue responses to manipulation in children, especially younger children, often differ from those in adults. The quality and quantity of change after the application of a technique may be less than usually felt in an adult. However, the child is more likely to incorporate this change into body movements sooner because they typically lack the compensatory adaptations present in the adult. Consequently, less is often more when treating children – or at least, less is often enough.

In the adult, somatic maps exist in the spinal cord, cerebellum and cortex which can reinforce normal muscular and articular relationships. When a muscle spasm relaxes, a restrictive barrier is removed or a fascial strain resolves, the map can then express itself. These maps do not exist at birth: they develop. When a child is born with a mechanical dysfunction, a congenital abnormality or a malposition, formation of the somatosensory maps may be distorted. This will influence motor patterning. Additionally, abnormal somatosensory and motor mapping may play a role in the cognitive issues seen in children with congenital motor problems. One needs to be cognizant of this when treating children. During times of growth, the musculoskeletal tissues undergo tremendous stress. Biomechanical strains and tissue stresses are often exacerbated. Children with chronic conditions should be treated close to times of growth. Furthermore, in very young children stresses that have apparently resolved with manipulative treatment may suddenly be exacerbated, albeit in a milder form, during growth periods. Parents should be forewarned of this. If the exacerbation does not resolve spontaneously over the course of a few days, then the child will probably need to be treated again. A simple way to think about this phenomenon is that a 4-month-old with congenital torticollis has had the dysfunction her entire life. Her body thinks it is normal. Although the biomechanical strain may be treated successfully, a portion of her somatosensory mapping has been created around the dysfunction. During a time of stress, such as growth, the mapping 'returns' to what it thinks is 'normal.'

BASIC PRINCIPLES OF OSTEOPATHIC MANIPULATIVE APPROACHES

Articulatory Technique

Background

The origin of articulatory techniques is unknown, although descriptions exist in ancient Greek, Egyptian and other

3

early cultures. Articulatory techniques are direct techniques that take a joint through its range of motion to engage and correct a restrictive barrier.

Principles of Diagnosis

Diagnosis is based upon range of motion changes at an articulation. The joint is moved slowly through all planes of motion and the restrictive barriers are identified. Tissue texture changes, such as muscle spasm, edema, and fibrosis, may be present and provide some clues as to the chronicity of the problem. The area may have an asymmetrical appearance compared to the other side. The presence of tenderness is a contraindication to articulatory techniques pending further evaluation.

Principles of Treatment

The affected joint is moved repetitively through the greatest and most complete range of motion possible, engaging but not moving through the restrictive barrier in each plane. The joint is first taken into its position of ease and then taken to the restrictive barrier. With each repetitive motion the restrictive barrier is engaged a bit more. For example, treatment of an internally rotated tibia would require the physician to flex the knee and internally rotate the tibia, and then immediately extend the knee and externally rotate the tibia. This sequence would be repeated several times. With each knee extension the tibia would be externally rotated a bit more.

Considerations when using Articulatory Techniques in Children

Articulatory techniques are quite useful in children of virtually all ages, except perhaps infants. Pain, swelling and tenderness are relative contraindications to articulatory techniques, pending further investigation. Joint instability, ligamentous laxity and connective tissue disease are absolute contraindications to this approach.

Balanced Ligamentous Technique (BLT)

Background

Balanced ligamentous and balanced membranous tension techniques were first described by William G. Sutherland in the early part of the 20th century (Lippincott 1949). Cranial osteopathy and osteopathy in the cranial field have their root in Sutherland's teachings. Balanced ligamentous tension (BLT) and membranous tension (BMT) techniques were described before the categorization of direct and indirect techniques was described. It is difficult to relegate this approach to either category because both direct and indirect forces can be used. Practitioners will categorize Sutherland's various techniques as balancing, involuntary mechanism, functional, biodynamic or cranial.

Ligamentous Articular Mechanisms

The principles of balanced ligamentous tension (BLT) are based on an understanding of ligamentous articular mechanisms. Ligaments regulate and guide movement between all the bones of the body. In most joints they act as checks to the voluntary actions of muscles. The wrist is a good example of a ligamentous articular mechanism. No muscles insert directly on the carpal bones. Flexion, extension, circumduction and other wrist motions result from the reciprocal movements of the carpal bones as they respond to the forces of the muscles of the forearm acting on the metacarpal and phalangeal bones. Motion at the wrist is initiated by the flexor and extensor carpi ulnaris and radialis muscles, and some of the muscles of the digits. However, the actual movements of the carpal bones are directed by the carpal ligaments. The specific insertion sites of the carpal ligaments create both fulcrums for movement and physiological barriers to movement. These checks and balances determine the complex movements of the carpal bones (Nordin and Frankel 1989, Norkin and Levangie 1992, Steinberg and Plancher 1995). For example, the carpi radialis muscles move the proximal phalanx of the thumb towards the radial side of the forearm. As the phalanx approximates to the radius, the trapezium, trapezoid and scaphoid accommodate this change in spatial relations by moving towards the midline of the wrist. The positions of the other carpal bones will adjust accordingly. None of the carpal bones are directed by muscular efforts: rather, they respond to distal muscular forces. This complicated movement is orchestrated and guided by the small ligaments lying between and around the carpal bones. All movements of the wrist are accomplished through a similar mechanism. Consequently, the carpal ligaments can be viewed as levers and pulleys and straps guiding the bones and the articular relationships. Sutherland described this arrangement as a ligamentous articular mechanism. Other examples of ligamentous articular mechanisms are the forearm (the intraosseous membrane of the radius and ulna), the intraosseous membrane of the tibia and fibula, and the foot. Sutherland also considered the internal dura as the intra-articular ligaments of the cranium and referred to the principles of balanced membranous tension to describe the mechanics in this area.

Balanced Tension

The positions of the carpal bones change, but the tensions on the carpal ligaments do not. In other words, when the wrist is flexed the dorsal ligaments are not stretched, nor do the palmar ligaments go slack. As long as the wrist is moved within its physiological range of motion, the tensions within the carpal ligaments remain balanced. Sutherland called this a balanced ligamentous articular mechanism. Although their range of motion is much less than that of the wrist, the ligaments of the foot are responsible for creating a system capable of weightbearing and mobility. Movements of the forefoot and hindfoot are dictated by the ligamentous arrangement. The sacroiliac joint is a yet another example of a ligamentous articular mechanism. Designed for weight-bearing and mobility, the sacroiliac joints must also be able to accommodate large changes in size, such as happen with labor and delivery, while maintaining stability. The ligaments of the sacroiliac and lumbosacral areas function with a reciprocal tension mechanism, responding to the moment-to-moment changes induced by gait (Magoun 1976, Snijders et al. 1993, Vleeming et al. 1995). According to Sutherland's model, all of the joints in the body are balanced ligamentous articular mechanisms. The ligaments provide proprioceptive information which guides the muscle response for positioning the joint, and the ligaments themselves guide the motion of the articular components.

Reciprocal Tension

Sutherland (1990) coined the terms 'reciprocal tension ligaments' and 'reciprocal tension mechanism' to describe the role of ligaments in joints. According his model, throughout the physiological range of motion of any given joint the associated ligaments maintain a constant level of tension. They do not stretch, nor do they become lax. The motion mechanics between the bones of a joint are a result of a change in the shape of the joint space, not because one set of ligaments becomes taut while another becomes slack. Think of the wrist moving in flexion and extension: as the wrist moves into flexion there is a displacement of the distal row of carpal bones towards the dorsal surface of the arm. During extension these same bones move towards the palmar surface. Accompanying these movements are rotations of individual bones. The sum total of these movements acts to maintain the tension of the carpal ligaments at a consistent level. This is a key concept in Sutherland's approach.

The type of motion that may take place at any given articulation is determined by the shape of the joint surfaces, the position of the ligaments, and the forces of the muscles acting upon the joint. Ligaments do not stretch and contract as muscles do; consequently, the tension in a ligament has very little variation. The tension distributed throughout the ligaments of any given joint is balanced. In normal movements, as the joint changes position the relationships between the ligaments also change, but the total tension within the articular mechanism does not (Fig. 1.1). However, when the joint is affected by injury, inflammation or mechanical forces etc., the distribution of tension between the ligaments is altered. This is what happens in somatic dysfunction. The

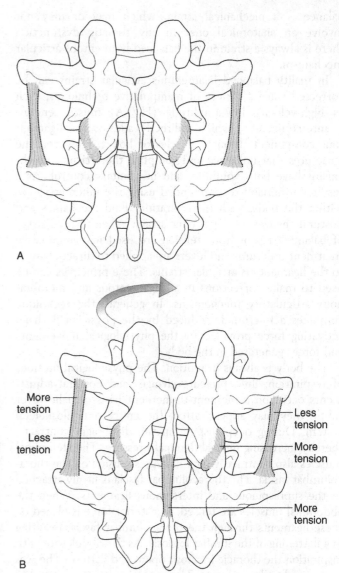

More tension

Less tension

Less tension

More tension

More tension

Fig. 1.1 • Schematic diagram of intervertebral segment in (A) a biomechanically neutral and (B) a right-rotated position. Note the variation in ligamentous tensions when the vertebra is rotated.

distribution and vector of tension within any given ligament will change according to the position of strain in the joint, but the shared tension within the ligamentous articular mechanism of any given joint remains constant as long as the ligament is not damaged. Sutherland called this a reciprocal tension mechanism. Of course, the balance within the ligamentous articular mechanism can be strained if the joint is inappropriately moved beyond its physiological range of motion. In the former case it is the balance of tension that is distorted. In the latter case, the fibers of the ligament are subjected to microscopic tears and stretch. Although this latter will most assuredly result in a strain to the balance of the articular ligaments, the ligaments do not need to be disrupted for the balance to be distorted. The distortion in balance is a mechanical strain, which may or may not involve an anatomical one. In any somatic dysfunction there is always a strain in the balanced ligamentous articular mechanism.

In reality balanced ligamentous articular strains can be corrected using a variety of manipulative techniques, such as high-velocity low-amplitude (HVLA) muscle energy, counterstrain, etc., which indirectly address the ligamentous component through muscles or bones. However, the structures that influence and comprise the articular mechanisms have both voluntary and involuntary control. As a result, Sutherland recommended using the inherent forces within the body, such as respiration, fluid mechanics and postural changes, to correct the strain. When the principles of balanced ligamentous tension are used in manipulative treatment, fulcrums and levers are applied to direct changes to the ligamentous articular strains. These principles can be used to make corrections in all ligamentous and membranous articulatory mechanisms. In general, the technique combines a fulcrum introduced by the physician with an activating force provided by the physiological movements and forces generated in the body.

The body is always in motion. The physiological motions of respiration, fluid pressure changes and postural adjustments occur on a moment-to-moment basis, and however subtle they may appear, affect the entire musculoskeletal system. During deep inspiration the diaphragm contracts, thereby increasing intra-abdominal pressure. The abdominal muscles also contract, which increases tension on the thoracolumbar fascia. The thoracolumbar fascia is firmly attached to the supraspinous and interspinous ligaments. When the abdominal muscles are tensed, a posterior force is placed on these ligaments through the thoracolumbar fascia, resulting in a flattening of the lumbar lordosis. As the ribs elevate with inspiration the thoracic kyphosis opens and flattens. The scalene muscles also contract. Their anterior attachment to the cervical vertebrae acts to flex the cervical spine. Thus the 'simple' act of respiration results in a response throughout the body (Fig. 1.2). This is an example of an inherent force – a physiological force acting within the body. The inherent forces within the body can be used as activating forces to assist the physician in the manipulative procedure. This is a very safe and effective method of treatment.

To be successful with balanced ligamentous and balanced membranous techniques, it is necessary to balance all the forces acting upon the ligamentous structures of the joint: this establishes a fulcrum that the inherent forces within the body can use to correct the strain.

Principles of Diagnosis

A strain in the balanced ligamentous articular mechanism of a joint creates an alteration in the permitted motion of

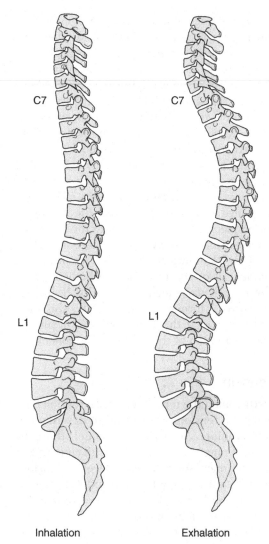

Inhalation   Exhalation

Fig. 1.2 • Schematic diagram depicting the changes in the sagittal spine curves during inhalation and exhalation.

that joint. This includes the normal motion that accompanies respiration and changes in position. Assessing the motion mechanics at a joint requires gentle tactile discrimination. Large movements are not necessary, nor are they useful when working with the ligamentous components. Patients may be examined sitting, supine or prone. The physician uses involuntary motion to determine the degree of restriction and the specifics of dysfunction. For example, we know that the thoracic kyphosis flattens slightly during inspiration. We can say that the upper thoracic vertebrae move toward extension (or backward bending) and the lower thoracic vertebrae move towards flexion as the anterior concavity straightens. Thus, if T3 is in a flexed lesion position – i.e. does not want to move into extension – it will resist the normal motion during inspiration. A strain in the balance of a ligamentous articular mechanism will produce exaggerated motion towards the position of the strain and restricted motion towards the neutral position. Ligamentous articular motion can be evaluated with quiet respiration and other inherent movements, but gentle motion testing may also be employed.

Principles of Treatment

The first and most important step in treatment is establishing balanced ligamentous tension in the articular mechanism so that the body's inherent forces can resolve the strain. The point of balanced ligamentous tension is 'the point in the range of motion of an articulation where the ligaments and membranes are poised between the normal tension present throughout the free range of motion and the increased tension preceding the strain…which occurs as a joint is carried beyond its normal physiology' (Magoun 1976).

All tensions between the ligaments of the articulation are equal. This may require the tension in any given tissues to be increased or reduced. Sutherland described five principles that can be applied to establish balanced membranous tension: exaggeration, direct action, decompression, opposing physiological motion, and molding. Each of these is described in the text. Exaggeration is an indirect approach. Balanced tension is achieved by slightly exaggerating the strain pattern or biomechanical dysfunction. Direct action established balanced tension by moving the strained articulation towards the restrictive barrier without engaging it. Decompression is used to reduce compressive forces on an area and thus establish balanced tension. Opposing physiological motion is created when the components of the articulation are moved in opposite directions to establish equal tension in the surrounding tissues, for example T4 is flexed as T5 is extended. Molding is a fluid technique that employs hydraulic forces to the tissue to create balanced tension. In most instances a combination of these principles is employed. Seldom is any one principle used in isolation.

As a joint reaches the extremes of its range of motion, the tensions within its ligaments increase; as the joint moves towards neutral, the tensions decrease so that in the neutral position the ligaments have the minimal amount of tension. When a joint is strained and normal motion restricted, the position of minimal tension within the joint is no longer its physiological neutral. Consequently, the point of balance for the ligaments will change in relation to the strain that is present. This new point of balanced tension exists somewhere between the tension created by the strain and the physiological neutral of the joint. We can look at this from a linear model (Fig. 1.3). When the articular mechanism is held at the precise (new) neutral position, all ligaments will be under the least possible strain. Then the physiological forces within the body become the activating forces to resolve the dysfunction.

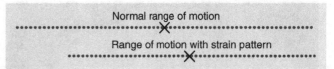

Fig. 1.3 • The upper diagram represents the range of motion in a vertebral joint with no somatic dysfunction. The lower diagram represents the range of motion in a vertebral joint that is rotated right. The midpoint or neutral of motion mechanics is represented by the 'x' in each diagram. The therapeutic point of balance is theoretically located somewhere between the neutral of the normal motion and neutral of the strain.

Initially the physician can learn to establish a neutral in a strained articular mechanism by assessing the degree of permitted motion in all planes. This is done by gently encouraging the joint first in one direction and then another. For example, to assess the degree of permitted motion in T3 extended and rotated right, the physician would encourage flexion and then extension. Next, she would assess rotation right then rotation left by applying a slow discriminating pressure to the spinous process. There will be a difference in the freedom of rotation in one direction as contrasted with another. The physician will easily discern a point in the motion of the joint where the tension in the articular mechanism is poised between the increased tension felt as the extremes of range of motion are approached. This is the point of balanced ligamentous tension. The physician will hold this position while the activating forces within the body, such as breathing, resolve the strain. When the strain corrects, the physician will feel a shift or change in the tension in the joint such that the neutral he created is no longer the point of minimal tension. In other words, the physician will often feel an increase in tension as the joint spontaneously moves towards its physiological neutral.

To establish the point of balanced ligamentous tension, the physician will need to assess the tension within the ligaments in all directions of motion. This is the most neutral position possible under the influence of all the factors responsible for the existing strain pattern. Thus, the balance point will change according to the pattern of the strain.

Osteopathy in the Cranial Field/Balanced Membranous Technique (for a complete description see Magoun, *Osteopathy in the Cranial Field* or Sutherland, *Teachings in the Science of Osteopathy*)

Background

Osteopathy in the cranial field was first described by Sutherland in the early part of the twentieth century. Sutherland's model has several key components: the fluctuation of the cerebral spinal fluid; the motility of the neural tube; the movement of the falx cerebri, tentorium cerebelli, and falx cerebelli as a reciprocal tension

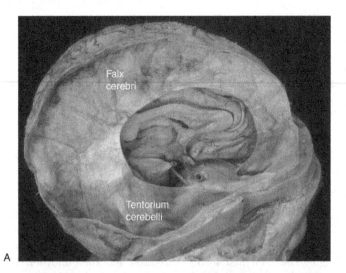

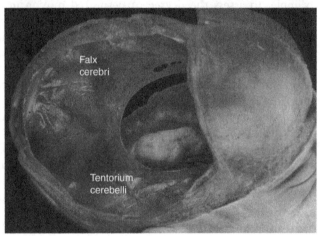

Fig. 1.4 • Lateral view of (A) adult and (B) infant cranium. The neural tissue has been removed. The falx cerebri and tentorium cerebelli are labeled.

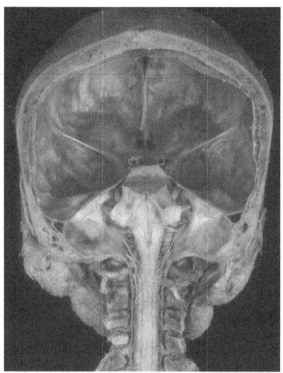

Fig. 1.5 • Posterior perspective into the cranium. The cerebellum and brain have been removed. The edge of the tentorium has been cut. The attachments of the falx cerebri at the crista galli and the tentorium cerebelli along the petrous portions of the temporal bone can be seen. The attachment of the falx cerebri along the meitopic suture (longitudinal septum) and the tentorium (transverse septum) and the lesser wings of the sphenoid (anterior septum) is sometimes referred to as the five-pointed star imprint of the dural septa.

membrane that influences the mechanics of the cranial bones; and the movement of the sacrum. Although there continues to be controversy regarding the physiological accuracy of Sutherland's model, it continues to be used throughout most of the world to discuss evaluation, diagnosis and treatment using this approach. Sutherland described the cranium as a balanced membranous mechanism because of the relationship of the cranial bones to the intra-articular ligaments, the tentorium cerebelli, the falx cerebri, and the falx cerebelli.

The internal membranes of the cranium, the tentorium and two falces act as the reciprocal tension mechanism for the cranium (Figs 1.4 and 1.5). This becomes apparent when examining newborns, especially premature infants. The mobility and deformability of the cranium are remarkable, yet in the majority of cases it will resume a normocephalic appearance within the first 48 hours of life. The ability of the newborn cranium to make such drastic changes is evidence of its responsiveness to the subtle forces

acting within the body. If a premature neonate is left in one position and not turned periodically, the infant will develop a flat spot over that area. The ability of the body to self-correct the deformity correlates with the length of time it has been present, and whether or not any external force, however subtle, has acted on the area. Another example of the deformability of the living skull is the molding that is often present in newborns. This molding occurs in response to the forces acting on the cranium during birth. Although the majority of these adaptations resolve, often a slight asymmetry remains. Cadaveric specimens can be examined for evidence of asymmetries in the cranial fossa. These asymmetries develop in response to the position of fluid-filled vessels and the custard-like substance we call the brain. The asymmetries that occur in response to the intrauterine pressures applied to the emerging cranium may also leave an impression. The shape of any given head is the product of genetics and mechanics. The difference in shape between individuals is readily appreciable through palpation.

The mechanics in the cranium, albeit subtle, can be used to ascertain areas of compression and stress within the membranous articular mechanism. This requires a good understanding of anatomy and a well-developed level of palpatory skill. The motions felt in the cranium are much more subtle than those palpated in the ligamentous mechanism of the spine or sacroiliac joint. Whereas in the majority of individuals the sutures remain cartilaginous with adjoining connective tissue (Pritchard), the articular surfaces in the cranium are generally serrated or beveled. This means that articular surfaces can only marginally glide or expand and contract in relation to each other. These movements are quite minimal, but they do allow for pliancy of the cranium.

Principles of Diagnosis

A strain in the balanced membranous articular mechanism of the cranial vault or base will alter its compliancy and permitted motion. Sutherland described a model of cranial function and motion comprising five components or phenomena, having involuntary motion: the motility of the central nervous system, the fluctuation of the cerebral spinal fluid, the movement of the reciprocal tension membrane, the mobility of the cranial bones, and the mobility of the sacrum. Each phenomenon has a unique quality and pattern of motion. Sutherland's model is widely used to describe qualitative and quantitative palpatory observations of the cranial mechanism and bones, and is used in this text as well.

Biomechanical Model

The movements of the bones of the cranial vault and base are described in relation to the sphenobasilar synchondrosis (SBS). This is described as being in a flexion or extension position. In flexion the position of the SBS is more towards the vertex and in extension it is more towards the feet. During SBS flexion all paired cranial bones are described as being in external rotation; during SBS extension all paired cranial bones are said to be in internal rotation. The parietals, temporals, zygomatics, maxillae, palatine, lacrimal, nasals and inferior conchae are all paired bones, and their mechanics are described as internal and external rotation. External rotation of the parietals will produce a feeling of widening between your two hands, whereas internal rotation will produce a feeling that your hands are coming together. All midline bones – the sphenoid, occiput, vomer and ethmoid – are described as being in positions of flexion or extension.

The morphology and motion at the suture are related. Serrated sutures are sawtoothed, with small toothlike projections like those found in the sagittal and coronal sutures. The size of the projections may vary depending on the stresses placed on the joint. Squamous sutures exist where bones overlap. There is a reciprocal beveling at the suture, such that the overlapping bone will be beveled internally and the underlying bone beveled externally. An example of this would be the temporoparietal suture. A harmonic or plane suture occurs where the irregular surfaces of two bones meet: an example would be the palatomaxillary and lacrimoethmoidal sutures. A gomphosis is a peg-and-socket arrangement like that found in the teeth with the maxillae. Finally, a synchondrosis is found in an area where two ossifying fronts are closely bonded by hyaline cartilage. The sphenobasilar junction is a synchondrosis.

Principles of Treatment

The structures of the head are treated using the principles of balanced tension previously described. The goal is to establish balanced or equal tension between all the tissues in the cranial mechanism. This does not mean less tension: in some cases the tensions may need to be increased. The five principles previously described are also used in the cranium: exaggeration, direct action, decompression, opposing physiological motion, and molding. Within the cranial mechanism opposing physiological motion may be created by opposing biomechanical position with the inherent cranial mechanism. For example, the temporal bone may be externally rotated during the inhalation phase, or may be externally rotated as the occiput is taken into extension. The principle of molding can be applied to the vault bone after all adjacent articulations have been released. As with the balanced ligamentous tension technique, some combination of the principles is usually used in treatment.

Considerations when using Balancing Technique in Children

The sutures do not exist at birth: during the first year of life they begin to develop in some areas, but continue to change until puberty. Many bones are composed of composite parts that are joined by cartilage bridges. The composites will unite at various times after birth (see Table 1.1, p. 3). Sutures provide protection against compressive forces. Because newborns and infants lack this protective mechanism, it is often safer to avoid indirect cranial techniques that exaggerate the strain pattern.

Facilitated Positional Release

Background

Facilitated positional release (FPR) is an indirect myofascial technique developed by Stanley Schiowitz (1990). Some osteopaths consider FPR a form of functional technique. In general, the indications for its use include hypertonic muscles and fascial restrictions. FPR can be used to treat segmental and group dysfunctions of the spine, as well as dysfunction of superficial and deeper myofascial tissue in the extremities, torso, pelvis and neck. Two models for the mechanism of action of this approach have been described. The first concerns the spinal reflex model and the second is based on the nociceptive model. The first model centers on the work of Irvin Korr (1977) and describes reducing or downregulating the γ motor neuron activity by repositioning the tissue. It is thought that the elevated γ activity, sometimes referred to as 'γ gain', is responsible for the characteristics of the somatic dysfunction. It is theorized that if the muscle is placed in a position whereby the fibers are passively shortened, the output of the muscle spindle will decrease and thus reduce the input to the motor neuron. The second model describes using the technique to reduce afferent drive to a facilitated spinal segment, thereby downregulating the reflex muscle spasm.

There are three basic steps for the technique: position the concerned area in neutral; position the area in the direction of ease, away from the restrictive barrier; and finally, add a facilitating force. The position of neutral is defined as the position midway between flexion and extension or medial and lateral rotation of the joint. The position of ease is the three-plane position away from the restrictive barrier. The facilitating force can be torsional, compressive or distracting, and will depend on the area being treated and the findings.

Principles of Diagnosis

Facilitated positional release uses the same principles of positional diagnosis used in the muscle energy technique to identify the position of ease and the restrictive barrier. Movement in three planes is assessed: the sagittal plane for flexion and extension; the coronal plane for lateral flexion (side-bending); and the transverse plane for rotation. The position of ease is identified. For example, a thoracic vertebra that is flexed, side-bent right and rotated to the right has a restrictive barrier in extension, side-bending left and rotation to the left. It will have ease of motion when flexed, side-bent right and rotated right.

Principles of Treatment

FPR is an indirect approach. The region to be treated (neck, thorax, lumbar spine) is placed into neutral, the specific vertebra is then positioned into the direction of ease, and a facilitating force is directed precisely to the segmental dysfunction. The sequencing of the addition of the facilitating force and the movement into the position of ease may vary for each specific technique.

In the example described previously a thoracic vertebra (T4) is flexed, side-bent right and rotated to the right. To treat this dysfunction using FPR, the area to be treated, the thorax, is placed into biomechanical neutral, that is, the natural thoracic kyphosis is flattened. The myofascial tissue surrounding T4 and the vertebra are then positioned in the direction of ease, away from the restrictive barrier. In this example the thorax would be flexed, rotated to the right and side-bent to the right at T4. A facilitating force – in this case compression – is added. The position is held for 3–5 seconds and then released. The area is reassessed and the technique may be repeated if necessary.

Considerations when using FPR in Children

Because joint architecture and structure is immature, the physiological end range of motion in many joints is much more subtle in children than in adults. In addition, depending on the area of the body, the adult morphology of some joints is not present until puberty. Consequently, with FPR, as with all indirect techniques, it is important to be very precise with positioning. Exaggerating the position of ease can stress the physiological barriers of the tissue and cause injury.

Muscle Energy

Background

The muscle energy approach was developed by Mitchell in the 1950s. In 1958 he published his work in the *Yearbook of the American Academy of Osteopathy*, and in the late 1970s his treatment approach was integrated into the curriculum of osteopathic institutions. Mitchell's principles of diagnosis and treatment incorporated his understanding of the principles of osteopathy described by Andrew Taylor Still, and the ideas of Carl Kettler and Thomas Ruddy (Mitchell et al. 1979). Muscle energy (ME) is a direct technique which engages the restrictive barrier and uses active muscle contraction to address the somatic dysfunction. The patient is asked to contract a specific muscle group from a specifically controlled position, in a particular direction and against a precisely executed counterforce. Muscle energy technique can be employed in one of five ways. These are classified according to the type of muscle contraction used: isometric, isotonic concentric, isotonic eccentric, isolytic or reciprocal inhibition.

During isometric contraction the contractile force of the muscle is met with an equal and opposite counterforce which prevents the muscle length from changing, i.e. the distance between the origin and the insertion remains constant (Fig. 1.6). However, the tone in the muscle may be increased. With isotonic contractions the muscle tone stays constant. During isotonic concentric contraction the muscle shortens, and with isotonic eccentric contraction the muscle lengthens. In the former case the resisting force is less than the contractile force of the muscle (Fig. 1.7). In the latter case the resisting force is greater then that of the muscle (Fig. 1.8). In both instances the change in muscle length occurs slowly. This is in contrast to isolytic contraction, where the counterforce meeting the muscle contraction quickly overcomes the muscle and rapidly lengthens it. Reciprocal inhibition is a physiological phenomenon involving inhibition of the antagonist muscle during isometric

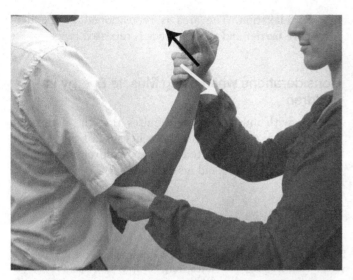

Fig. 1.6 • The biceps contracts against an equal counterforce. There is no change in the length of the muscle.

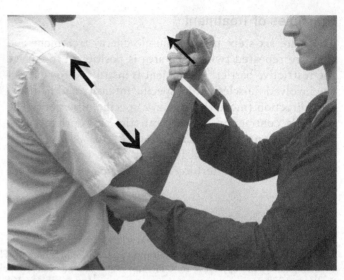

Fig. 1.8 • The biceps contracts against a counterforce that gradually increases, lengthening the muscle.

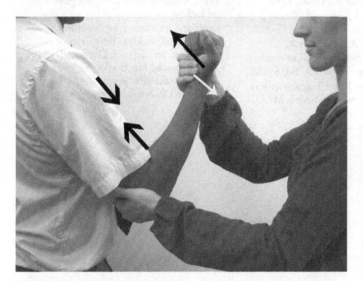

Fig. 1.7 • The biceps contracts against a counterforce that gradually weakens, allowing the muscle to shorten.

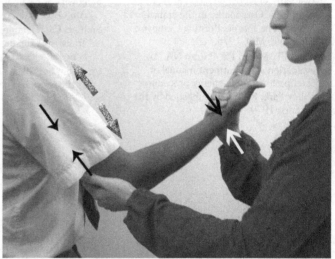

Fig. 1.9 • The triceps contracts against an equal counterforce. The biceps is reciprocally inhibited (stippled arrow).

contraction of an agonist (Fig. 1.9). For example, during isometric knee extension the knee flexors are inhibited.

In general, the muscle energy technique may be used to improve motion in a joint, strengthen weak muscles, increase the resting length of shortened muscles, stretch tight myofascial tissue, influence reduced muscle tone, and improve respiratory/circulatory function in an area. Each of these types of muscle contraction can be used for a different clinical purpose. For example, isometric contraction can be used to address a muscle strain or spasm. Isotonic concentric contraction may be used to treat articular problems with a myofascial component, or to strengthen a weak muscle. Isotonic eccentric contraction may be used to retrain firing patterns in an injured muscle or lengthen a chronically shortened muscle. Isolytic contraction can be employed to

address fibrosis or edema, or to mobilize a joint. Reciprocal inhibition may be used to indirectly treat a painful area, address severe or chronic muscle spasm, or to retrain firing patterns.

Principles of Diagnosis

Muscle energy assesses tissue texture changes, asymmetry and range of motion of an area in flexion, extension and neutral. This is called three-positional diagnosis. The restrictive barrier is identified and the dysfunction is named for the position of ease of motion. For example, if the femur has restricted motion in internal rotation, the dysfunction is named external rotation of the femur, and the restrictive barrier is internal rotation.

Principles of Treatment

There are six steps used in muscle energy treatment and they are repeated twice. The area is positioned to engage the restrictive barrier. The patient is instructed to contract the involved muscles with a specific intensity and in a specific direction (move the area in a specific direction). The patient's contraction is met with the appropriate counterforce (isometric, isotonic, isolytic) for 3–5 seconds. The patient is instructed to slowly relax, and the physician relaxes the counterforce. There is a pause to allow for muscle relaxation. The area is repositioned to the new restrictive barrier and the sequence is repeated twice.

Considerations when using Muscle Energy in Children

Success with muscle energy requires that the patient be able to follow directions precisely. Because of this, the use of muscle energy is limited to older children and adolescents who can understand instructions.

References

Korr IM. The neurobiological mechanisms in manipulative therapy. New York: Plenum Press, 1977.

Lippincott HA. The osteopathic technique of Wm G Sutherland, DO. Kirksville, MO: Academy of Applied Osteopathy, 1949.

Magoun HIS. Osteopathy in the cranial field, 3rd ed. The Journal Printing Company, Kirksville, MO, 1976.

Mitchell FL, Moran PS, Pruzzo NA. An evaluation and treatment manual of osteopathic muscle energy procedures. Valley Park, MO: Self-published by the authors, 1979.

Nordin M, Frankel VH. Basic biomechanics of the musculoskeletal system. Philadelphia: Lea & Febiger, 1989.

Norkin CC, Levangie PC. Joint structure and function. Philadelphia: FA Davis, 1992.

Schiowitz S. Facilitated positional release. J Am Osteopath Assoc 1990; 901: 145–155.

Snijders CJ, Vleeming A, Stoeckart R. Transfer of the lumbosacral load to iliac bones and legs. Clin Biomech 1993; 8: 285.

Steinberg BG, Plancher KD. Clinical anatomy of the wrist and elbow. Clin Sports Med 1995; 14: 299.

Sutherland WG. Teachings in the science of osteopathy. Portland, OR: Rudra Press, 1990.

Vleeming A, Snijders CJ, Stoeckart R, Mens JMA. A new light on low back pain: The selflocking mechanism of the sacroiliac joints and its implication for sitting, standing and walking. In: Vleeming A, Mooney V, Snijders CJ, Dorman T, eds. The integrated function of the lumbar spine and sacroiliac joints. Rotterdam: European Conference Organisers, 1995.

Chapter Two

Head and neck

2

CHAPTER CONTENTS

OVERVIEW

In newborns the head and neck generally bear the brunt of the mechanical forces encountered during labor and delivery. In spite of this, most babies go on to be productive and well-adjusted adults. The passage through the vaginal canal and subsequent emergence into the light of day is an age-old process for which most humans are extremely well adapted. The flexibility of the cartilaginous neurocranium produces a folding of the vault bones, similar to the arrangement of petals in a rose bud. After delivery, the mechanical forces and movements associated with breathing, crying and suckling expand the cranium and correct the sutural overlap. In some cases the normal forces of life are unable to resolve these strains, and we then have a baby who may present with irritability, problems suckling, abnormal posturing, delayed postural patterning, or myriad other vague clinical symptoms. Establishing a clinical diagnosis and understanding its etiology are probably the most difficult tasks faced by a clinician caring for such an infant. As a result, one's index of suspicion must remain high for a broad differential diagnosis.

The head and neck play an important role in the establishment of posture and balance mechanisms. Strains and mechanical dysfunction may present immediately after birth, or with the expression of new developmental milestones. Along with a thorough history, the symmetry and execution of new movement patterns can provide the clinician with clues about somatic dysfunction in the infant. Basic reflexes linking head and neck control with eye movements, mastication and suckling, vestibular activity, and control of the torso and extremities exist at birth. These influence and are in turn influenced by mechanical function in the craniocervical junction and the neck.

TORTICOLLIS

Clinical Notes

Torticollis is a malposition of the neck such that there is limited range of motion in one direction. The child prefers to hold the neck side-bent. Torticollis may be congenital or acquired. The most common etiology is biomechanical (functional), but other etiologies need to be considered. Congenital deformities of the cervical or upper thoracic spine may present as congenital torticollis. Injury to the cervical musculature with hemorrhage or scarring will also present as torticollis. Rarely, torticollis may occur as a result of neurological damage to the spinal cord or brain. Magoun (1973) describes congenital torticollis as a sign of accessory nerve irritation (not damage) secondary to strains of the cranial base. In infants and young children torticollis may develop secondary to strabismus. In newborns, torticollis is sometimes described as a component of a larger postural condition called infantile postural asymmetry (see below).

Congenital torticollis due to a mechanical etiology may be primarily cervical, involving the scalene or the sternocleidomastoid muscles; or it may be compensatory to changes at the craniocervical junction resulting from a cranial base strain pattern. In either case the mechanical dysfunction is due to abnormal uterine lie or acquired birth strain. When uterine lie is the underlying cause, there is often a history of abnormal lie or early engagement. There may be a history of a difficult or prolonged labor and/or assisted delivery. The neonatal review of systems may reveal difficulty with nursing, or more difficulty nursing on one breast than the other. There may be associated signs of infantile postural asymmetry, such as newborn reflexes that are present but not symmetrical. Congenital torticollis due to uterine lie typically involves the scalene muscles, with dysfunction of upper rib mechanics and compensatory changes in the thoracic area. Findings in the cranial base are often mild. Accommodative molding, which develops during labor and resolves rather quickly, is typically limited to the cartilaginous vault bones and does not extend to the supra-occiput.

There may also be a history of abnormal lie or early engagement in newborns with torticollis arising secondary to cranial base strain. However, these babies typically have molding that does not resolve quickly. There is obvious asymmetry in the head and face. Molding deformity is present, with obvious asymmetry of the supra-occiput parts. The primary areas of dysfunction are the craniocervical junction and the cranial base, rather than the cervical spine. In these children the base strain changes the condylar relationship of the occiput and atlas. Condylar compression may or may not be present, depending on the specific strain pattern. Congenital torticollis is often not diagnosed until the child is 4–6 weeks old, at which time the parent or physician notices an awkward positioning of the head or the early development of a flat spot on the skull. Plagiocephaly tends to present sooner in newborns with torticollis secondary to base strain than in those with primary cervical torticollis.

Torticollis may also result from bleeding within the belly of the sternocleidomastoid, trapezius or scalene muscle secondary to trauma. In the neonatal population this may be associated with shoulder dystocia, a prolonged second stage of labor and assisted delivery. When the torticollis is due to intramuscular hemorrhage, there is a palpable swelling in the muscle and bruising may be seen. Complications include fibrosis, scar formation and shortening of the muscle. In addition to osteopathic treatment the infant should receive physical therapy or at least an at-home stretching program to address the fibrosis and muscle contracture. Myositis ossificans occurs when the scar tissue forms a calcification. It and other structural problems in the muscle belly can be diagnosed with ultrasonography. In severely affected children surgical release is occasionally necessary.

In older children and young athletes the most common cause of torticollis is muscular strain related to trauma, such as whiplash or acceleration sports injuries (see Whiplash). In most cases the sternocleidomastoid is involved; however, injury to the digastric, scalene and paraspinal musculature may also present as torticollis. Changes at the craniocervical junction are usually compensatory. Microtrauma or bleeding into the muscle belly places the child at risk for scarring and myositis ossificans. Torticollis can also develop in association with respiratory tract infections, especially pharyngitis. The pathophysiology is thought to be lymphadenopathy and subsequent neuromuscular irritation or virally mediated neuritis.

INFANTILE POSTURAL ASYMMETRY
(Figs 2.1 and 2.2)

Clinical Notes

The term infantile postural asymmetry (IPA) has been used to describe a complex of asymmetrical positioning in infants that includes reduced cervical rotation and/or idiopathic infantile scoliosis (Philippi et al. 2006). Asymmetrical posturing in infants may be due to neurological, mechanical or structural etiologies. Of these, mechanical etiologies are the most common, and the condition is considered postural and idiopathic (Hamanishi and Tanaka 1994). Neurological causes of abnormal positioning and appearance include cerebral infarction, nerve injury and neuromuscular abnormalities. Structural etiologies include bony malformations and skeletal deformities. The most common presentations of postural asymmetry are plagiocephaly, torticollis, scoliosis and foot malpositioning. There is some concern that asymmetries of posturing in infancy may influence functional development (Konishi et al. 2002) and scoliosis (McMaster 1983, Brunetaeu and Mulliken 1992, Cheng and Au 1994). These children may also have subtle asymmetries in infantile reflexes.

From an osteopathic perspective, postural asymmetries in infants should not be treated or evaluated in isolation. Strains and adaptations in one area require compensations in other areas. Within the osteopathic concept, infantile asymmetries in positioning and movement have the potential to affect the body systems, their development and cognitive processes through their influence on proprioceptive mapping, motor planning development, respiratory–circulatory function and myofascial relationships.

Philippi et al. (2006) described a method of measuring two of the components of this complex: reduced cervical rotation and truncal convexity. Her nomenclature may be useful for clinicians to describe and document findings in children with postural asymmetries (Table 2.1).

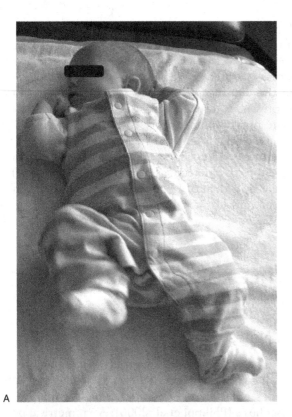

A

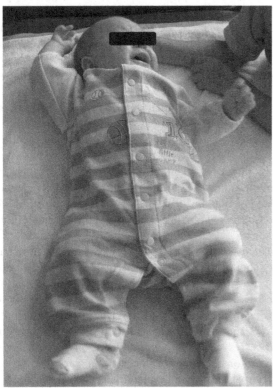

B

Fig. 2.1 • A, B Two-month-old infant with signs of infantile postural asymmetry. Note asymmetry in cervical rotation. When supine, the infant would only raise her head to the right. Trunk is side-bent left (convex right) and resisted passive motion to side-bending right (convex left).

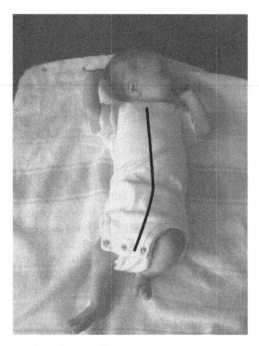

Fig. 2.2 • Infant with significant asymmetry and truncal convexity to the left.

Table 2.1 Typical patterns of postural asymmetry in infants (Adapted from Philippi H, Faldum A, Jung T, et al. Patterns of postural asymmetry in infants: a standardized video-based analysis. Eur J Pediatr 2006; 165: 158–164)

Category	Description of spinal convexity
1	Equal convexity or no convexity
2	Convexity can be resolved to neutral and flexibility in other direction is present but slightly decreased
3	Convexity can be resolved to neutral and flexibility in opposite direction is present but obviously decreased
4	Convexity can only be resolved to neutral, resists movement to other directions
5	Convexity cannot be resolved to neutral, only a flattened curve
6	Convexity cannot be resolved
Category	**Description of active cervical spine rotation**
1	No restriction in motion
2	Slight decrease in active rotation in one direction, no preferential head position
3	Obvious decrease in active rotation to one side, but beyond midline. Able to overcome
4	Obvious decrease in rotation to one side, not beyond midline but may occasionally be overcome
5	Decrease in rotation to one side not beyond midline and difficult to overcome

ASSESSING ACTIVE CERVICAL ROTATION

Supine and Prone Infant

The assessment is performed with the infant in both the supine and the prone position.

1. The infant is supine. The head and body are held in alignment for several seconds. Without touching the infant, the examiner then attempts to stimulate the infant to look to the left by calling his name or using a toy. The examiner notes the range of cervical rotation, the coupling with side-bending, and at what point the contralateral shoulder engages. The examiner also notes the position of the trunk (Fig. 2.3A).

2. The sequence is repeated with the infant looking towards the right. The range of cervical rotation, the coupling with side-bending, engagement of the contralateral shoulder and position of the trunk are compared with the previous findings (Fig. 2.3B). In this example, the infant engages his right shoulder with active left cervical rotation.

3. If the infant is more than 2 weeks old he is placed in the prone position and the sequence is repeated comparing the two sides.

4. Restricted rotation in the supine position suggests dysfunction in the sternocleidomastoid or trapezius muscles, the upper cervical complex (C1/C2) or atlantoaxial junction. Restricted rotation in the prone position indicates dysfunction of the lower cervical complex (C3–C7) (Pang and Veetai 2004, Phillipi et al. 2006).

5. The presence of asymmetry of cervical motion and trunk posturing suggests infantile postural asymmetry.

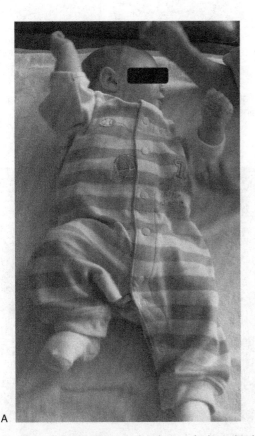
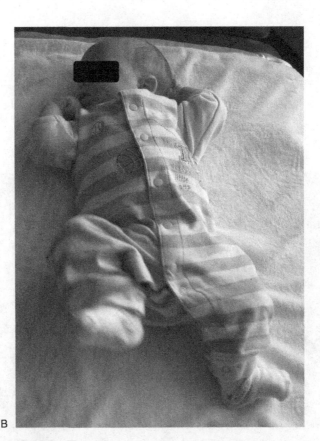

A　　　　　　　　　　　　B

Fig. 2.3 • A,B Assessment of active cervical rotation in a 2-month-old boy. The infant engages his right shoulder with left cervical rotation, indicating restricted motion. The trunk is convex left, although his striped jumper makes it difficult to see.

ASSESSING PASSIVE CERVICAL ROTATION

Supine Infant

When assessing cervical motion in infants, it is essential that the child be lying on a flat surface and not be engaged or distracted by the parents, sounds, or any other entity. If the child is stimulated to look with his eyes he will engage cervical muscles, which will result in an inaccurate assessment of motion mechanics.

1. The physician stands at the head of the table with the infant lying supine in front of her. The physician gently holds the infant's head, keeping the neck in a neutral position. The physician slowly rotates the head to the right and left (Fig. 2.4), assessing passive myofascial resistance.

2. The physician notes when and whether the infant engages the opposite shoulder during the rotation.

3. Rotation to the left that is accompanied by movement of the right shoulder indicates resistance, and vice versa.

4. Segmental testing can then be performed. The physician contacts two adjacent vertebrae on opposite sides. For example, C4 is contacted on the right and C5 is contacted on the left (Figs 2.5 and 2.6).

5. The physician induces left rotation of the superior vertebra (C4) by lifting anteriorly and to the left with her contacting finger. The response of that vertebra and the vertebra below (C5) are noted. The physician changes her contact (left contact on C4 and right on C5) and introduces right rotation to C4 by lifting anteriorly and to the right.

6. This procedure is repeated throughout the lower cervical vertebrae to locate the area of primary dysfunction.

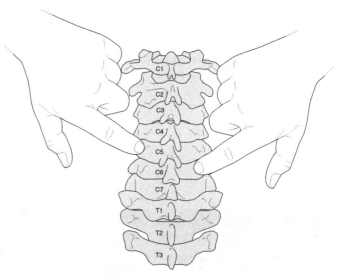

Fig. 2.5 • Schematic diagram of finger contact for segmental testing in the cervical spine.

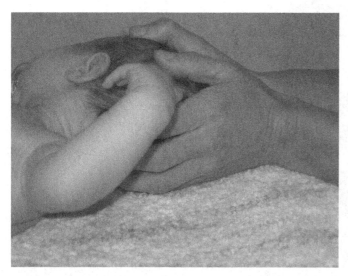

Fig. 2.4 • Gross motion testing of passive cervical rotation in a neonate.

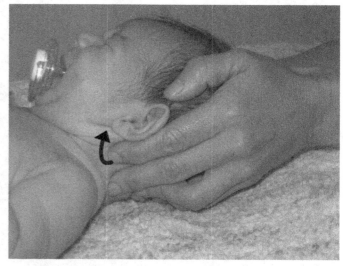

Fig. 2.6 • Segmental testing of cervical motion mechanics in a 1-week-old neonate.

ASSESSING PASSIVE CERVICAL SIDE-BENDING

Supine Infant

The physician can assess cervical side-bending using a similar procedure as that described above.

1. Gross motion is assessed by gently and slowly side-bending the head and neck towards each shoulder and noting when and whether there is engagement of the shoulder on the convex side. This indicates the end range of motion.

2. As the head is moved into the side-bending position, note the reflex response of the extremities. An alternating pattern of upper and lower limb extension is expected on the side contralateral to the side-bending. In Figure 2.7A and B the infant extends the contralateral upper extremity but the lower extremity response is dulled. Figure 2.7A also demonstrates that the torso and pelvis adapt to left cervical side-bending earlier than to right cervical side-bending. This indicates restriction to left cervical side-bending.

3. Segmental motion can be assessed by gently testing compliancy to translation in both directions in each cervical vertebra.

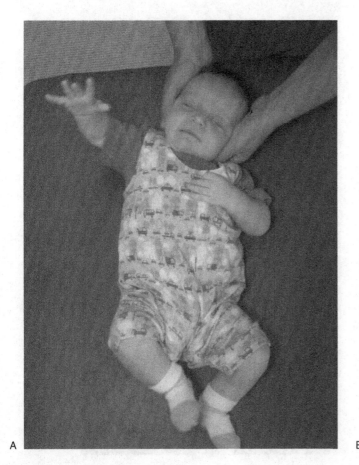
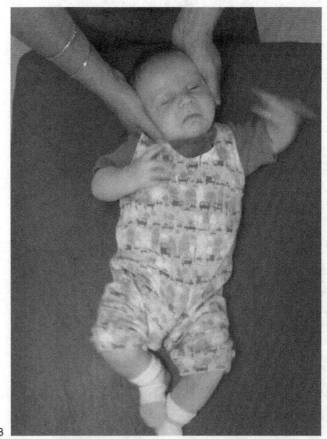

A

B

Fig. 2.7

ASSESSING MYOFASCIAL RESISTANCE TO BODY ON HEAD MOTION

Supine Infant (Figs 2.8 and 2.9)

This technique can be used to assess flexibility in the spine and visual control of posture.

1. The infant is supine on a flat surface. The examiner stands directly over the infant.

2. The baby's attention is attracted so that her gaze is directed forward.

3. The pelvis is slowly rotated to the right. The infant should continue to keep her head in the midline as the rotation progresses from the pelvis into the lumbar and thoracic spines. This infant (Fig. 2.8) immediately turns his head to the right when the pelvis begins to rotate to the left.

4. Motion is assessed in both directions. When the pelvis is rotated to the right (Fig. 2.9), the torso and neck engage simultaneously and the infant 'log rolls' to the right.

5. Asymmetry of head and neck movement in relation to the body rotation is indicative of motion restriction, which may be neurological or mechanical. When the restrictive barrier is met, there is simultaneous rotation of several vertebral segments. Depending on the location of the barrier, the entire upper thorax and cervical spine may rotate as a unit.

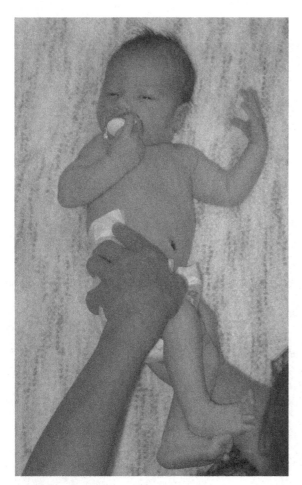

Fig. 2.8

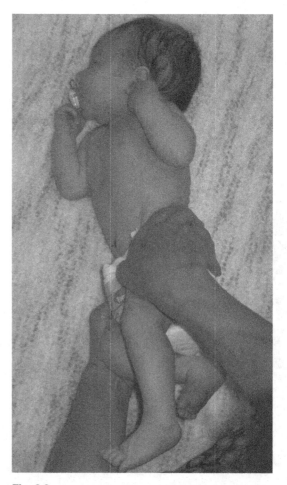

Fig. 2.9

ASSESSING SIDE-BENDING IN THE TORSO

Supine Infant (Figs 2.10 and 2.11)

1. The infant is supine on a flat surface. The examiner stands directly over the infant.

2. The baby's attention is attracted so that her gaze is directed forward.

3. The pelvis is gently side-bent to the right (Fig. 2.10). The side-bending is exaggerated to produce left side-bending in the lumbar and thoracic spines (white arrow and line, concave left). This infant immediately turned his head to the right, with side-bending of the lumbar spine to the left.

4. This is repeated (Fig. 2.11) with side-bending of the pelvis to the left, creating lumbar side-bending right (white arrow and line, concave right). The same infant shows considerably less irritability in this position, although the head once again is turned to the right.

5. The lumbar and thoracic spines should side-bend while the head and shoulders remain level on the table. A restrictive barrier will cause the shoulders to side-bend or the head to rotate.

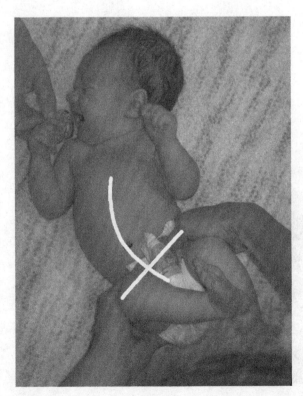

Fig. 2.10

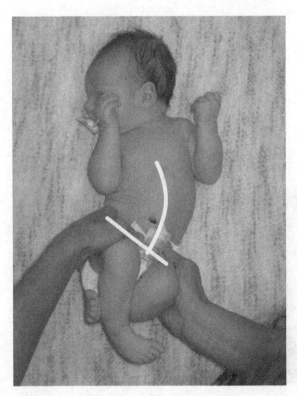

Fig. 2.11

THREE-POSITION SEGMENTAL DIAGNOSIS

Cervical Spine

Supine Child/Athlete

1. The patient is supine. The physician sits or stands at the head of the table, supporting the patient's head with both hands (Fig. 2.12).

2. With the neck relaxed, the physician places her index fingers bilaterally on the articular pillars of the segment to be evaluated. The physician gently lifts the segment anteriorly to induce extension.

3. With the segment in a semi-extended position the physician will assess motion restriction. This is done by introducing a lateral translatory force first from one side and then from the other. Lateral translation of the vertebra produces contralateral side-bending. A translatory force introduced from the left will translate the vertebra to the right and induce left side-bending.

4. The physician begins at C7 and moves superiorly (C7–C3), positioning each segment in a semi-extended position and making note of any motion dysfunctions. If restriction is found, the segment is then tested with the neck in flexion (Fig. 2.13).

5. The diagnosis is named according to the direction of greatest freedom in three planes of motion; flexion, side-bending and rotation.

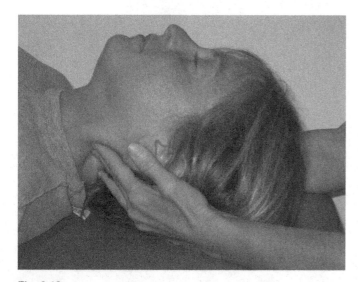

Fig. 2.12

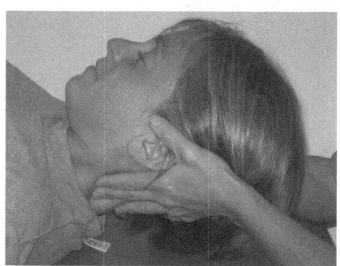

Fig. 2.13

TORTICOLLIS/INFANTILE POSTURAL ASYMMETRY

Treatment Notes

Congenital torticollis is usually associated with cranial base strain and dysfunction at the craniocervical junction. These findings may be primary or secondary to the torticollis. Often, the cranial findings will not respond to treatment until the cervical dysfunction is resolved, which suggests that the cranial strain is probably secondary to the torticollis. If the cranial findings are primary, they must be addressed prior to any improvement in the neck. It is sometimes difficult to determine which problem is primary; however, there are certain clues one can look for.

When the torticollis is primarily cervical there is often palpable, frank spasm in the sternocleidomastoid or scalene muscles. The child may become irritable when the injured or strained muscles are palpated, but palpation of other adjacent muscles produces no such response. The upper ribs on the involved side are elevated and markedly restricted, with scalene involvement. Motion mechanics in C2 and C3 will be markedly impaired. The clavicle and shoulder will be restricted with sternocleidomastoid etiology, and a temporal bone dysfunction is more likely on the involved side. The cranial base strain is mild or secondary. Glide (lateral translation) at the craniocervical junction is fairly symmetrical, although tilt and rotation may be limited. The child is usually able to engage postural reflexes with visual stimulation when the head is supported (see Visual–motor integration in Chapter 5).

When the primary problem is the cranial base the most significant findings of the cranial base strain pattern will be in the occipital and condylar parts rather than the sphenoid. There is mild facial asymmetry and the child is more likely to have asymmetry of the two supra-occipital parts at birth or soon after. The mastoid portions are often unleveled and lie on different anteroposterior planes. The greatest restriction to motion testing is found at the craniocervical junction and involves restriction to glide or lateral translation. The infant may have more difficulty stabilizing her posture with head support than the previously described infant, because the occipitoatlantal muscles are under greater strain and the oculocephalic reflex may be affected.

Torticollis may be diagnosed early in infants by closely assessing the baby's response to the Moro reflex, asymmetrical tonic neck reflex (ATNR) or a rolling maneuver. During the Moro reflex the arm on the affected side will often remain more flexed than the contralateral arm. During the ATNR, the response will occur much more quickly when the head is turned away from the side of the mechanical strain. When the rolling and side-bending maneuvers are performed, there will be asymmetry of passive rotation in the thorax and lumbar spines.

Treatment of the torticollis should focus on the primary strain within the complex. Various manual modalities are thought to be effective and are often used in combination. Balanced ligamentous techniques can be used to address the articular dysfunction of the cervical area. Myofascial or facilitated positional release can be helpful in treating the myofascial components. The occipitoatlantal and cranial base strains should respond to the balanced membranous techniques described for plagiocephaly. Input from the craniocervical junction may maintain abnormal postural reflexes and patterning via the cervicospinal, cervicocolic and other reflexes. Postural tone that is unresponsive to treatment with osteopathic approaches may respond to the Atlas Impulse technique, especially if the primary dysfunction involves the craniocervical junction.

DIRECT MYOFASCIAL RELEASE

Cervical Tissue

Supine Athlete

This technique focuses on the lateral myofascial structures of neck: the scalenes, levator scapulae, clavicular portion of the sternocleidomastoid (SCM), and the anterior portion of the upper trapezius (Trap).

1. The patient is supine. The physician stands or sits at the head of the table and cradles the occiput in the hand contralateral to the side to be treated. The physician uses a firm contact. The other hand contacts the superior aspect of the thorax, including the clavicle, upper ribs and scapula (Fig. 2.14A, B).

2. The physician introduces a caudad force into the upper thorax, loading the myofascial tissues of the neck. With the head and neck in neutral, the physician side-bends the head and neck to the restrictive barrier.

3. This oppositional tension is maintained as the patient breathes. The physician can adapt the position of the head and neck to best load the restrictive barrier.

4. With each inhalation, the physician resists movement of the head and upper thorax. With each exhalation, the physician moves to the next restrictive barrier. As the tissue is loaded, the restrictive barrier will move.

5. This is continued for several breaths, until there is a change in tissue texture.

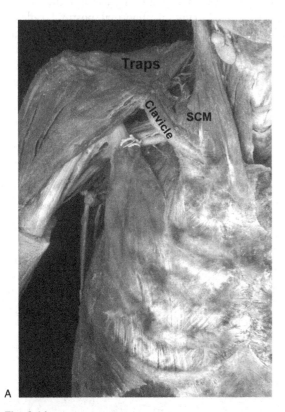

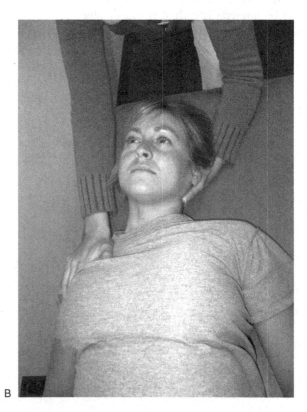

A   B

Fig. 2.14

BALANCED LIGAMENTOUS TENSION

Lower Cervical Spine

Seated Toddler/Infant

Although this approach can be taken with an athlete or child, the patient is more likely to relax if the supine approach is used. The example given is for a C6 dysfunction, side-bent right (translated left).

1. The child is seated facing away from the physician. The physician controls the head with one hand. The other hand contacts the vertebra to be treated at each transverse process (Figs. 2.15, 2.16A and B).

2. A stacking technique is used whereby the head is gently positioned into flexion, extension and rotation as the vertebra is translated laterally to the right and left to achieve balanced ligamentous tension. In this example, the tissues are being moved towards the restrictive barrier to achieve balanced tension.

3. Once balanced tension is present, the position is maintained until there is a change in tissue texture or an improvement in function.

BALANCED LIGAMENTOUS TENSION

Lower Cervical Spine

Supine Infant/Child/Athlete

See Cervicogenic Cephalgia, this chapter.

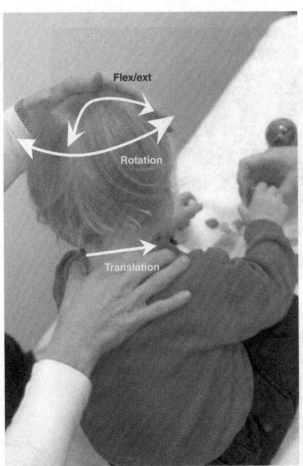

Fig. 2.15

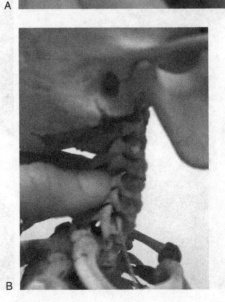

Fig. 2.16

FACILITATED POSITIONAL RELEASE (FPR)

Lower Cervical Spine – Superficial Tissues

Seated Toddler/Infant

FPR techniques can be especially useful in acute situations where the child is in pain and guarding or splinting the area.

In this technique the palpatory focus is the superficial and deep cervical fascia, and the upper trapezius, splenius capitus, longissimus capitus and cervicus, and semispinalis capitus and cervicus muscles, rather than the articular relationships, the segmental muscles or the ligaments.

1. The child is seated. The physician contacts the cervical area and monitors the superficial tissues to be treated.

The physician's other hand is placed upon the head (Fig. 2.17A, B).

2. The child's head and neck are positioned in postural neutral.

3. The physician applies a steady and gradual axial compression of less than 2.5 kg until there is a softening of the monitored tissues (white arrow).

4. While maintaining the compression, the physician gently positions the head to place the tissues in the direction of ease (away from restrictive barrier). In the example, side-bending to the left reduces the tissue tension (black arrow).

5. This position is held for 3–5 seconds and released. The area is reassessed.

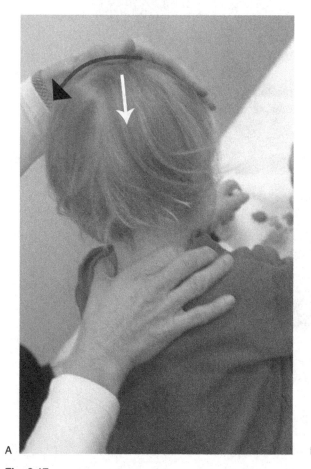

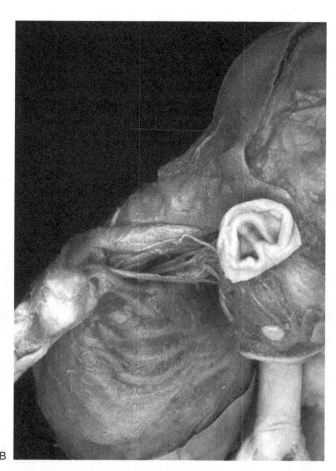

A · B

Fig. 2.17

FACILITATED POSITIONAL RELEASE

Lower Cervical Spine – Segmental Strain

C4 Extended Side-bent Rotated Right (Translated Left)

When treating a segmental dysfunction with FPR the palpatory focus is on the articulation, joint mechanics and the connective tissues involved.

Seated Toddler/Infant

1. The child is seated. The physician contacts the cervical area and monitors the articular facet at the involved level (C4/C5). The physician's other hand is placed upon the head (Fig. 2.18A, B).

2. The child's head and neck are positioned in postural neutral.

3. The physician applies a steady and gradual axial compression of less than 2.5 kg until there is a softening of the monitored tissues.

4. While maintaining the compression, the physician gently extends C4 on C5 and translates C4 to the left, producing right side-bending. This is the direction of ease.

5. This position is held for 3–5 seconds and released. The area is reassessed.

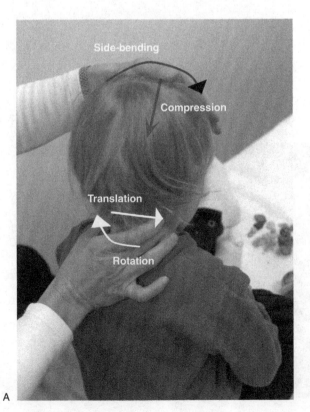
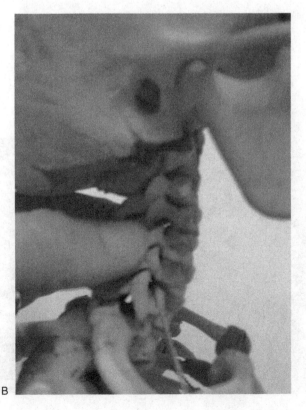

Fig. 2.18

FACILITATED POSITIONAL RELEASE

Lower Cervical Spine – Segmental Strain

C4 Flexed Side-bent Rotated Left (Translated Right)

When treating a segmental dysfunction with FPR the palpatory focus is on the articulation, joint mechanics and the connective tissues involved.

Seated Toddler/Infant

1. The child is seated. The physician contacts the cervical area and monitors the articular facet at the involved level (C4/C5). The physician's other hand is placed upon the head (Fig. 2.19A, B).

2. The child's head and neck are positioned in postural neutral.

3. The physician applies a steady and gradual axial compression of less than 2.5 kg until there is a softening of the monitored tissues.

4. While maintaining the compression, the physician gently flexes C4 on C5 and translates C4 to the right, producing left side-bending. This is the direction of ease.

5. This position is held for 3–5 seconds and released. The area is reassessed.

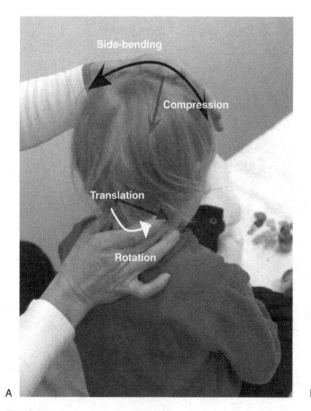

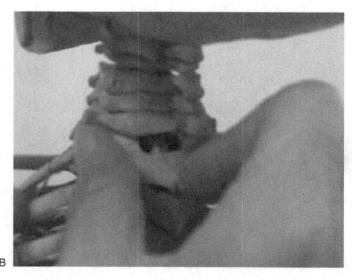

A   B

Fig. 2.19

MUSCLE ENERGY ISOMETRIC CONTRACTION

Lower Cervical Spine – Flexed

Supine Child/Athlete

A flexed dysfunction will have the greatest restricted motion when tested in extension. Muscle energy is a direct technique that engages the restrictive barrier. A flexed segment is treated in extension.

1. The athlete is supine with the physician seated at the head of the table. The physician contacts the dysfunctional segment with the thumb and finger of one hand. In the example, the diagnosis is C5 FSRr. The left hand is used to contact the dysfunction (Fig. 2.20). The head and upper neck are extended to the level of the dysfunction.

2. Maintaining extension at the level of the dysfunction, the physician uses her right hand to cup the chin. The physician introduces the coupled motion of left side-bending and left rotation at the level of the dysfunction to engage the restrictive barrier. This is done by gently pushing on the left articular pillar, much as was done for diagnosis.

3. Once the restrictive barrier has been engaged in all three planes (flexion, side-bending and rotation), the athlete is instructed to gently push her chin into the physician's hand (black arrow).

4. The physician resists this motion with an equal and opposite counterforce (white arrow). This is maintained for 3–5 seconds. The athlete is then instructed to relax as the physician simultaneously relaxes her counterforce.

5. The physician waits 3–5 seconds for the post-isometric relaxation phase to occur. Then the physician uses her left hand to introduce left side-bending and rotation (right translation) to the new restrictive barrier as the right hand introduces more extension.

6. The sequence is repeated two more times. Then the motion mechanics are reassessed.

Fig. 2.20

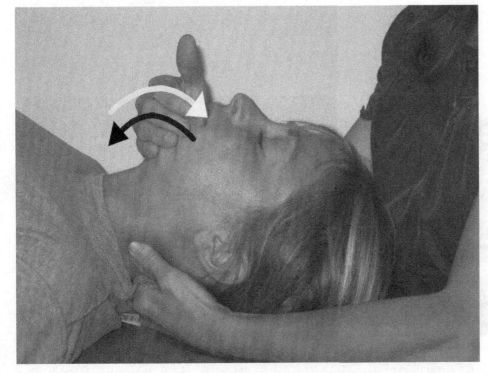

MUSCLE ENERGY ISOMETRIC CONTRACTION

Lower Cervical Spine – Extended

Supine Child/Athlete

An extended dysfunction will have greatest restricted motion when tested in flexion. Muscle energy is a direct technique that engages the restrictive barrier. An extended segment is treated in flexion.

1. The athlete is supine with the physician seated at the head of the table. The physician contacts the dysfunctional segment with the thumb and finger of one hand. In the example the diagnosis is C5 ESRl. The right hand is used to contact the dysfunction (Fig. 2.21A, B).

2. The left hand cups the occiput and the head is gently flexed in a sequential manner from the occiput down to C5 until motion is localized.

3. Maintaining flexion at C5, the right hand introduces the coupled motions of side-bending and rotation to the restrictive barrier. This is done by gently pushing on the right articular pillar to induce left translation, similar to the procedure used for diagnosis. Both side-bending and rotation are to the right, the opposite of the described dysfunction.

4. Once the restrictive barrier has been engaged in all three planes (flexion, side-bending and rotation) the athlete is instructed to gently push her neck into the physician's hand (black arrow).

5. The physician resists this motion with an equal and opposite counterforce (white arrow). This is maintained for 3–5 seconds. Then the athlete is instructed to relax as the physician simultaneously relaxes her counterforce.

6. The physician waits 3–5 seconds for the post-isometric relaxation phase to occur. Then the physician uses her left hand to introduce a bit more flexion as the right hand introduces right side-bending and rotation (left translation) to the new restrictive barrier.

7. The sequence is repeated twice more, then the motion mechanics are reassessed.

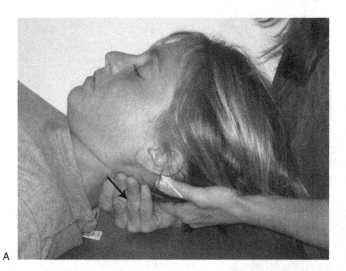
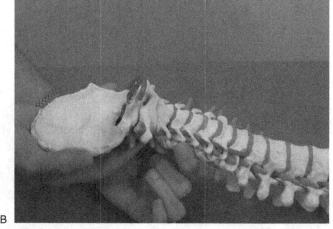

Fig. 2.21

CERVICOGENIC VERTIGO

Clinical Notes

Posture and balance are dependent on input from three systems, the vestibular, the visual and the proprioceptive. Minute by minute, these three systems interact to orchestrate the complex process of keeping each of us in the appropriate postural relationship with our surroundings. Problems in any one of the systems can affect the accuracy and reliability of the whole. This is the case in cervicogenic vertigo, a condition where the child or athlete feels unsteady, 'lightheaded' or dizzy because of abnormal signaling from the cervical proprioceptive fibers. The cervical somatic tissue is densely innervated with proprioceptive fibers that provide information about head position and neck position. The potency of the input from the neck is so significant that it can be used to retrain balance mechanisms in stroke patients with infarcts affecting the vestibular system. Somatic dysfunction and mechanical dysfunction are probably the most common causes of cervicogenic vertigo.

Cervicogenic vertigo typically occurs in older children as a result of trauma, but can be seen in infants and toddlers as part of conditions such as sporadic spastic torticollis or sporadic spastic vertigo. The areas of densest proprioceptive innervation are in the upper neck and at the craniocervical junction. As would be expected, these are also the areas of greatest somatic dysfunction in patients with cervicogenic vertigo. In toddlers, the problem often includes a lateral strain at the cranial base; in older children and athletes, the primary somatic dysfunctions are at the craniocervical junction and in the upper neck. Cervicogenic vertigo may develop after head trauma involving collision, as might be seen in soccer, football or basketball players. Cervicogenic vertigo can also develop as a component of whiplash, and must be differentiated from post-concussion symptoms secondary to contrecoup injury.

Treatment Notes

Manipulative treatment can employ techniques such as those described for whiplash injury and cervicogenic cephalgia, as the areas of greatest dysfunction are similar.

WHIPLASH

Clinical Notes

Whiplash is caused by a rapid acceleration–deceleration movement of the head on the neck. Although classically associated with motor vehicle accidents, whiplash injury also occurs in sports injuries, shaken baby syndrome and head injuries. The mechanism of injury may be rapid linear displacement of the head and neck in any plane. The speed of the displacement and the position of the cervical spine at initiation determine the extent of the injury, which typically involves the paraspinal soft tissues but may also include the articular surfaces of the vertebrae. When the linear displacement occurs while the neck is rotated, there is an increased incidence of injury to the facets, the joint capsule and the annulus fibrosis. The linear displacement of the head does not create a consistent hyperflexion or hyperextension in the cervical spine. In very rapid or high-impact displacement the cervical spine will simultaneously flex and extend, producing an 'S'-shaped curve. Stretching of ligaments, muscles and articular capsules results in microtrauma, and in severe cases connective tissue tears, rupture or disc injury. At the endpoint of motion, the compressive contact of the articular surfaces can produce microfractures in the cartilaginous surface of the facet or uncovertebral joints. The reflexive shortening of the stretched muscles causes spasm that may impede tissue repair processes. The rapid stretch can irritate branches of the recurrent meningeal or somatosympathetic nerves. Localized swelling or facet damage may irritate the nerve root or dorsal ramus.

Infants and young children lack the protective reflexes and muscular strength to control rapid head displacement. This puts them at greater risk for contrecoup injury, intracerebral vascular injury, soft tissue rupture and avulsion fracture. Infants and young children who sustain whiplash injury should be evaluated for evidence of vertebral instability and neurological injury. In older children and young adults, the most common complaints related to whiplash are neck pain, headache and dizziness. Generalized cervical pain and stiffness are probably due to soft tissue injury. Deep aching pain presenting in the posterior neck and across the upper back at the level of the shoulders suggests anterior strain and somatosympathetic nerve irritation, most often due to direct stretch of the anterior structures or chemical irritation secondary to annular tears. Burning or radiating pain presenting in a dermatome distribution may represent irritation of the nerve roots or dorsal rami. Pain localized to the area without radiation suggests localized somatic dysfunction or recurrent meningeal irritation (a more complete discussion of mechanical pain patterns in the spine can be found in *An Osteopathic Approach to Children*). Patients may also present with headache, especially if the primary area of injury is the upper cervical complex. The headache typically has a cervicogenic presentation. Older children with whiplash may complain of difficulty focusing, or unsteadiness. This may represent a mild form of cervicogenic vertigo, whereby proprioceptive input from the upper cervical spine is distorted by the soft tissue injury, altered mechanics and tissue swelling. These symptoms may also be due to mild concussion.

Treatment Notes

In whiplash injuries, one or two vertebrae are often found out of pattern with the remainder of the neck. For example, the cervical lordosis is flattened but two vertebrae are in marked extension; or the neck is hyperlordotic but one or two vertebrae are flexed. The associated soft tissue is tender, with specific tender points and/or trigger points. Evaluation of involuntary motion reveals marked compression between the involved segments. The non-pattern segments may represent the junctional areas of maximum strain when the neck moved through the plane of linear displacement. The muscle energy techniques described under Torticollis may be an effective modality when treating older children with whiplash.

Changes in cervical muscle tone influence lumbar tone and postural strategies, and vice versa. As a result, compensatory changes in lumbosacral mechanics may play a role in maintaining cervical strain patterns in patients with chronic whiplash complaints.

ASSESSMENT OF ACTIVE MOTION

First Rib

Supine Athlete (Fig. 2.22)

1. The patient is supine with the physician standing at the head of the table. The physician contacts the posterior lateral margins of the first ribs bilaterally.

2. The patient is instructed to inhale and exhale.

3. The physician evaluates the quality and excursion of motion of the first ribs. If the posterior margin of the rib has reduced motion during exhalation, the rib is depressed because the anterior aspect will not rise.

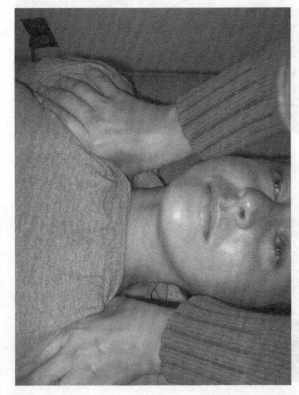

Fig. 2.22

BALANCED MEMBRANOUS TENSION

First or Second Rib

Supine Child/Athlete

1. The child is supine. The physician sits beside the child on the affected side. The physician places the hand closest to the child's head beneath the upper thorax, contacting the spinous process of T1 with her middle finger and the shaft of the first rib with her index finger (Fig. 2.23).

2. If the second rib is being treated, the physician contacts the spinous processes of T1 and T2 using her middle and ring fingers and the shaft of the second rib with her index finger.

3. The other hand is placed on the anterior chest wall, contacting the same rib at its costocartilaginous junction (Fig. 2.24A, B). In the example, only the first rib is being treated.

4. Thinking of the rib as a caliper (black line), the physician introduces a compressive force through her anterior and posterior contacts on the rib to engage its articulatory ends (small black arrows). Then she gently distracts the rib from its midline attachments (large black arrow) using the contact on the vertebrae to monitor and control the vertebral response.

5. The physician can then introduce torsion, side-bending, elevation, depression, translation etc. into the rib and its corresponding vertebra (in the case of the first rib) to achieve balanced tension in the associated structures.

6. Once balanced tension is achieved, the physician maintains that position until there is a change in tissue texture, a correction of the strain or an improvement in the somatic dysfunction.

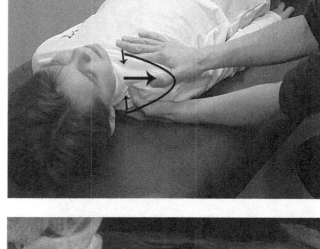

A

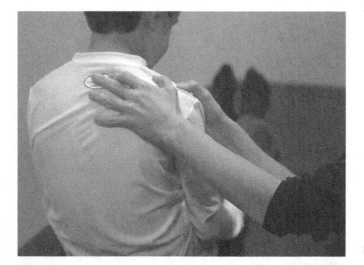

Fig. 2.23

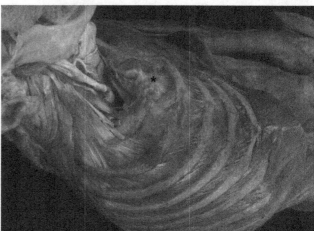

B

Fig. 2.24

ACTIVE RESISTANCE REDUCTION TECHNIQUE

Cervical Spine

Supine Young Athlete/Child

Example C3 FSRr

This technique works well in traumatic injuries with significant intra-articular compression and on areas where opposing dysfunction is present, for example a hyperextended cervical spine with a single-segment flexed vertebral dysfunction. The child must be able to cooperate with the physician. The technique is a combination of indirect muscle energy and direct technique. The physician uses translation to address the side-bending and rotation of the vertebrae.

1. The athlete is supine and the physician sits at her head. The physician places her hands under the neck, contacting the articular processes of the dysfunctional vertebra with the thumb and index finger of one hand (Figs 2.25, 2.26 and 2.27). In the example, the skeletal spine is rotated away from the camera and the spinous process (SP) of C3 is labeled. The middle finger and thumb of the other hand contact the articular processes of the vertebra below (Fig. 2.28).

2. In this example, the diagnosis is C3 FSR. The physician carries C3 away from the restrictive barrier into the direction of ease, but not to the physiological barrier. (For purposes of illustration, the movements used on C3 and C4 are depicted separately without the presence of the other hand, which in each case obstructed the view.) To produce C3 flexion, the physician uses both her contacts on C4 to lift the vertebra anteriorly and bring it into extension (Fig. 2.28 black arrow), while simultaneously flexing C3 with her other hand (Fig. 2.27 black curved arrow).

3. The physician uses her inferior hand to translate C4 to the right, while the superior hand translates C3 to the left. In this example, the middle finger on C4 in Figure 2.28 is used to translate C4 to the right (out of the picture). Meanwhile, the middle finger on C3 in Figure 2.27 would translate the vertebra to the left

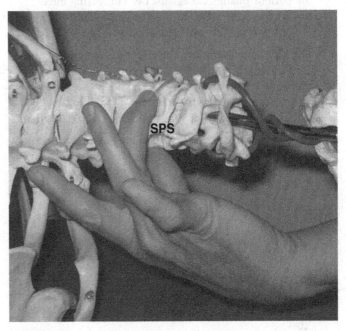

Fig. 2.26

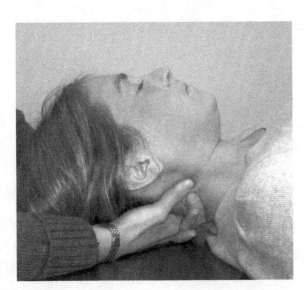

Fig. 2.25

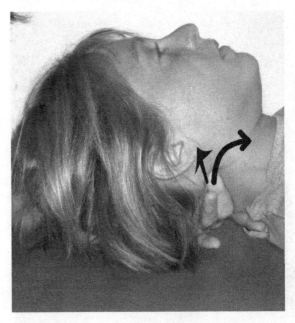

Fig. 2.27

(Fig. 2.27: the straight black arrow is meant to be pointing into the picture, towards the patient's left side).

4. The patient is asked to engage the muscles around C3. The following direction will help the patient accomplish this: the physician presses her middle finger against the right articular process of C3 (the ipsilateral side to the dysfunction) and asks the patient, 'Can you feel my finger?' 'Push just this part of your neck into my finger.'

5. The physician stabilizes the right articular process as the patient pushes C3 against her contacting finger, so that the right articular process is prevented from moving but the left articular process is not.

6. The physician maintains the counterforce against the right articular process for 2–3 seconds, until a slight change in tissue texture is felt on the left side. It is important that the patient employs and localizes extensor muscles to push C3 into the physician's hand.

7. Then the physician asks the patient to stop her motion. As the patient is relaxing her muscles, the physician stabilizes C4 and carries C3 into left rotation (by

translating it to the right with her thumb and lifting anteriorly with the middle finger only).

8. In this example, C3 FSRr, the left facet is restricted in flexion and resists extension. The left facet is the problem. The physician presses against the right articular process and holds that facet in a flexed position as the patient loads the muscles by pushing C3 into extension. The patient's forces are directed onto the left side because the physician is stabilizing the right side of C3.

9. As the patient relaxes, the physician carries C3 into left rotation, through its restrictive barrier, thereby 'closing' the left facet joint.

10. If, for example, the dysfunction had been C3 ESRr, then the left facet would be the problem because it would be resisting extension. The physician would contact C3 and extend and translate it to the left (position of ease) while translating C4 into the opposite direction. The physician needs to stabilize the right side so that the patient's forces summate on the restricted facet joint on the left.

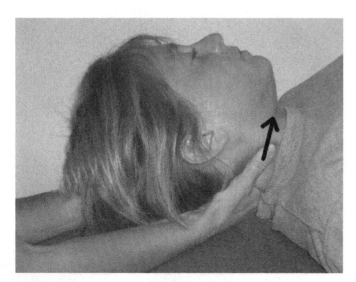

Fig. 2.28

FACILITATED POSITIONAL RELEASE (FPR)

Cervical Flexed Dysfunction

Supine Athlete/Child

Three-positional diagnosis of the segmental dysfunction is carried out to identify the positions of freedom of motion. In this example, the diagnosis is C5 FSRr (flexed, side-bent and rotated right).

1. The athlete is supine with the physician sitting at her head. The physician contacts the dysfunctional vertebra bilaterally using her thumb and middle or index finger. In this example, the physician is contacting C5. The physician uses her other hand to contact and control the position of the head (Fig. 2.29).

2. The neck is placed into postural neutral. The physician flexes the head and upper neck to the level of C5, to the point that a softening in tissue texture is noted.

3. Using both hands simultaneously the physician brings the head and upper neck, including C5, into right rotation and right side-bending until a softening in tissue texture is noted.

4. Using the hand that is on the head, the physician applies a gentle compression in the direction of the restricted area, to the point where a softening in tissue texture is noted. This is the facilitating force.

5. This is held for 3–5 seconds and then released. Motion is reassessed.

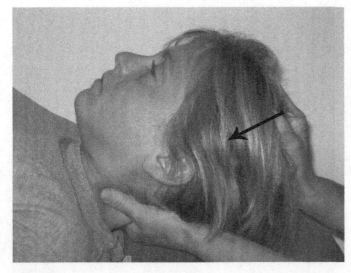

Fig. 2.29

FACILITATED POSITIONAL RELEASE (FPR)

Cervical Extended Dysfunction

Supine Athlete/Child

Three-positional diagnosis of the segmental dysfunction is carried out to identify the positions of freedom of motion. In this example, the diagnosis is C5 ESRr (extended, side-bent and rotated right).

1. The athlete is supine with the physician sitting at her head. The physician contacts the dysfunctional vertebra bilaterally using her thumb and middle or index finger. In this example, the physician is contacting C5. The physician uses her other hand to contact and control the position of the head (Fig. 2.30)

2. The neck is placed into postural neutral. The physician extends the head and upper neck to the level of C5, to the point that a softening in tissue texture is noted.

3. Using both hands simultaneously the physician brings the head and upper neck, including C5, into right rotation and right side-bending until a softening in tissue texture is noted.

4. Using the hand that is on the head, the physician applies a gentle compression in the direction of the restriction, to the point that a softening in tissue texture is noted. This is the facilitating force.

5. This is held for 3–5 seconds and then released. Motion is reassessed.

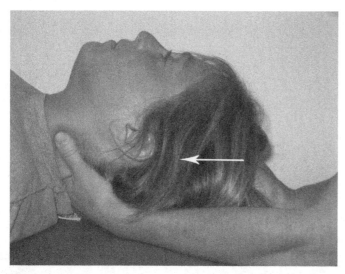

Fig. 2.30

DIRECT MYOFASCIAL RELEASE

Anterior Cervical Fascias

Seated Athlete

This technique is used to improve motion of the supraclavicular myofascial tissues and assist fluid movement through the cervicothoracic junction.

1. The athlete is seated on the table facing the physician. The table height should be set so that the patient's shoulders are slightly higher (above) the physician's. The physician places her hands over the patient's thoracic inlet so that the thumbs rest on the superior medial margin of the clavicles and the fingers drape over the shoulders (Fig. 2.31).

2. The patient then drapes his arms over the physician's so that his wrists and forearms rest in the crook of her elbow (Fig. 2.32). The physician asks the patient to flex his head. This relaxes the supraclavicular fasciae, allowing the physician to gently sink her thumbs into the supraclavicular space.

3. The patient is instructed to take a deep breath in, and as he exhales to allow his head to 'fall' between the physician's arms. As his head drops, the physician moves to the new restrictive barrier in the anterior fasciae by sinking her thumbs into the supraclavicular space.

4. This sequence is repeated three times. With each exhalation, the patient drops his head and the physician moves her thumbs to the new restrictive barrier in the fasciae. With each inhalation the physician resists the tightening of the fasciae.

5. At the end of the third sequence, the patient is instructed to take a deep breath and sit up straight as the physician maintains her tension on the anterior fasciae. The patient's change in posture stretches the fascial tissues.

6. Once the patient is sitting upright, he drops his arms and the physician slowly and gently releases her contact. Fascial motion is reassessed.

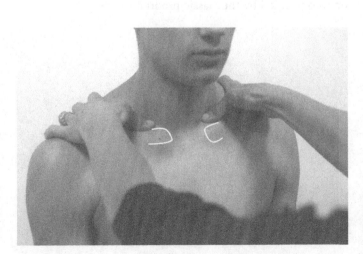

Fig. 2.31

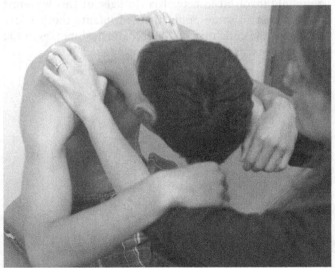

Fig. 2.32

MIGRAINE CEPHALGIA

Clinical Notes

Migraine cephalgia is less common in children than cervicogenic or 'muscular' headache. Depending on his age, the child may or may not describe a prodrome. The headache is typically unilateral and associated with photophobia and nausea. However, any headache of sufficient intensity and duration can evolve to include these symptoms. Classic migraine is often described as a vascular phenomenon whereby a change in vasomotor tone is the primary trigger for inflammatory-mediated irritation of trigeminal primary afferent fibers. There is a reported association between colic in infancy and migraine headaches in adults. In children with migraine it is important to address dysfunction in the thorax, which may play a role in sympathetically mediated changes in vasomotor tone and function.

COLIC

Clinical Notes

Although colic may represent a 'wastebasket' of multiple etiologies presenting with a similar clinic picture, a plausible explanation for infantile colic in some children is that it is a variant of cephalgia. The common gastrointestinal manifestations such as nausea and vomiting that often accompany cephalgia may account for the GI symptoms we see in infants. Vagally mediated symptoms are a common accompaniment to cephalgia. The osteopathic literature includes much discussion of strain patterns common to colic. These include dysfunction in the cranial base, craniocervical junction, and upper and mid-thoracic areas. These areas are also commonly involved in cephalgia. In light of this we must consider that in some populations of infants the primary etiology of the colic may be the somatic dysfunction in the head and neck, as it is in cervicogenic headache.

In some children colic may also be a disease of the immature nervous system. An inability to screen out afferent input may lead to sensory overload, agitation and irritability. The fact that most children 'grow out' of colic at approximately the same time as they achieve developmental milestones in the brain and gut supports this argument. The presence of somatic dysfunctions in these infants may be a contributing factor, but not necessarily the primary cause of the child's symptoms. Lastly, colic may be a clinical manifestation of immature gut function, whereby the gut is responding to new antigenic materials. Regardless of the etiology, there appears to be a commonly accepted involvement of the vagal and trigeminal systems. As such, anything that could be deemed as irritating to these systems should be addressed in an attempt to give the baby and the family some peace.

CERVICOGENIC CEPHALGIA

Clinical Notes

Cervicogenic cephalgia is trigeminally mediated pain that arises as a result of a combination of spinal facilitation and referred pain patterns (for a more complete discussion see *An Osteopathic Approach to Children*). The actual pain generators may be structures in the upper cervical or craniocervical areas. The pain is mapped to V3 sclerotomes, dermatomes and myotomes (Fig. 2.33). The child may or may not complain of associated neck pain or stiffness. The headache classically begins in the occipital area and may progress across the vertex and behind the eyes. The pain is bilateral, often described as a feeling of tightness or a vice on the head. When severe, photophobia and nausea may be present and the headache may take on a throbbing or pounding quality, similar to migraine cephalgia. However, unlike migraine, cervicogenic cephalgia is rarely unilateral or accompanied by the classic prodrome.

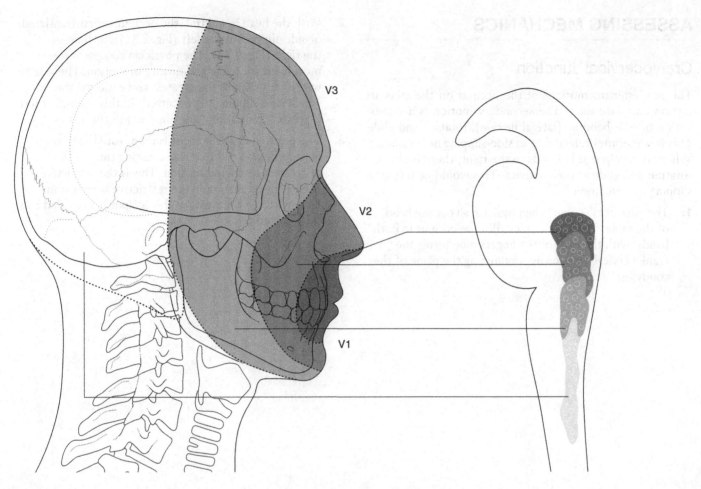

Fig. 2.33 • Schematic diagram of the trigeminal sclerotomes, myotomes and dermatomes.

ASSESSING MECHANICS

Craniocervical Junction

The predominant motions of the occiput on the atlas are flexion and extension. The secondary motion is a combination of side-bending (lateral flexion), rotation and glide. This is sometimes referred to as side-slipping or translation. When the occiput side-bends to the right, there is also left rotation and glide at the condyles. This would be left side-slipping or translation.

1. The patient is supine. The physician sits at the head of the table. The physician cradles the occiput in both hands, with the pads of the fingers monitoring the craniocervical junction approximating the plane of the condyles.

2. With the head in neutral, the occiput is first translated or side-slipped to the left (Fig. 2.34) and then to the right (Fig. 2.35). The physician compares the movement for range and quality of motion. The side to which excursion is the greatest and easiest is the side to which side-slipping has occurred. In this example there is greater translation (side-slipping) to the left.

3. The position of the occiput is then tested with the head in flexion and extension, noting the position of greatest restricted motion. This is the restrictive barrier. In this example the restrictive barrier is in flexion and to the right, so the occiput is extended and side-slipped left.

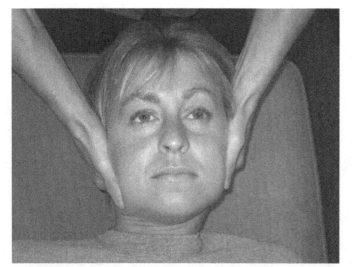

Fig. 2.34

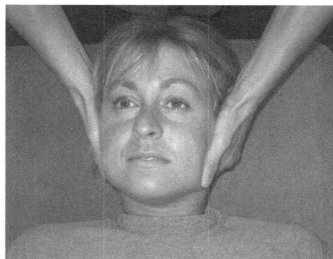

Fig. 2.35

ASSESSING SEGMENTAL MECHANICS

Lower Cervical Spine

Supine Athlete, Child, Infant (Fig. 2.36)

1. To assess the articular and myofascial mechanics in the cervical spine the child is supine. The physician sits at the head of the child, cradling the neck between her hands.

2. The physician places the pads of her index or middle fingers along the articular pillars of the lower cervical vertebrae. The left and right articular pillars of C7 are contacted with the physician's left and right middle fingers, respectively.

3. The physician slowly applies a lateral force from the left finger, translating the vertebra towards the right. The translation induces side-bending and rotation towards the finger. The response to this motion is assessed.

4. The physician slowly applies a lateral force from the right finger, translating the vertebra towards the left.

The translation induces side-bending and rotation towards the finger. The physician assesses tissue response to this motion.

5. The physician compares the tension created within the articular mechanism during the two motion tests.

6. The physician then assesses freedom of motion with respiration.

7. If restriction is present, the physician then assesses the tissue response of the vertebra against that of the vertebra above and below to identify the primary strain (Fig. 2.37).

ALTERNATE METHOD OF ASSESSMENT

Lower Cervical Spine

Alternatively, the cervical spine can be diagnosed using the muscle energy model of three-positional diagnosis described earlier.

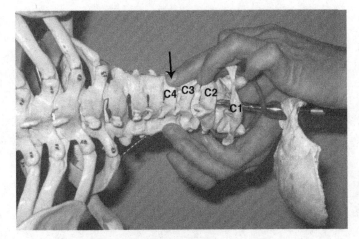

Fig. 2.36

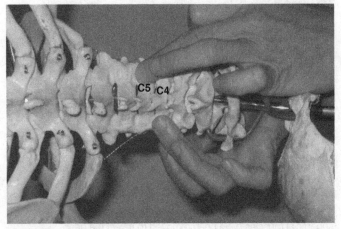

Fig. 2.37

CERVICOGENIC CEPHALGIA

Treatment Notes

A patient with cervicogenic cephalgia will typically have altered mechanics in the upper cervical and occipito-atlantal complexes on physical examination. The strain pattern usually involves articular compression in one plane with minimum movement in the myofascial components. The compression is typically found in an articular relationship of the occipitoatlantal or atlantoaxial joints. Occasionally, the 'primary lesion' may be the biomechanical transition at C3. Depending on the chronicity of the problem, there may or may not be trigger points in the deep short extensors of the head, but tender points are commonly present. Sphenobasilar synchondrosis (SBS) compression is frequently found and may be the primary pain generator, or compensatory to primary upper cervical dysfunction (Fig. 2.38). There is also marked compression and restriction of normal mechanics in the general area of the cranial base (occipitomastoid, petrobasilar), which is often compensatory in older children with no previous history of headache. Dysfunction in the vault is also usually secondary, except in those cases with a history of severe head trauma involving the vault, such as fracture. In some children tender points over the lambdoidal and occipitomastoid sutures will reproduce the pain pattern and a feeling of light-headedness. Fascial restriction is present throughout the cervical and upper thoracic area. In patients in whom the headache has a tendency to evolve into a migraine, there is often paraspinal muscle spasm in the area of T4. Hypertonic changes in the muscles of mastication will occur as a reflexive adaptation to the trigeminal irritation. When this is present the child may have bruxisms.

Reflex patterns exist between the muscles of mastication and those in the cervical area. Head posture and jaw mechanics can influence each other to the extent that one area can maintain dysfunction in the other, and vice versa. For example, dysfunction of the craniocervical junction or upper cervical complex can be associated with hypertonicity in the muscles of mastication. Clinically, this may present as jaw complaints such as temporomandibular joint (TMJ) syndrome, bruxisms, or trouble latching during breastfeeding. Treatment of the tissues of the mandible, temporal bones and cranial base may improve the complaints, but if the concomitant dysfunction in the cervical spine is not addressed the improvement will be temporary.

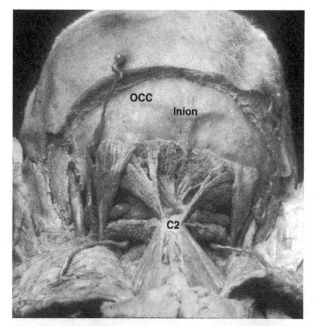

Fig. 2.38 • Posterior view of the craniocervical junction. The superficial muscles have been removed to reveal the deep suboccipital muscles extending from the occiput to C2.

BALANCED LIGAMENTOUS TENSION

Cervical Spine (Fig. 2.39)

Supine Infant

1. The infant is supine. The physician sits at the baby's head. The physician places her hands under the baby's upper neck, contacting the transverse articular processes of the vertebrae with the pads of her index and middle fingers.

2. The physician applies a gentle force with the index finger of one hand to translate the vertebra laterally, testing for tissue response (Fig. 2.40, black arrow). Resistance to translation is indicative of segmental somatic dysfunction.

3. Once the physician has identified a level of dysfunction she contacts the articular process of that vertebra on the side of the dysfunction and either the vertebra above or below (depending upon the tissue response) on the opposite side. For example, if the vertebra resists translation to the left (it will not side-bend right), then the right articular pillar is contacted. In Figure 2.41 the primary dysfunctional level is between C4 and C5.

4. The physician uses her contacts on C4 and C5 to introduce motion in the sagittal, coronal and horizontal planes to achieve balanced tension within the tissues.

5. Once balanced tension is achieved, the position is maintained until there is change in tissue texture, a resolution of the dysfunction or an improvement in mechanics.

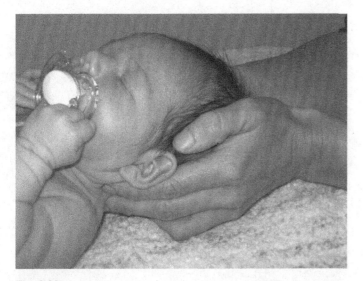

Fig. 2.39

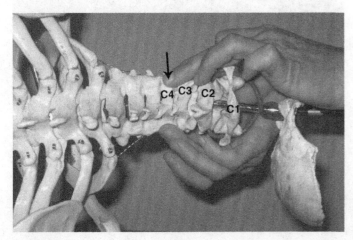

Fig. 2.40

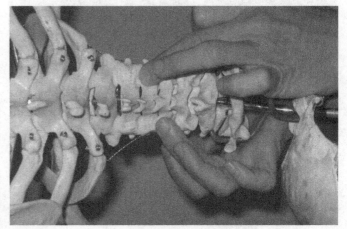

Fig. 2.41

BALANCED LIGAMENTOUS TENSION

Occipitoatlantal Junction

Supine Infant (Fig. 2.42)

1. The infant is supine and the physician sits at the baby's head. The physician cradles the occiput with one hand. The middle finger of the other hand contacts the inion and then slides inferiorly and anteriorly, curling around the occiput to rest at the craniocervical space slightly above the spinous process of C2 (Fig. 2.43).

2. The physician uses the hand contacting the occiput to bring the occiput posteriorly and into postural flexion while stabilizing C1 and C2 with her index finger.

3. The physician can introduce side-bending, translation and rotation into the occiput to achieve balanced tension in the suboccipital tissues.

4. The physician introduces these movements to the point of balanced tension. These movements are not used to engage the restrictive barrier, nor are these positions introduced in the direction of ease.

5. Once balanced tension is achieved, the position is maintained until there is a change in tissue texture, an improvement in mechanics or a resolution of the strain.

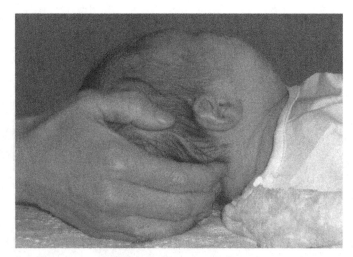

Fig. 2.42

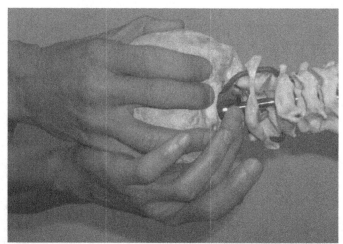

Fig. 2.43

BALANCED MEMBRANOUS TENSION

Condylar Decompression (Fig. 2.44A, B)

Supine Infant

The focus of this technique is the condylar compression between the occiput and atlas. This is an articular dysfunction rather than a muscular dysfunction involving the sub-occipital muscles. Condylar compression is often found in infants with colic, torticollis or plagiocephaly.

1. The neonate is supine and the physician sits at the baby's head. The physician cradles the baby's head in her two hands.

2. The physician curls her fingers into the craniocervical space so that the ring fingers lie on the approximate plane of the occipital condyles and the middle fingers approximate the plane of the atlas. Each index finger monitors the ipsilateral temporal bone at the mastoid portion.

3. The physician uses the ring fingers to introduce a firm but gentle force in a lateral direction to 'lift and spread' the tissues posteriorly and away from the atlas (Fig. 2.45). This is done towards but not up to the restrictive barrier. The middle fingers may be used to decompress the atlas from the occiput.

4. This decompression is performed until balanced tension is felt between the occiput and the atlas. The position is maintained until there is a change in tissue texture or improved freedom of motion between the occiput and atlas.

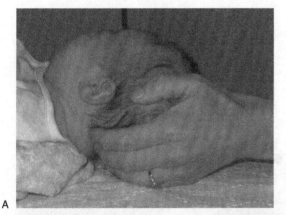

A

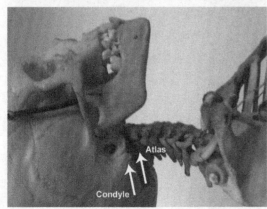

B

Fig. 2.44

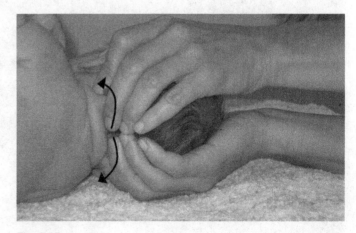

Fig. 2.45

Direct Condylar Decompression (Fig. 2.46)

Supine Infant

This technique is described as a direct because the vector of contact approaches but does not move through the restrictive barrier. The amount of force used is MINIMAL. The force used should match and not exceed the tension in the tissues. **If the reader is uncertain as too how much force that should be, then they should not attempt this technique until they can be properly supervised by someone with experience in using the direct approach in infants.**

1. The neonate is supine. The physician sits at the baby's head. The physician cradles the head in a similar manner to the contact used in the previous technique. The middle fingers approximate the plane of the atlas and the ring fingers approximate the plane of the occipital condyles.

2. The physician assesses mechanics at the condyles and notes which side feels more restricted. In the figure, the left side is restricted.

3. The physician stabilizes both the atlas and the occiput on the contralateral side (the right side in this example). The physician uses the middle finger on the side ipsilateral to the dysfunction (the left side in this example) to stabilize the atlas (the asterisk represents finger contacts).

4. The physician uses the ring finger on the ipsilateral side to carry the ipsilateral condyle posteriorly and laterally to the restrictive barrier, but not through it (black arrow). The infant may be irritable with this approach. It is imperative that the physician avoid using too much force.

5. This position is maintained until there is a change in tissue texture, a release of the compression, or an improvement in motion at the condylar junction.

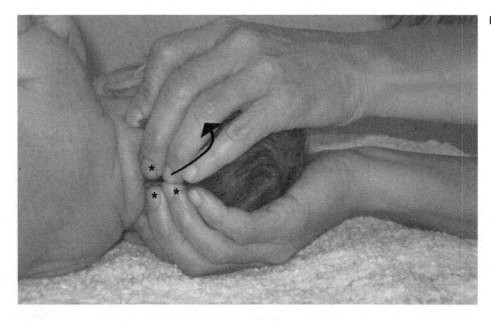

Fig. 2.46

BALANCED MEMBRANOUS TENSION

Base Spread

Supine Infant

1. The infant is supine or held in the parent's arms. The physician sits at the infant's head with her forearms supported. The physician places her hands beneath the infant's head, with a contact very low (inferior to inion) on the occiput (Fig. 2.47).

2. The physician places her fingers so that the smallest fingers meet in the midline of the occiput just inferior to the inion along the sagittal plane of the occiput. The ring fingers curve along the surface of the occiput to approximate the plane of the condyles. The middle fingers contact C2 posterior and medial to the transverse processes, and the index fingers contact the temporal bones at the occipitomastoid sutures (Figs 2.48 and 2.49).

3. The following motions are performed simultaneously (Fig. 2.48):

   a. The ring fingers introduce a curvilinear traction to the occiput in a postural flexion motion to disengage the occipital condyles.

   b. As this is being done the middle fingers contacting the plane of the condyles introduce a cephalad–lateral force in such a direction to prevent the atlas from being carried posteriorly with the occiput.

   c. The temporal bones are decompressed from the condylar parts by being 'lifted' anteriorly and cephalad.

4. The physician can vary the vector of her forces slightly to achieve balanced membranous tension in the associated structures and tissues.

5. Once balanced membranous tension is achieved, the position is held until there is a release of tissue tension or a sense of opening of the composite cranial base.

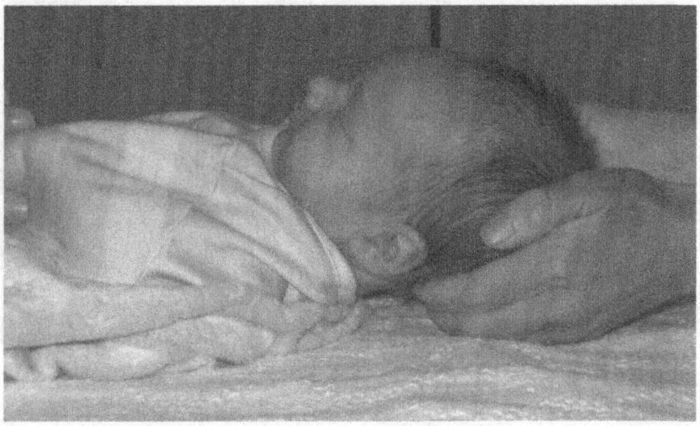

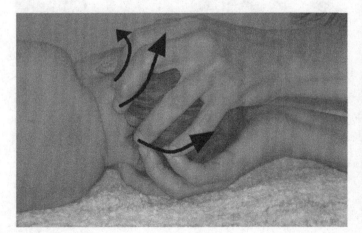

Fig. 2.47

Fig. 2.48

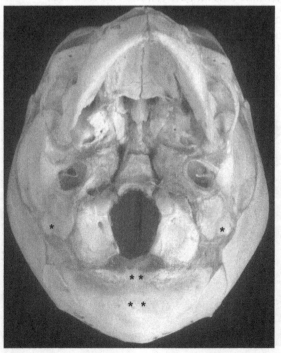

Fig. 2.49

BALANCED LIGAMENTOUS TENSION

Lower Cervical Spine

Supine Young Athlete/Child

In many cases, especially chronic presentations, the mechanics in the lower cervical complex, thoracic spine and pelvis will need to be addressed before the upper cervical spine, occipitoatlantal (OA) joint and cranial base. The hand placement is the same as described above in Assessing Lower Cervical Spine; the example used is a C4/C5 dysfunction.

1. The patient is supine and the physician sits at the head of the table. The physician places both her hands under patient's the neck, with her fingers lying alongside the lateral aspects of the vertebrae (Figs 2.50 and 2.51).

2. The physician positions her fingers such that the pads of her middle or index fingers contact the articular pillars of C5 and C6 on opposite sides (Fig. 2.52). In a C5 rotated left dysfunction the pad of the right middle finger would be placed on the right articular pillar of C6 and the pad of the left middle finger on the left articular pillar of C5.

3. The physician then applies a gentle anterior pressure to the left articular pillar of C5, encouraging C5 to rotate to the right while simultaneously applying pressure to the right articular pillar of C6, encouraging C6 to rotate towards the left. As this is being done, the physician pays close attention to the changing ligamentous tension between the two vertebrae.

4. The articular mechanism is only rotated to the point where the tension within the ligaments is felt to be equal and in a point of balance.

5. The physician uses this contact to simultaneously introduce various vectors of motion: lateral translation, compression, decompression, flexion and extension into the two vertebrae to bring the structures around the vertebrae into balanced tension.

6. The physician then holds the joint in this position of balanced ligamentous tension while the child breathes quietly. The child's breathing is the activating force.

7. The position is held until there is a change in tissue texture or improvement in function.

8. The remainder of the cervical spine can be treated in the same manner. The physician can 'walk' her fingers up along the articular processes, assessing the mechanics of each vertebra and treating her findings.

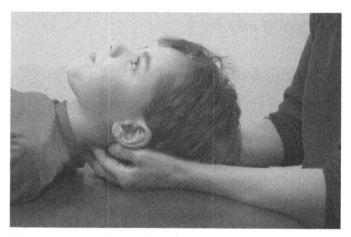

Fig. 2.51

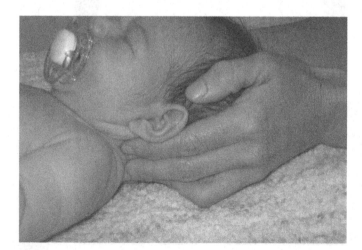

Fig. 2.50

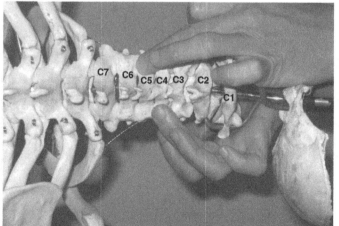

Fig. 2.52

BALANCED LIGAMENTOUS TECHNIQUE

Occipitoatlantal Junction

Supine Young Athlete/Child

1. The child is supine and the physician sits at the head of the table. The physician cradles the occiput in one hand so that the pad of the middle finger slides inferiorly towards the opisthion (Fig. 2.53). The index and ring fingers are placed slightly lateral to the midline, approximating the plane of the occipital condyles (Fig. 2.54, asterisk).

2. The other hand is placed under the upper cervical complex with the pad of the middle finger just above the spinous process of C2 and contacting the ligaments between the occiput and cervical spine (Fig. 2.55).

3. The head must rest, relaxed, upon the physician's hands.

4. The physician then applies a gentle traction in a circumlinear vector, taking the occiput into postural flexion. The physician will feel a change in the tension under her hands.

5. The physician uses the contact between C1 and C2 and the contact on the occiput to establish balanced ligamentous tension between the condylar parts, the occiput, C1 and C2.

6. Once balanced ligamentous tension is achieved, the position is held until there is a release in tissue tension. Often the physician will feel the occiput 'drop' into her hands, or the cervical processes lift out of her hands as the occipital condyles disengage from those of the atlas.

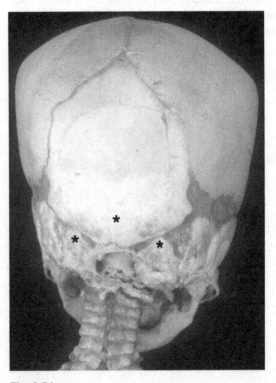

Fig. 2.54

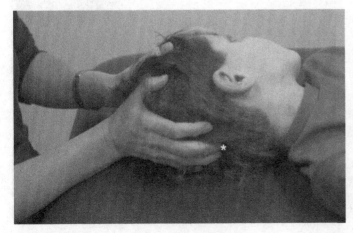

Fig. 2.53

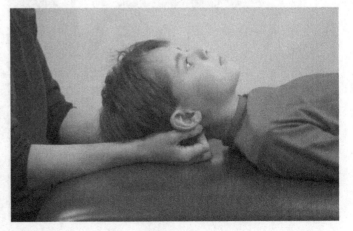

Fig. 2.55

FACILITATED POSITIONAL RELEASE

Occipitoatlantal Joint

Supine Young Athlete/Child

In this example, the occiput is side-slipped right, i.e. it is side-bent left.

1. The patient is supine with the physician sitting at her head. The physician cradles the head with her left hand such that the base of her hand lies over the vertex (Fig. 2.56). The right hand is placed under the craniocervical junction so that the palmar surface of the middle finger contacts the OA junction on the left (Fig. 2.57).

2. The physician flexes the head slightly to position the OA in biomechanical neutral.

3. A compressive force is introduced through the hand contacting the vertex (Fig. 2.56, white arrow) until there is some freedom of motion noted with the finger contacting the left OA.

4. The physician uses her right middle finger to introduce a lateral shearing force towards the right across the OA junction (Fig. 2.56, black arrow). This movement exaggerates the left side-bending and right side-slipping.

5. This position is held for 3–5 seconds and then released. The area is reassessed.

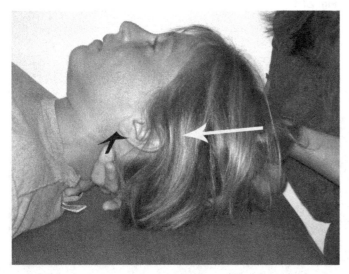

Fig. 2.56

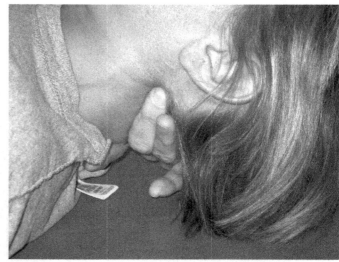

Fig. 2.57

MUSCLE ENERGY

Oculovestibulo-cephalic Reflex

The following three techniques use the oculovestibulo-cephalic (OVC) reflex to correct the strain at the cranio-cervical junction. The OVC is a primitive reflex that coordinates head and eye movements. When the eyes move, the OVC stimulates the short restrictor muscles of the craniocervical junction to move the head and follow the direction of the eyes. The child must be able to follow directions accurately for this technique to succeed. It may be used in conjunction with the FPR and/or BLT techniques described above.

OCULOVESTIBULO-CEPHALIC REFLEX

Occipitoatlantal Junction – Extended Dysfunction

Supine Child/Athlete

1. The child is supine. The physician sits at the child's head with her forearms supported. The physician places her hands under the child's head, cradling the occiput with the pads of her fingers on the suboccipital muscles (Fig. 2.58).

2. The physician flexes the child's head to the restrictive barrier for flexion (black arrow). Then the physician induces side-slipping – a combination of side-bending, translation and rotation – to the restrictive barrier. In Figure 2.58 the OA is ESSr (extended side-slipped right); it is side-bent to the left, and rotated and translated to the right. The restrictive barrier is side-bending to the right and rotation and translation to the left. This is also called side-slipping left.

3. The physician stabilizes the head in the side-slipped left position. The child is instructed to look with his eyes only over his head (white arrow). He should not consciously extend his head or lift his chin. As the child does this, the physician should feel the tension in the suboccipital muscles change. The physician resists the motion by stabilizing the occiput.

4. The child maintains this position for 4–5 seconds and is then instructed to relax or look straight and close his eyes. The physician pauses for 3–5 seconds until she feels the post-isometric relaxation phase.

5. Then the physician flexes the head to the new restrictive barrier and engages the new restrictive barrier to side-slipping (translation).

6. This procedure is repeated twice.

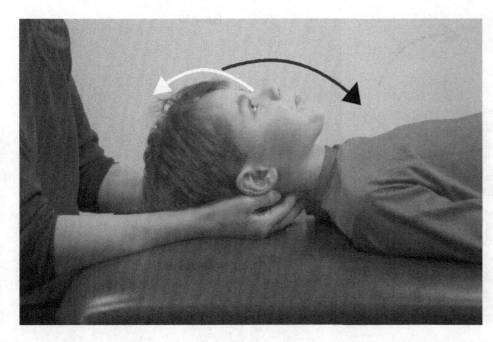

Fig. 2.58

OCULOVESTIBULO-CEPHALIC REFLEX

Occipitoatlantal Junction – Flexed Dysfunction

Supine Child/Athlete

1. The child is supine. The physician sits at the child's head with her forearms supported. The physician places her hands under the child's head, cradling the occiput with the pads of her fingers on the suboccipital muscles (Fig. 2.59).

2. The physician extends the child's head to the restrictive barrier for extension (black arrow). Then the physician induces side-slipping – a combination of side-bending, translation and rotation – to the restrictive barrier. In Figure 2.59 the OA is FSSR (flexed side-slipped right); it is side-bent to the left, and rotated and translated to the right. The restrictive barrier is side-bending to the right and rotation and translation to the left. This is also called side-slipping left.

3. The physician stabilizes the head in the side-slipped left position and the child is instructed to look with his eyes towards his feet (white arrow). He should not consciously flex or lift his head. As the child does this, the physician should feel the tension in the suboccipital muscles change. The physician resists the motion by stabilizing the occiput.

4. The child maintains this position for 4–5 seconds and is then instructed to relax or look straight and close his eyes. The physician pauses for 3–5 seconds until she feels the post-isometric relaxation phase.

5. Then the physician extends the head to the new restrictive barrier and engages the new restrictive barrier to side-slipping.

6. This procedure is repeated twice.

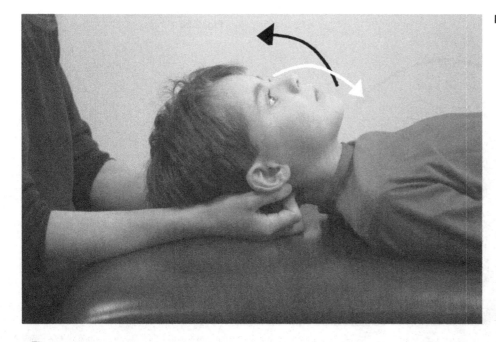

Fig. 2.59

OCULOVESTIBULO-CEPHALIC REFLEX

Atlantoaxial Junction

Supine Child/Athlete (Fig. 2.60)

1. The patient is supine. The physician sits at the patient's head with her forearms supported. The physician places her hands under the patient's head, cradling the occiput with the pads of her fingers on the suboccipital muscles (Fig. 2.61).

2. With the athlete's neck in a neutral position, the physician rotates the head to the restrictive barrier for rotation. In this example, the diagnosis for the atlantoaxial joint is right rotation; the restrictive barrier is to left rotation.

3. The physician induces flexion at the occipitoatlantal joint to lock out that joint and rotates the head to the restrictive barrier, in this case left.

4. The physician stabilizes the head in this position and the athlete is instructed to look with her eyes only in the opposite direction (in this case towards the left). She should not move her head. As the patient does this, the physician should feel the tension in the suboccipital muscles change. The physician resists the motion by stabilizing the occiput.

5. The patient maintains this position for 4–5 seconds, and is then instructed to relax her eyes or look straight ahead, and close her eyes. The physician pauses for 3–5 seconds until she feels the post-isometric relaxation phase.

6. Then the physician gently rotates the head to the new restrictive barrier.

7. This procedure is repeated twice.

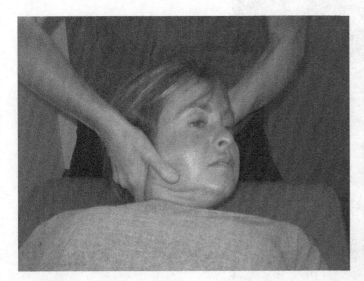

Fig. 2.60

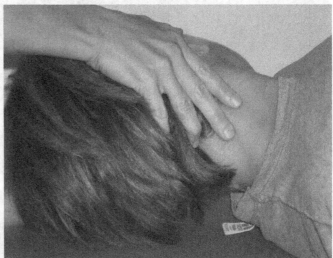

Fig. 2.61

MUSCLE ENERGY ISOMETRIC CONTRACTION

Atlantoaxial Junction

Supine Athlete

1. The patient is supine. The physician sits at the patient's head with her forearms supported. The physician places her hands under the patient's head, cradling the occiput with the pads of her fingers on the suboccipital muscles (Fig. 2.62).

2. The physician induces flexion at the occipitoatlantal joint to lock out that joint, and rotates the head to the restrictive barrier. In this example the diagnosis for the atlantoaxial joint is right rotation; the restrictive barrier is to left rotation.

3. The physician stabilizes the head in this position and the athlete is instructed to turn her head to the right (white arrow). The physician resists this motion with an equal and opposite force (black arrow).

4. This isometric contraction is maintained for 4–5 seconds. The patient is then instructed to relax as the physician simultaneously relaxes her counterforce. The physician pauses for 3–5 seconds until she feels the post-isometric relaxation of the suboccipital muscles.

5. Then the physician gently rotates the head to the new restrictive barrier. This sequence is repeated twice more.

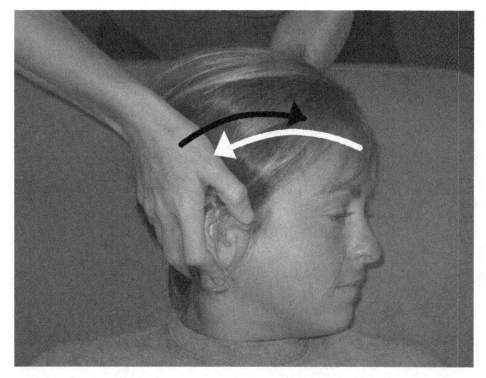

Fig. 2.62

BALANCED MEMBRANOUS TENSION

Direct Temporal Lift

Supine Child/Athlete (Fig. 2.63)

1. The athlete is supine and the physician is seated at her head. The physician places her hands under the patient's head so that her hyperthenar eminence contacts the mastoid process and mastoid portion just lateral to the occipitomastoid suture.

2. The patient's head should rest comfortably so that its weight is poised along the mastoid process and the mastoid portion of the temporal bones.

3. The physician positions her hands so that they introduce an anterolateral vector at the point of contact to decompress the forces at the occipitomastoid juncture. There is no internal or external rotation.

4. The position is maintained as the weight of the patient's head falls between the physician's points of contact until there is a change in tissue texture.

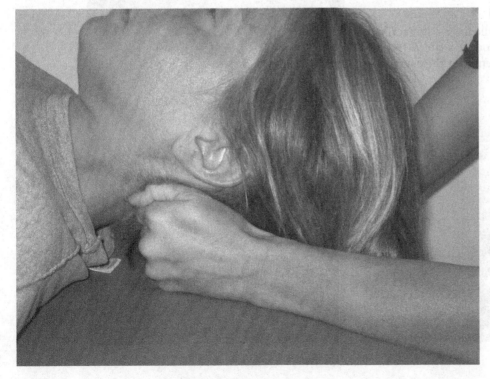

Fig. 2.63

BALANCED MEMBRANOUS TENSION

Base Spread

Supine Child/Athlete

This is a direct approach to balanced tension.

1. The child is supine. The physician sits at the child's head with her forearms supported. The physician places her hands beneath the child's head with a contact very low (inferior to inion) on the occiput (Fig. 2.64).

2. The physician places her fingers so that the smallest and ring fingers (Figs 2.65 and 2.66, asterisk) meet in the midline of the occiput just inferior to the inion along the sagittal plane of the occiput. The middle fingers (M) curve along the surface of the occiput to approximate the plane of the condyles. The index fingers contact C1 posterior and medial to the transverse processes, and the mastoid process rests on the lateral aspect of the thumb (T).

3. The following motions are performed simultaneously (Fig. 2.64):

   a. The index fingers stabilize C1.

   b. The thumbs introduce an anterolateral force into the mastoid process to decompress the occipitomastoid area.

   c. Simultaneously the ring and smallest fingers introduce a curvilinear traction into the occiput in a postural flexion motion to disengage the occipital condyles.

   d. As this is being done the middle fingers contacting the plane of the condyles introduce a lateral force in a direction that would decompress the condylar parts.

4. The physician can vary the vector of her forces to decompress and achieve balanced membranous tension in the associated structures and tissues.

5. Once balanced membranous tension is achieved, the position is held until there is a release of tissue tension or a sense of opening of the composite cranial base.

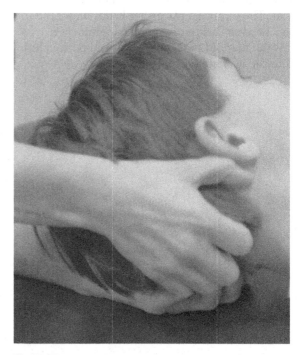

Fig. 2.65

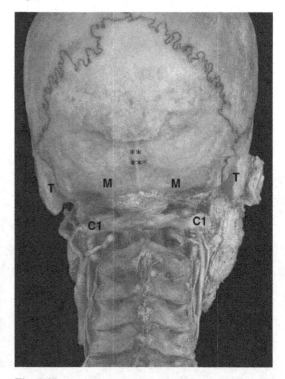

Fig. 2.66

Fig. 2.64

PLAGIOCEPHALY

Clinical Notes

Plagiocephaly is a general term used to describe an abnormal shape of the skull. It differs from the normal adaptive molding that accommodates the newborn head to the maternal pelvis in that molding resolves spontaneously within the first day of life and plagiocephaly persists or even worsens. The term plagiocephaly can also be used more specifically to describe a parallelogram-shaped head that displays prominence in one quarter of the skull and flattening of the ipsilateral side. Other specific terms, such as brachycephalic and scaphocephalic, exist to describe the other deformities seen in the skull (Fig. 2.67). The brachycephalic skull is wider from ear to ear and narrower from frontal to occiput. This is the opposite of the scaphocephalic head, which is very narrow from ear to ear and broader from occiput to frontal. Throughout this section we will use the term plagiocephaly in its general sense.

Plagiocephaly may or may not be associated with craniosynostosis, i.e., premature fusion of the sutures (Kane 1996). Most children with plagiocephaly have patent cranial sutures, and head circumference is not affected by the deformity. Plagiocephaly may be present at birth as a result of abnormal uterine lie or a complication of labor and delivery. This is called primary plagiocephaly. Secondary plagiocephaly develops after birth and is often not diagnosed until after the first month of life.

Primary plagiocephaly may or may not be associated with a significant cranial base strain pattern. When there is no cranial base strain pattern and there is suture overlap, it is probably adaptive molding and will resolve within 1 or 2 days.

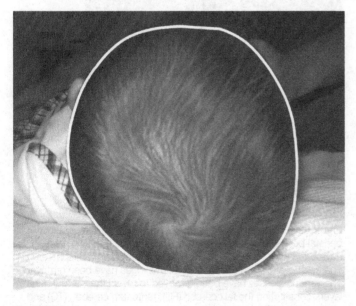

Fig. 2.67

If it does not resolve, the suture overlap persists, and there is no detectable cranial base or cervical strain pattern, one must consider premature closure (craniosynostosis) or congenital malformation. If the plagiocephaly is due to intrauterine lie, the deformity may not involve changes in relationships at sutures, but there are changes in the morphology of the bone, which may even include the cranial base and mandible. There may or may not be a history of prolonged or difficult labor and delivery, and a significant cranial base strain pattern may or may not be present. Plagiocephaly due to uterine lie has a bony quality to the strain even in the vault, whereas in plagiocephaly due to the forces of labor or delivery the strain has a membranous quality in the vault. If the primary plagiocephaly arose during labor and delivery, there may be overlap of the sutures and deformation of the vault bones (molding), but not the bones of the base or mandible. Cranial base strain patterns, especially SBS compression, are common in these children. As the child grows the deformation may be exacerbated by the abnormal tissue forces influencing the bone. The presence of facial asymmetry suggests that the primary point of entry of the strain was the sphenoid. Facial symmetry with significant cranial base unleveling suggests that the primary point of entry was the occiput. Typically, when the occiput is the primary lesion there is malpositioning of the head on the neck, which gives the appearance of a torticollis. This is more likely in lateral strains that are primarily posterior (occipital) than in those that are primarily anterior (sphenoid). The presence of significant facial asymmetry warrants a work-up for craniosynostosis or congenital malformation.

Secondary plagiocephaly typically develops as a result of abnormal tensile forces in the cervical tissues or at the craniocervical junction. It is often not noticed until the infant is a few months old. Secondary plagiocephaly may develop in premature infants due to intubation and positioning in the isolette. In the former case a scaphocephalic deformity is common, and in the latter a brachycephalic deformation. In full-term infants secondary plagiocephaly may develop as a result of persistent supine positioning or torticollis. When it is purely a result of positioning the vault bones will be misshapen but there is no significant cranial base strain. These deformities often resolve spontaneously once the child attains head control and begins sitting. Secondary plagiocephaly that develops secondary to a cranial base strain pattern or torticollis typically does not resolve spontaneously, and often worsens as the infant grows. This is because the vault bones are responding to abnormalities in the tensile forces in the myofascial tissues of the cranial and cervical areas, as well as the persistent head position when supine. In the case of torticollis, the child has a preferential posture of the head and neck that may have been dismissed as inconsequential. The abnormally increased tensile forces on the involved side alter growth patterns. In some cases head movement may be restricted to the point where the head constantly rests on one side. In both cases the cranial deformity is compensatory, and although present in the squamal portion of the occiput and the ipsilateral parietal bone, there may be only a mild compensatory SBS strain. Secondary plagiocephaly that is due to cranial base strain presents with a significant cranial base strain pattern and the primary postural adaptation is at the craniocervical junction, not in the neck.

Treatment Notes

Treatment of plagiocephaly, especially secondary plagiocephaly, requires two things: resolution of any mechanical strains or abnormal tensions that are contributing to maintaining the distortion of the cranial bones; and – most importantly – somehow getting the child to stop lying on the flat spot. The timing of treatment in infants and newborns with plagiocephaly appears to play a role in outcome. Resolving tissue strains and balancing tensile forces just prior to a growth phase seems to allow the body to re-establish tissue balance in the distorted area. As the child grows the

untreated plagiocephaly exerts influence over the cervical spine, torso and postural strategies, and it becomes much more difficult for these strains to resolve.

In plagiocephaly, the distortion of the vault is often due to the membranous strain through the reciprocal tension membrane (RTM) system of the head. Depending on your point of view, this may or may not be adaptive to the strain in the cranial base or cranial cervical junction. All components (membranous, articular and ligamentous) need to be addressed before the distortion will resolve. Often the fluid mechanics in these newborns and infants are not significantly affected by the distortion. To release the membranous strain, a modified venous sinus technique can be used. The focus of this approach is the membranous structure in which the sinus has formed, rather than the relationship between the sinus and the suture, or the fluid within the sinus (Figs 2.68 and 2.69). This is a direct approach to achieving balanced membranous tension between the components of the reciprocal tension membrane. The following sequence describes a treatment approach that begins at the craniocervical junction and progresses into the vault, addressing first the membranous, then the osseous, and finally the fluid components. This sequencing reflects the

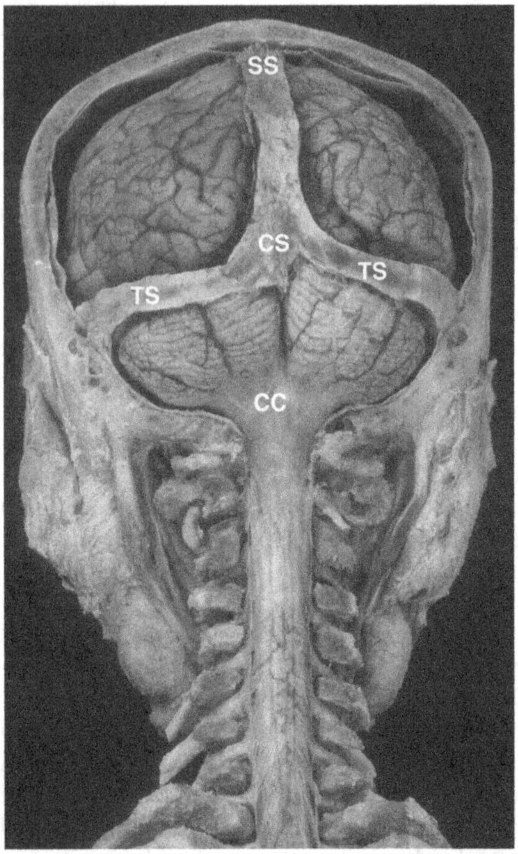

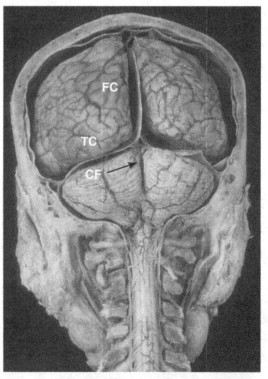

Fig. 2.68 • Posterior view of the occipital squama. The posterior parietal bones have been removed. The cerebellar cistern (CC) is exposed as well as the dural meninges extending into the neck. The external and internal dura have been removed over the cortical and cerebellar hemispheres, leaving the venous sinuses intact. TS, transverse sinus; CF, confluence of sinuses; SS, straight sinus.

Fig. 2.69 • Posterior view of the occipital squama. The posterior parietal bones have been removed. The external and internal dura have been removed over the cortical and cerebellar hemispheres. The cerebellar cistern (CC) and dural meninges have been removed. The venous sinuses have been removed to reveal the internal dural layers constituting the falx cerebri (FC), tentorium cerebelli (TC) and cerebellar falx (CF and arrow).

most likely developmental sequencing of the strain pattern. During engagement and labor, forces would be directed through the membranous vault to the craniocervical junction, the only true joint in the neonatal head. This joint is typically locked out in a flexed position as the head enters the maternal pelvis. With the occiput flexed upon the atlas, rotational and side-bending forces are not easily accommodated at the occipitoatlantal joint. Torsional and rotational stresses transmitted through the membranous vault must be absorbed by the junctional areas of the composite cranial base and vault. The membranous quality of the vault provides it with a relatively flexibility that is able to accommodate to these forces compared to the structures of the base. When the degree of stress through the vault exceeds the accommodation of the base, the osseous and cartilaginous structures of the cranial base will develop a base strain pattern. The vault will then adapt to the base strain, resulting in the plagiocephaly.

The only truly functional joint in the neonatal head is the occipitoatlantal joint. Consequently, the condylar area is commonly involved in plagiocephaly that originates in the cranial base. Although true condylar compression may not be present, more often than not there will be some strain between the occiput and the atlas, which may or may not involve C2 and C3. Mechanically, C3 is a junctional area of the cervical spine, resolving the forces occurring in the upper complex (occiput, atlas, axis) with those of the lower complex. The other area not to be forgotten is the cerebellar falx, which extends inferiorly from the tentorium along the midline of the inner table of the supraocciput to anchor into the periosteum of the neural arches of C1, C2 and C3. This is the continuation of the dural attachment to the cervical spine.

Overlap and ridging at the sutures need to be resolved before the molding deformation of the vault bones can change. The strain at the suture can be maintained by unresolved membranous forces within the reciprocal tension membrane, or by external myofascial forces from the neck and craniocervical junction. The molding technique as described by Sutherland (Magoun 1976) is often not effective until these other influences are addressed.

Treating the neck and thoracic cage before the head is the preferred way to proceed in most children with plagiocephaly. This allows for several things. First, respiratory mechanics can be addressed and the inherent forces of respiration can further assist in the treatment. Second, the child can see the physician and become somewhat accustomed to the treatment before having his head and craniocervical junction touched – areas that are often tender. Correcting the compensatory or adaptive changes in other areas of the body removes those influences from the somatic condition in the head, and in effect creates a bit more slack in the tissues involved in the primary strain.

The 'at-home assignment' for baby and parents is to encourage the infant to engage the cervical muscles symmetrically and to avoid lying on the more convex side of the head. The first, which is done to reinforce normal postural relationships, can be accomplished by increasing the amount of time the infant spends prone. Most infants with plagiocephaly, especially if there is cervical involvement, dislike the prone position. Propping the prone infant up on pillows (so she is not flat), or laying her prone on a parent's chest, allows her to look up into her surroundings. When supine, the infant can be encouraged to turn her head away from the affected side by positioning toys and mobiles on the unaffected side, or by placing her in the crib so that she turns away from the affected side to view her mother or the doorway. Helmets or dynamic cranial orthotic devices may prevent the child from exacerbating the deformity by stopping him from lying on the flattened aspect. These cranial helmets are generally made of a lightweight substance and can be appropriately integrated into the therapeutic plan to support the changes made by the osteopathic treatment.

Children with plagiocephaly that does not respond to treatment should be evaluated for suture patency with X-ray or CT. Abnormal hair patterns, persistent ridging or overlap of the sutures, and significant facial asymmetry which worsens with growth are all signs that further evaluation is warranted. Surgery is the definitive treatment for premature closure of the sutures. In the immediate postoperative period (first week) the child may benefit from osteopathic treatment of the torso, pelvis and extremities. However, osteopathic evaluation and treatment of the neck or head should be delayed at least 8–12 weeks, unless the practitioner is well skilled in treating post-craniotomy heads. It takes many weeks for the post-craniotomy head and neck to re-establish a functional relationship and integrate any surgical implants. Biomechanical findings during this time can be very misleading, and improper treatment may have deleterious effects on the healing process.

BALANCED MEMBRANOUS TENSION

Cerebellar Falx

Supine Infant (Figs 2.70 and 2.71)

This technique uses a similar approach to a venous sinus spread technique but the intention is directed at the membranous structure, the cerebellar falx. Studies have show that fibers from the cerebellar falx are continuous with dural ligaments extending into the upper cervical complex as low as C3. This technique is used to balance membranous strains in the cranial base that involve these connections. This may need to be performed prior to condylar decompression or base spread. This approach can also be used in older children with cervicogenic cephalgia.

1. The infant is supine or held in the parent's arms. The physician sits at the infant's head with her forearms supported. The physician places her hands beneath the infant's head with a contact very low (inferior to inion) on the occiput (Fig. 2.70).

2. The physician places her fingers so that she is contacting the midline of the occiput just inferior to the inion along the sagittal plane of the occiput. This approximates the location of the cerebellar falx (Figs 2.71 and 2.72).

3. The ring fingers meet in the midline and contact just inferior to the inion (Fig 2.72, circle). The middle fingers approximate each other and lie just inferior to the ring fingers (asterisks). The index fingers contact the second cervical vertebra medial and posterior to its transverse processes.

4. A gentle, steady anterior and lateral pressure (Fig. 2.71, black arrows) is introduced through the ring and middle fingers and directed into the deep connective tissues of the cerebellar falx. The index fingers monitor C2.

5. As the tissue texture under the ring and middle fingers begins to change, the index fingers can control C2 to establish balanced membranous tension through the cerebellar falx and its dural connections to the upper cervical complex.

6. Once balanced membranous tension is established the position is maintained until there is a softening, a change in tissue texture or a correction of the strain.

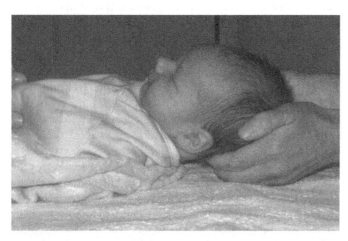

Fig. 2.70

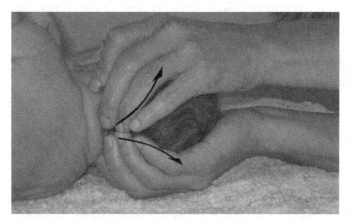

Fig. 2.71

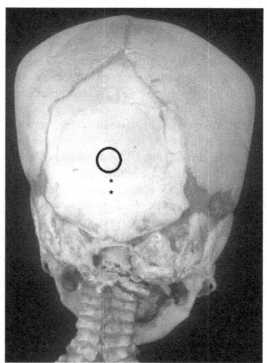

Fig. 2.72

BALANCED MEMBRANOUS TENSION

Temporal Lift/Tentorium Cerebelli

Supine Infant (Figs 2.73 and 2.74)

This technique is used to decompress the temporo-occipital junction. The mastoid process is not present at birth, and takes several years to develop. There is no occipitomastoid suture per se. This technique focuses on the posterior aspect of the petrobasilar junction and the relationship between the basiocciput and the mastoid portion of the temporal bone (Figs 2.75 and 2.76).

1. The infant is supine or held in the parent's arms. The physician sits at the infant's head with her forearms supported. The physician places her hands beneath the infant's head. The middle or index fingers contact the temporal bone just anterior to the occipitomastoid junction approximately on the same plane as the external auditory meatus. In the picture (Fig. 2.74), the middle finger is contacting the appropriate area, which is indicated by an asterisk in Figures 2.77 and 2.78 (BO, basiocciput).

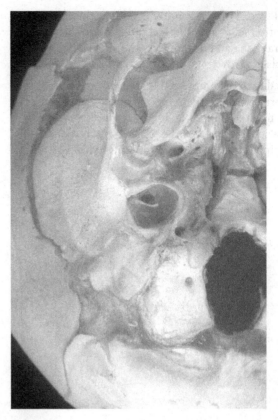

Fig. 2.75

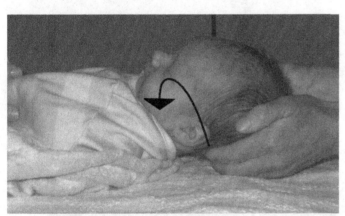

Fig. 2.73

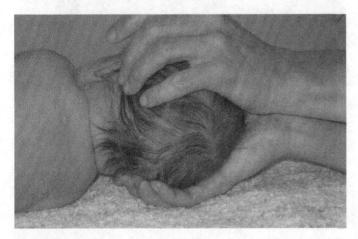

Fig. 2.74

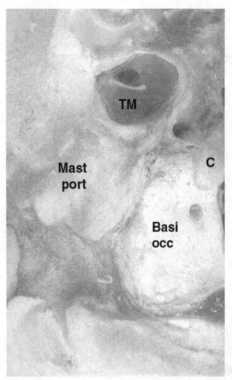

Fig. 2.76

2. A gentle steady force is introduced into the temporal articulation in an anterolateral direction to 'lift' the temporal bone and decompress the articulation (Fig. 2.73, black arrow).

3. The goal is to decompress this area, not to internally or externally rotate the temporal bone. Care must be taken initially that the 'lift' decompresses the articulation and engages the tissues. The responses of the occiput and tentorium are monitored.

4. As the tissue texture under the fingers begins to change, the physician can slightly vary her force vector to achieve balanced tension along the articulation and through the tentorium.

5. Once balanced membranous tension is established, the position is maintained until there is a softening, a change in tissue texture or a correction of the strain.

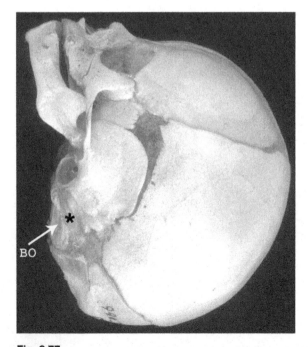

Fig. 2.77

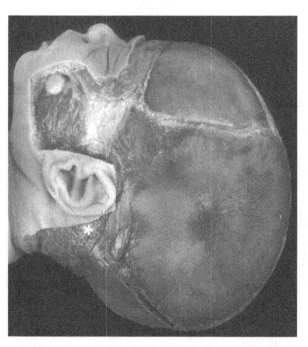

Fig. 2.78

BALANCED MEMBRANOUS TENSION

Falx Cerebri

Supine Infant (Figs 2.79, 2.80 and 2.81)

This technique uses a similar approach to a venous sinus spread technique to the sagittal sinus, but the intention is directed at the membranous structure, the falx cerebri (Fig. 2.82).

1. The infant is supine or held in the parent's arms. The physician sits at the infant's head with her forearms supported. The physician places her hands on the vault, with her thumbs crossed over the sagittal suture just anterior to lambda (Fig. 2.80).

2. The physician places her thumbs so that she has a contact with the contralateral thumb on each side of the sagittal suture (Fig. 2.79). This approximates the location of the falx cerebri.

3. A gentle steady traction is applied across the across the sagittal suture by introducing slow steady pressures from the thumbs away from each other (Fig. 2.81, white arrows). The intention is to introduce the force into the deeper tissues.

4. As the tissue texture begins to change, the physician may alter the vector of her force slightly to achieve balanced membranous tension.

5. Once balanced membranous tension is established the position is maintained until there is a softening, a change in tissue texture, or a correction of the strain.

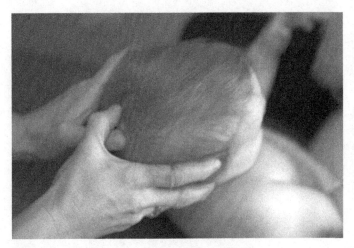

Fig. 2.79

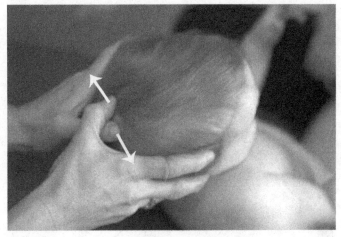

Fig. 2.81

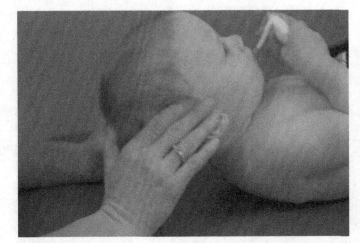

Fig. 2.80

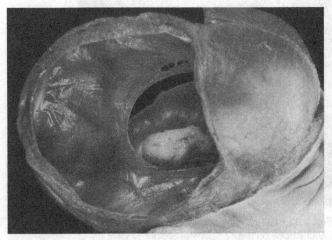

Fig. 2.82

DECOMPRESSION LAMBDOIDAL SUTURE

Supine Infant

This technique can be used in infants with persistent overlap at the lambdoidal suture. Typically, the intraparietal occiput (IPO) is inferior to the parietal bones (Fig. 2.83) at the lambdoidal suture (LS). The posterior fontanelle may be quite small or not palpable. The physician provides a fulcrum for the weight of the baby's head. The weight of the head and the inherent motions of respiration are the activating forces in this technique. The physician is essentially passive.

1. The infant is supine. The physician sits at the infant's head. The physician spreads her index and middle fingers apart, making a large V shape (Fig. 2.84).

2. The physician places her hand under the infant's occiput so that the V formed by her two fingers rests along the parietal side of the sutures (black line), NOT the occipital side.

3. The infant is placed supine so that the weight of his head is nestled in the V formed by the physician's fingers.

4. The physician allows the weight of the infant's head to fall between her fingers. The physician does not introduce any force into the infant's head.

5. If necessary, the physician may tilt or turn her fingers to redistribute the weight of the infant's head evenly across both fingers.

6. The physician maintains this position until there is a change in tissue texture.

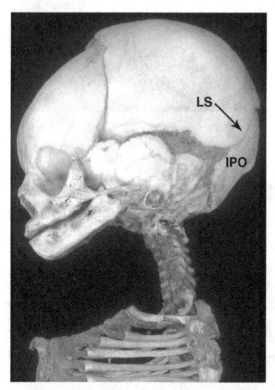

Fig. 2.83 • Lateral view of an infant skeleton. The overlap of the parietal bone on the intraparietal occiput (IPO) at the lambdoidal suture (LS) is indicated by the black arrow.

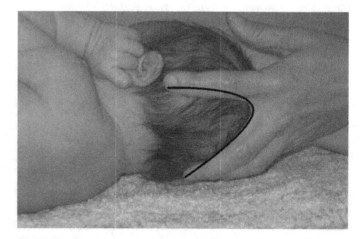

Fig. 2.84

BALANCED MEMBRANOUS TENSION

Reciprocal Tension Membrane

Supine Infant

In infants and toddlers cranial base strains typically have a significant membranous component. The mechanism of injury usually involves forces transmitted through the vault to which the craniocervical junction cannot adapt because of its flexed position. The SBS and cranial base are 'caught' between the forces loading on the vault and the locked-out craniocervical junction. The resulting strain pattern is a compensatory response of the tissues, which then maintains the abnormal relationships throughout the vault. This approach is used to balance the forces within the reciprocal tension membrane, taking into account the strain pattern at the cranial base. It should be used prior to addressing the SBS strain pattern in infants and young children. This approach takes into account the five-pointed star model of the RTM relationship with the cranial base (Carreiro 2009).

1. The infant is supine. The physician is seated at the infant's head with her forearms supported (Fig. 2.85). The physician places one hand under the infant's head; the middle finger lies along the sagittal plane of the cerebellar falx, the metacarpophalangeal junction lies along the plane of the tentorium cerebelli, and the thumb and the smallest or ring finger contact just below the asterion.

2. The other hand is placed over the vault; the middle finger lies along the plane of the sagittal sinus or falx cerebri, and the metacarpophalangeal joints lie over the coronal suture with the thumb and the index or smallest finger contacting just above the pterion. The latter component of this contact replicates the plane of the anterior dural girdle (Fig. 2.86).

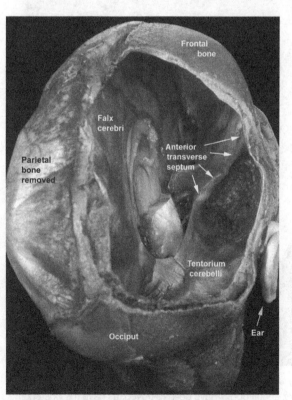

Fig. 2.86 • Dissection of a term infant. The view is from a posterosuperior perspective looking down into the right side of the head. The parietal bone, external dura and right hemisphere have been removed to expose the superior layer of the tentorium, the anterior cranial fossa. The RTM is still intact and labeled.

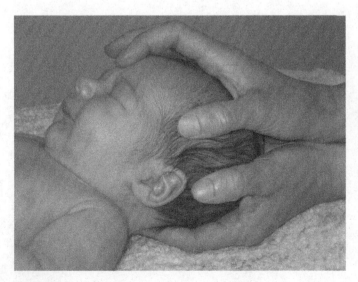

Fig. 2.85

3. The physician notes the tissue tensions in the membranous components and their relationship and influence to their attachments at the median axial stem (Fig. 2.87).

4. The physician balances the forces within the RTM around its attachments at the median axial stem. These structures do not attach at the SBS, but rather around the sella turcica at the anterior and posterior clinoid processes and the crista galli. The crista galli is located much more posteriorly in infants than in adults, and is significantly closer to the anterior clinoid processes.

5. The physician maintains balanced tension until there is a change in tissue texture and increased freedom of motion in the vault and base structures.

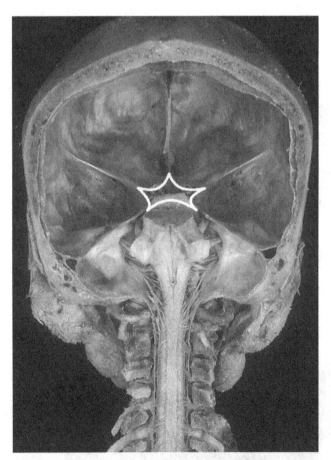

Fig. 2.87 • Posterior view into an adult skull. The occiput and posterior parietal bones have been removed, as have the posterior elements of the cervical spine. The brain and cerebellum have been removed, leaving the medulla and cerebellar peduncles exposed as well as the fourth ventricle. The attachments of the RTM have been highlighted in white as the center of the five-pointed star (Carreiro 2009).

BALANCED MEMBRANOUS TENSION

Sphenobasilar Synchondrosis (SBS)

Supine Infant

In infants the SBS is cartilaginous, the greater wings are poorly developed, and the lateral angles of the intraparietal occiput are not yet fused with the supraocciput or the basicranium. Membranous strains influencing the SBS from above, or articular strains influencing the SBS from below need to be addressed before treating the SBS strain.

1. The infant is supine and the physician is seated at the baby's head. The physician places her hands on the head, contacting the area of the greater wing of the sphenoid and the lateral angle of the occiput with each hand (Fig. 2.88).

2. As can be seen (Fig. 2.89), these areas are quite small even in a toddler's skull.

3. The physician monitors the membranous tensions oriented around the SBS. The physician may then choose to use either active or passive assessment.

4. Active assessment involves the physician gently introducing movement patterns into the cranial base and assessing the tissue response.

5. Passive assessment involves the physician observing involuntary motion and discerning the strain pattern implied by it.

6. The area should be treated using a direct approach to balanced tension.

7. After noting the strain pattern, the physician introduces the appropriate force vectors towards, but not into, the restrictive barrier to achieve balanced tension in the associated tissues.

8. Once balanced tension is achieved, the position is maintained until there is a change in tissue texture, an improvement in function or a correction of the strain.

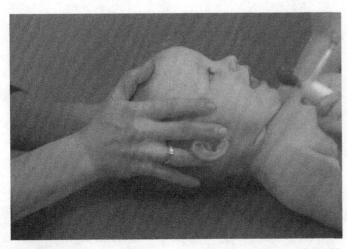

Fig. 2.88

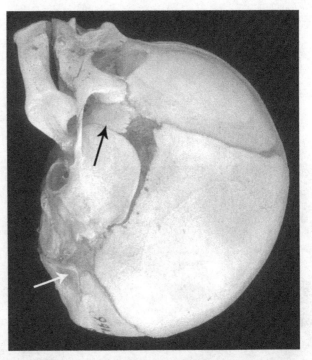

Fig. 2.89 • Lateral view of a skull at approximately 2 years of age. The greater wing of the sphenoid (black arrow) and the lateral angle of the intraparietal occiput (white arrow) are still poorly developed.

MOLDING TECHNIQUE

Supine Infant (Fig. 2.90)

This technique is most effective in very young infants. The goal of the technique is to rebalance the tensile forces acting on the squamous portion of the bone. Somatic dysfunctions in the cranial base and vault need to be treated prior to using this approach. All the articular relationships surrounding the bone must also be free of restriction. The parietal bone is used in this example.

1. Decompressing the articulations: The neonate is supine. The physician sits beside or at the infant's head. The physician uses the finger pads of one hand to contact the parietal bone along the coronal suture. The other hand contacts the frontal bone on the opposite side of the suture. Typically the parietal bone overlaps the frontal bone: in many children this will resolve spontaneously in the first day or so.

2. The physician introduces a gentle but steady traction on the parietal and frontal bones (Fig. 2.91, white arrows). This acts to decompress the articulation, taking the frontal bone anteriorly and the parietal bone posteriorly.

3. The position is maintained for 3–5 seconds until there is slight change in tissue texture. The physician then 'walks' her fingers along each articulation, repeating this procedure at the temporoparietal (Fig. 2.92), sagittal and lambdoid sutures.

4. Once the tissue stresses at the articulations have been addressed, the molding technique can be introduced.

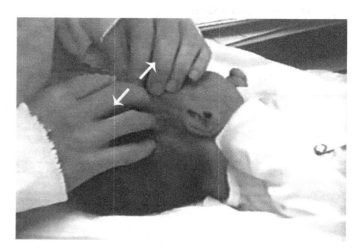

Fig. 2.91

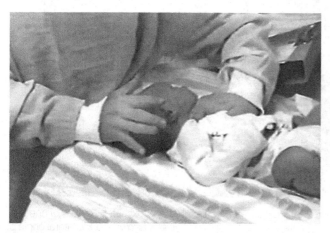

Fig. 2.90

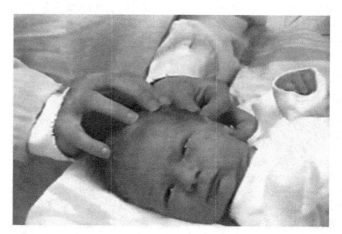

Fig. 2.92

5. The parietal bone is quite malleable during the newborn phase (Fig. 2.93): it lacks true bony articulations with its neighbors, and the sutures are instead thickened membranous bands between the bones. The development of the parietal leaves its imprint in the neonatal bone as lines radiating from the boss, the primary ossification center.

6. The physician takes the palm of her hand and places it over the parietal bone so that the boss or prominence lies in the center of her palm (Fig. 2.90). The physician then very slowly spreads her hand so that her palm flattens. As she does this the response of the tensile forces in the tissues surrounding the parietal and the response of the parietal bone itself are observed. The physician repeats the movement, this time changing the position of her palm, its contacts with the head, and the tensions in the intrinsic muscles of her hand to accommodate the tissue response in the child.

7. The goal is to achieve balanced tension within the tissues.

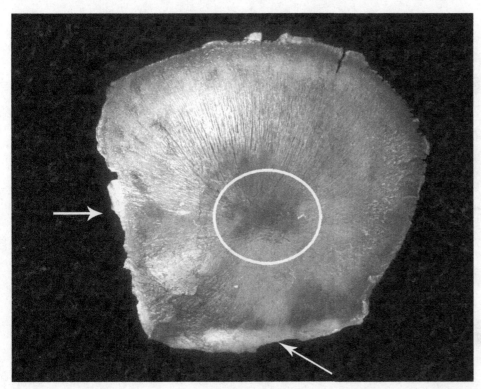

Fig. 2.93 • External view of a neonatal parietal bone that was removed by cutting the membranous bands of the immature sutures (white arrows). The boss, the primary ossification center, is identified by the white circle. The lines of development radiate from the boss towards the periphery.

DACRYOSTENOSIS

Clinical Notes

Dacryostenosis is a condition whereby the nasolacrimal duct is narrowed or blocked and the glandular secretions into the eye are prevented from draining properly. The secretions collect around the orifice of the duct and in the corner of the eye, where they thicken, resulting in a gooey, sticky substance that further clogs any drainage route. Dacryostenosis is common in newborns, and most children 'grow out of it' as the face grows and the narrow lumen of the duct enlarges. In rare cases the problem is structural and unresponsive to conservative treatment. A simple surgical procedure is then performed to correct the problem. Children with congenital conditions affecting the face and head are at a slightly higher risk for dacrostenosis that is recalcitrant to conservative treatment. Parents and caregivers are told to apply warm compresses to the area to relieve some of the congestion and improve drainage.

Treatment Notes

From an osteopathic perspective dacryostenosis is a mechanical problem involving the structures in the upper third of the face. It is often seen in prolonged labors and in neonates with early engagement of the head into the maternal pelvis. Newborns with dacryostenosis often have somatic dysfunction in the areas corresponding to the ethmoid notch, nasion, frontal and/or maxilla, in addition to that found at the lacrimal ethmoid area (Fig. 2.94). Treatment of these areas can be followed by a gentle decompression technique that may be taught to capable parents.

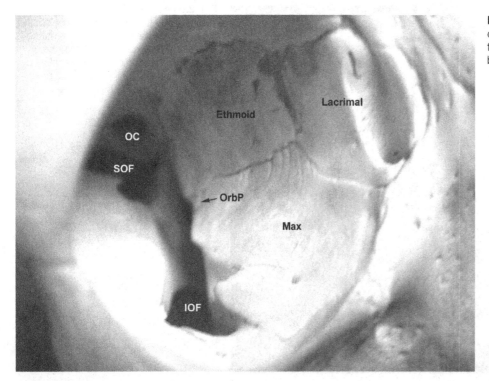

Fig. 2.94 • Anterior view into the right orbit of an adolescent skull, focusing on the medial wall. The lacrimal and ethmoid bones are clearly labeled.

DECOMPRESSING THE LACRIMALS

This is a direct technique that should be performed after the somatic dysfunctions in the cranial base, vault, frontal and ethmoid have been addressed. It is similar to a parietal or frontal lift in that the response of the associated membranous and myofascial tissues is observed as the decompression is performed, and the endpoint is a sensation of the structure being lifted and carried away from the physician's contact.

1. The infant is supine. The physician sits beside the child at his head. The physician gently places one hand over the frontal bones with the middle finger along the metopic suture and resting at the glabella. The other hand contacts the lacrimal bones bilaterally using the index finger and thumb (Fig. 2.95).

2. The physician monitors mechanics at the frontal and the ethmoid notch with the superior hand.

3. The physician gently introduces external rotation into the frontal area as she carries the frontal cephalad to decompress the ethmoid notch (white arrows).

4. Using the other hand, the physician gently introduces a caudad and lateral motion simultaneously into the lacrimals to decompress and lift them from the ethmoid (black arrows).

5. The physician monitors the response of the affected membranous and myofascial tissues for balanced tension and waits for a resolution of the compressive dysfunction.

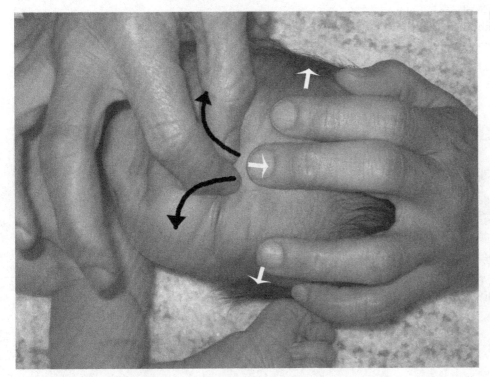

Fig. 2.95

SUCKLING DYSFUNCTION/ OROPHARYNGEAL DYSFUNCTION

Clinical Notes

Suckling dysfunction may involve latching on, maintaining contact, or generating sufficient pressure to successfully obtain breast milk. From an osteopathic perspective, problems with latching are most likely due to inability to open the mouth wide enough or failure to control the lips to form a seal. Inability to maintain contact can arise because the infant fatigues or cannot position her head appropriately. When the problem is due to the latter, the infant will typically nurse better on one breast than the other. Problems generating sufficient force are often due to mechanical dysfunction of the hyoid stabilizers, the tongue or the muscles controlling the mandible.

Oropharyngeal dysfunction may present as difficulties feeding, stuttering, or speech abnormalities. The problem may be neurological or mechanical. Mechanical etiologies typically involve the ability to properly position and control the tongue. The structures influencing the base of the tongue, the hyoid and mandible need to be addressed.

ASSESSING INFANT SUCKLING

Tongue/Coordination of the Tongue and Hyoid

1. The infant is supine. The physician places her gloved smallest finger into the infant's mouth so that the palmar surface contacts the palate. This position should stimulate the infant to begin suckling. The other hand monitors first the cranium (Fig. 2.96).

2. Both sides of the tongue should approximate the infant's palate simultaneously. The physician should feel equal pressure on her finger. Movement between the mandible, tongue and palate should be smooth and coordinated.

3. The physician then places her free hand on the anterior cervical tissues and the hyoid (Fig. 2.97). The hyoid can be palpated within the arch of the mandible. It should be seated in the midline and move in synchrony with the mandible as the tongue moves against the palate.

4. If the hyoid deviates laterally, there may be involvement of the digastric or omohyoid muscle on the ipsilateral side. If the cornua do not lie on the same horizontal plane, then the sternohyoid muscle and clavicle should be evaluated on the inferior side, and the stylohyoid muscle, temporal bone and cranial base mechanics on the superior side.

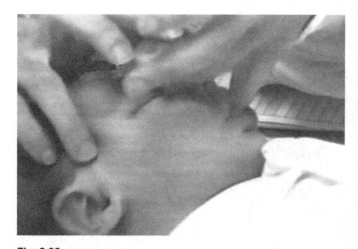

Fig. 2.96

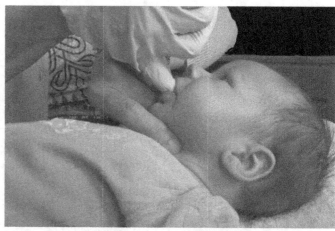

Fig. 2.97

ASSESSMENT

Hyoid Stabilizers – Omohyoid

Supine Infant

The omohyoid should be assessed in children with oropharyngeal dysfunction, especially if there is a history of prolonged second stage of labor, shoulder dystocia or large size for gestational age.

1. The infant is supine or held by the parent. The physician sits beside or at the head of the infant. The physician uses one hand to gently contact the hyoid and the other to contact the scapula and the clavicle (Fig. 2.98A, B).

2. The physician monitors the positions and tensions in the associated tissues as the infant suckles. The hyoid should move symmetrically.

3. If strain in the shoulder is influencing the hyoid through the omohyoid then the hyoid may deviate laterally and the physician will feel increased stress in the myofascial tissues or movement of the scapula.

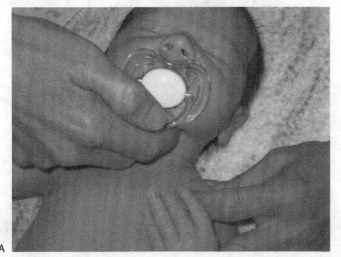

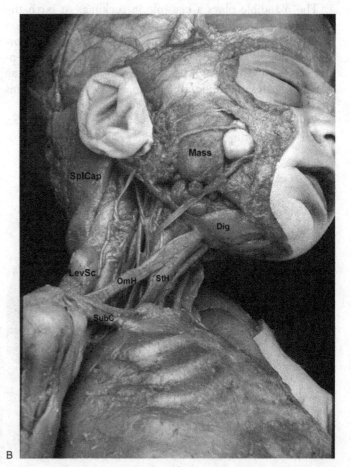

A

B

Fig. 2.98

SUCKLING DYSFUNCTION/ OROPHARYNGEAL DYSFUNCTION

Treatment Notes

When there is an abnormal or ineffective sucking pattern the infant should be evaluated and treated osteopathically, and consultation with a lactation specialist should be initiated. Often maternal posture, nipple characteristics and poor technique can play a role in suckling problems. Recommendations to keep the child nursing on one breast for the entire feed should be considered to afford maximum opportunity for the infant to obtain high-fat breast milk (Woodward et al. 1989). Studies suggest that the 'hind breast milk' has a higher fat content than the 'fore breast milk' (Jensen et al. 1978, Woodward et al. 1989, Boersma et al. 1991).

The stabilizers of the hyoid and tongue need to be evaluated and treated. This often requires initial treatment of the cranial base, cervical spine, upper torso and/or shoulders. Once the stabilizers have been addressed then the base of the tongue should be treated using an intraoral inhibition technique described by Miller (1996, personal communication).

The mandible plays a key role in suckling. At birth the mandible is in two parts, joined by a cartilaginous junction at the mental. Intraosseous strains are possible with abnormal uterine lie or abnormal presentation. The petrosphenoid articulation passes through the posterior aspect of the mandibular fossa of the temporal bone. Cranial base strains may alter mechanics at the temporomandibular joint.

The following techniques may be beneficial in treating an infant with suckling dysfunction.

BALANCED LIGAMENTOUS TENSION

Hyoid Stabilizers – Omohyoid

Supine Infant

1. The infant is supine or held by the parent. The physician sits beside or at the head of the infant. The physician uses one hand to gently contact the hyoid and the other to contact the scapula and the clavicle (Fig. 2.99).

2. The physician uses the contacts on the hyoid and scapula to balance the tensions in the omohyoid and associated tissues (Fig. 2.100).

3. Once balanced tension is achieved, the position is maintained until there is a change in tissue texture, an improvement in motion mechanics or a resolution of the strain. The hyoid should move more symmetrically after treatment.

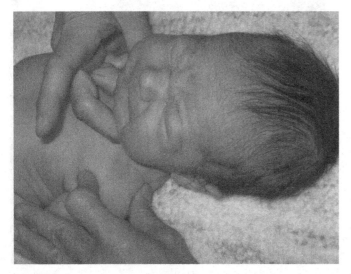

Fig. 2.99

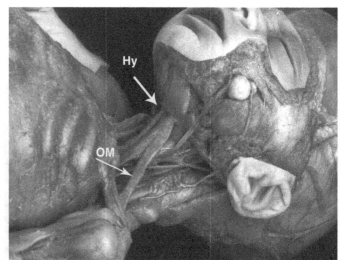

Fig. 2.100

BALANCED LIGAMENTOUS TENSION

Mandible

Supine Infant

The mandible is not fused at birth. There is a cartilaginous juncture at the mental (Fig. 2.101).

1. The infant is supine or held in parent's arms. The physician sits at the infant's head and contacts the mandible bilaterally. The middle fingers contact the submandibular tissues (Fig. 2.102).

2. The myofascial elements of the submandibular area are assessed for strain, and the mandible is assessed for intraosseous strain patterns.

3. The physician uses her contacts to bring the myofascial tissues and mandible into balanced tension.

4. Once balanced tension is achieved the position is maintained until there is a change in tissue texture, an improvement in motion mechanics or a resolution of the strain.

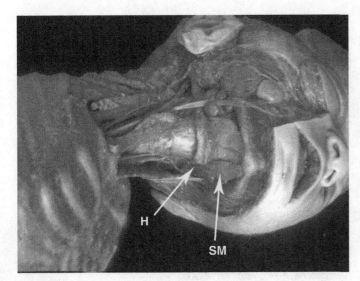

Fig. 2.101

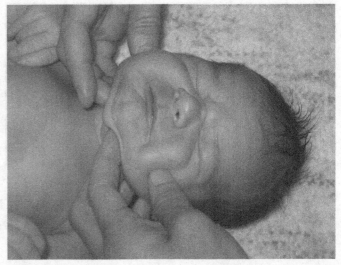

Fig. 2.102

INHIBITION TECHNIQUE

Tongue

Infant Supine

This technique should be performed after dysfunctions of the hyoid and mandible have been treated. This technique may also be of benefit in older children with bruxisms or temporal mandibular joint issues.

The tongue is part of a postural reflex loop that includes the cervical spine and jaw. The muscles controlling the tongue are densely innervated with proprioceptive fibers that influence the muscles of mastication and suboccipital muscles. Primitive reflexes exist between these structures as well, so that persistent dysfunction at the craniocervical junction or temporomandibular area may alter tongue mechanics and vice versa.

1. The child is supine. The physician monitors the cranium with one hand. The physician places the gloved smallest finger of her other hand under the infant's tongue superior to the sublingual fold and at the root of the genioglossus (Fig. 2.103).

2. This is an inhibition technique. The physician will sequentially contact the genioglossus and hyoglossus muscles on each side of the tongue and apply a gentle pressure (Figs 2.104 and 2.105).

3. The physician begins by making contact just lateral to the frenulum on the side opposite to which she is seated. The physician slowly sweeps the pad of her finger along the root of the tongue (an area of approximately 1.2 cm in a newborn) assessing tissue tension in the genioglossus muscle. A small, palpable pea-sized area of muscle spasm or bogginess may be present.

4. The physician places her finger on this area and gently uses a tissue unwinding technique until there is a change in tissue tension.

5. The physician then moves her finger posteriorly along the root of the tongue to the anterior edge of the hypoglossus and perhaps the most anterior aspect of the styloglossus as it interdigitates into the genioglossus. Again tissue tension is assessed. A small, palpable pea-sized area of muscle spasm or bogginess may be present.

6. The physician places her finger on this area and gently uses a tissue unwinding technique until there is a change in tissue tension.

7. The procedure is repeated on the opposite side of the tongue.

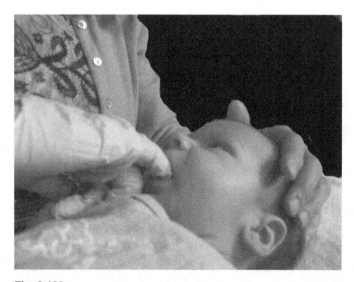

Fig. 2.103

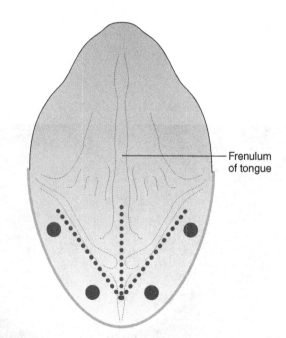

Frenulum of tongue

Fig. 2.104 • Schematic diagram looking into the opened mouth with the tongue raised. The black dots indicate the approximate points of contact. (Adapted from Williams P. Gray's anatomy. London: Churchill Livingstone, 1995, with permission.)

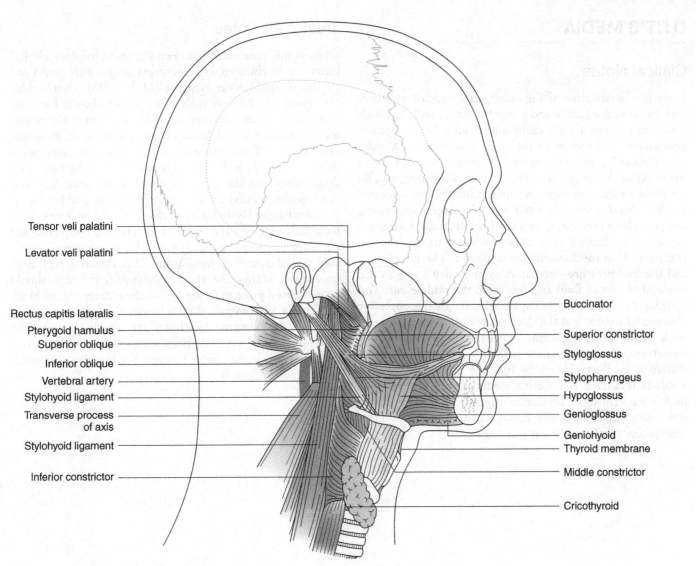

Tensor veli palatini

Levator veli palatini

Rectus capitis lateralis

Pterygoid hamulus

Superior oblique

Inferior oblique

Vertebral artery

Stylohyoid ligament

Transverse process of axis

Stylohyoid ligament

Inferior constrictor

Buccinator

Superior constrictor

Styloglossus

Stylopharyngeus

Hypoglossus

Genioglossus

Geniohyoid

Thyroid membrane

Middle constrictor

Cricothyroid

Fig. 2.105 • Diagram showing the muscles of the tongue and pharynx. (Adapted from Williams P. Gray's anatomy. London: Churchill Livingstone, 1995, with permission.)

OTITIS MEDIA

Clinical Notes

From the perspective of the osteopathic models of structure and function, acute and recurrent otitis media has both a respiratory–circulatory component and a biomechanical component in addition to the infectious process. Middle ear effusion is a normal response of the eustachian tube to irritation in the upper respiratory tract. Persistent middle ear effusion alters pressure within the middle ear, increases the likelihood of insufflation of nasopharyngeal secretions, and provides a hospitable medium for infectious organisms. Middle ear effusion may persist when normal drainage and resorption mechanisms are impaired. The lymphatics and the low-pressure circulatory system play a role in the removal of serous fluid and pus from the middle ear. The lymphatics of the middle ear travel through the posterior pharyngeal tissues and the deep prevertebral fasciae of the neck. From there, respiratory mechanics play a role in the movement of low-pressure circulatory fluids into the subclavian vein. Eustachian tube function is thought to play a role in recurrent acute otitis media as well as persistent middle ear effusion. The biomechanical relationships of the structures adjacent to the eustachian tube will influence tube patency and middle ear pressures.

Treatment Notes

Osteopathic treatment has been shown to improve clinical outcomes in children with recurrent acute otitis media and persistent middle ear effusion (Mills 2003). Osteopathic treatment of children with otitis media should focus on addressing somatic dysfunction in the context of the respiratory–circulatory and biomechanical models of structure and function. Tissue strains in the pelvis or junctional areas may interfere with the pumping functions of the associated diaphragms and the thoracoabdominal cylinder. Thoracic cage mechanics play a role in arterial, venous and lymphatic fluid exchange. Dysfunction in the head and neck may have local influences on the eustachian tube, its lymphatic and circulatory components. Within the respiratory–circulatory model described by Gordon Zink (Ward 2003), fluid movement within the thoracoabdominal cylinder should be addressed prior to treatment of the extremities or head. The thoracoabdominal cylinder houses the largest collecting channels for venous and lymphatic fluids. The pelvic, abdominal and cervical diaphragms and the muscles of respiration provide the motor to move the low-pressure fluids within these channels.

BALANCED LIGAMENTOUS TENSION

First Rib/Thoracic Inlet

Seated Infant

In addition to the technique previously described under Whiplash, there are also several techniques described in detail in Chapter 4 on the shoulder.

BALANCED LIGAMENTOUS TENSION

First Rib/Thoracic Inlet

Seated Toddler Alternative Approach

This is a general approach to the ligamentous, myofascial and articular relationships in the thoracic inlet (Fig. 2.106A, B).

1. The child is seated facing away from the physician. The physician places her hands over the first ribs. The middle and index fingers contact the first ribs bilaterally at the costosternal junctions. The hands rest on the superior margin of the shaft of the ribs and the thumbs contact the ribs posteriorly at the costovertebral junctions (Fig. 2.107).

2. A gentle but steady posterolateral vector is applied from the anterior contact through both ribs, such as one would use to open a caliper (white arrow). This engages the adjacent tissues and the articular mechanisms.

3. The contacts on the superior margins (black outline) are used to simultaneously bring the two ribs through multiple planes of motion – inhalation, exhalation, elevation and flaring – to establish balanced tension in the associated tissues.

4. Balanced tension is maintained until there is a change in tissue texture and an improvement in mechanics.

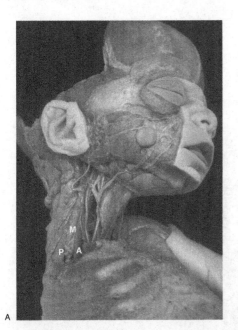
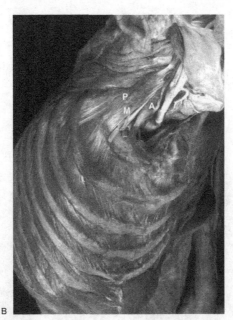

Fig. 2.106 • A, B Superolateral view of the thoracic inlet. The upper extremity and clavicle and their associated tissues have been removed to expose the upper ribs. The anterior (A), middle (M), and posterior (P) scalene muscles are identified. Note the curvilinear form of the adult ribs compared to neonatal ribs, which lie on a more horizontal plane.

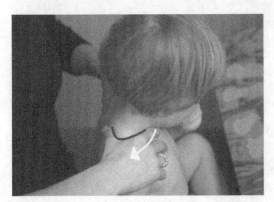

Fig. 2.107

BALANCED LIGAMENTOUS TENSION

Costosternal Junction/First Rib

Seated Toddler

When there is significant compression at the costosternal junction, this area may need to be treated before the thoracic inlet can be balanced. A direct approach is used to establish balanced tension.

1. The child is seated or supine. The physician's thumb and finger of one hand contact each first rib at the costosternal junction. The other hand monitors the shafts of the first ribs anterior to the trapezius (Fig. 2.108).

2. A steady, lateral tension is placed on the anterior articulation, spreading the ribs from the manubrium (black arrows) until there is balanced tension.

3. This position is maintained until there is a change in tissue tension or an improvement in function.

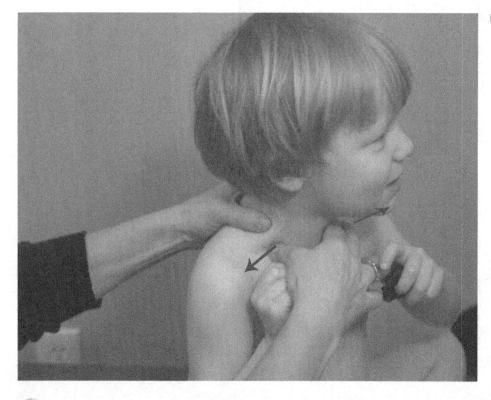

Fig. 2.108

BALANCED LIGAMENTOUS TENSION

Craniocervical Junction

Seated Toddler

This is a general approach treating the relationship between the occiput, atlas and axis. This approach uses the child's natural movements to balance the occiput, C1 and C2.

1. The child is seated. With one hand the physician contacts the occiput bilaterally at the occipitomastoid junctions using the middle finger and thumb. The ring finger of this hand monitors C2 at the transverse process ipsilateral to the dysfunction. The other hand stabilizes the child's head (Fig. 2.109A,B).

2. The physician then applies a slow, gentle traction in a circumlinear vector, taking the occiput into postural flexion until balanced tension is achieved. This is a direct approach to decompress the OA and achieve balanced tension.

3. Once the physician feels a change in tissue tension under her hands, the traction is released. The physician may use the contact between C1 and C2 and the contact on the head and occiput to establish balanced ligamentous tension between the occiput, C1 and C2. Alternatively, the physician may transition into a temporal lift technique.

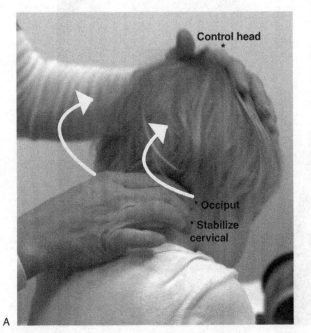

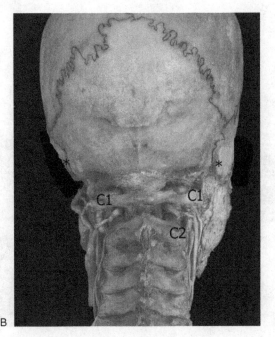

A   B

Fig. 2.109

BALANCED LIGAMENTOUS TENSION

OA/Condylar Decompression

Seated Toddler

This technique uses a direct approach to decompress and balance the tensions of the occipital condyles on the atlas (Fig. 2.110).

1. The child is seated. The physician cradles the occiput in one hand so that the pad of the middle finger slides inferiorly towards the opisthion. The index and ring fingers are placed slightly lateral to the midline, approximating the plane of the occipital condyles (OC). The middle finger is placed just superior to the posterior tubercle of C2 (PCT) (Fig. 2.111, asterisks).

2. The other hand monitors the frontal area.

3. The physician then applies a gentle traction in a circumlinear vector (Fig. 2.110, white arrow), taking the occiput into postural flexion while stabilizing C1 and C2.

4. The physician uses the hand contacting the occiput and C1 and C2 to vary the vector of her force to establish balanced ligamentous tension between the condylar parts of the occiput and C1.

5. This position is maintained until the physician feels a change in the tension under her hands, a correction of the strain pattern or improved freedom of motion in the occiput.

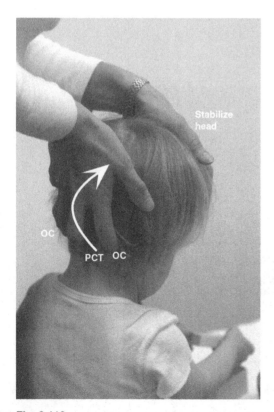

Fig. 2.110

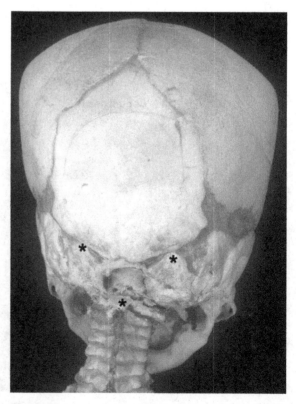

Fig. 2.111

VENOUS SINUS TECHNIQUE

(Figs 2.112, 2.113 and 2.114)

Venous sinus techniques can be performed from various perspectives: as osseous techniques to decompress suture tension; as fluid techniques to promote venous drainage; or as membranous techniques to improve function in the reciprocal tension membrane. Depending on the condition, one or more of these perspectives may be appropriate. With cranial base strain and plagiocephaly the osseous and membranous approaches seem to be helpful. With congestive headache, allergies, sinusitis and infectious processes, the fluid perspective should be added.

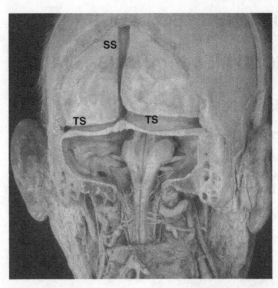

Fig. 2.113 • Posterior view. The occiput and posterior parietals have been removed, exposing the external dura as it lies over the cortical hemispheres. The cerebellum has been removed, exposing the brain stem and the inferior surface of the tentorium. The external walls of the sagittal and transverse sinuses have been removed, exposing the inner surfaces of the lateral walls.

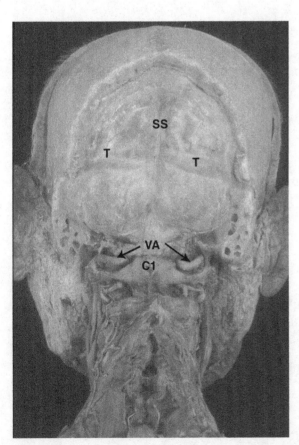

Fig. 2.112 • Posterior view. The occiput and posterior parietals have been removed, exposing the external dura as it lies over the brain. The external walls of the sagittal (SS) and transverse sinuses (TS) can be discerned. The neural arch of C1 is intact, with the vertebral artery (VA) above it.

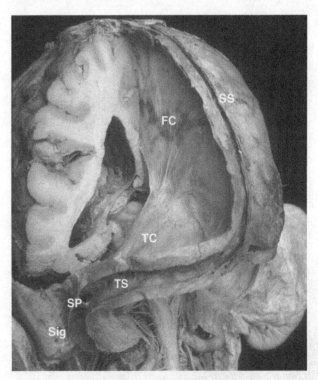

Fig. 2.114 • Posterolateral view of the left posterior cranium. The vault, occiput, posterior parietal cortex and cerebellum have been removed. The internal dural layers and venous sinuses are left intact. This perspective is as though you were standing behind and to the left of the cadaver. The left layer of the falx cerebri (FC) sweeps laterally to become the superior layer of the tentorium (TC). The sagittal sinus flows inferiorly and to the left into the transverse sinus (TS), which flows into the sigmoid sinus (Sig). The entrance into the superior petrosal sinus (SP) is also visible.

VENOUS SINUS TECHNIQUE

BALANCED MEMBRANOUS TENSION

Cerebellar Falx

Seated Toddler

1. The child is seated. The physician stands or sits alongside the child. The physician places the fingers of one hand along the region of the cerebellar falx inferior to the inion and superior to the occipitoatlantal junction. The other hand stabilizes the head (Fig. 2.115).

2. A gentle anterior force is introduced in the direction of the crista galli. This is accompanied by a gentle spreading of the fingers until a change in tissue texture is appreciated. Care must be taken that no compressive force passes into the OA or condyles. This is an intraosseous technique, not an intra-articular one.

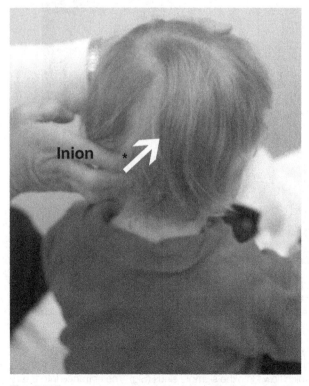

Inion

Fig. 2.115

VENOUS SINUS TECHNIQUE

BALANCED MEMBRANOUS TENSION

Transverse Sinus/Tentorium

Seated Toddler

This technique is intended to affect fluid drainage through the transverse sinus and membranous strain in the tentorium. These components need to be addressed simultaneously. The fluid congestion may influence lymphatic and venous drainage (Fig. 2.116). The membranous strain has the potential to influence temporal bone mechanics (Fig. 2.117).

1. The child is seated. The physician places the pads of her fingers against the intraparietal occiput, starting above and below the inion. The other hand stabilizes the head (Fig. 2.118).

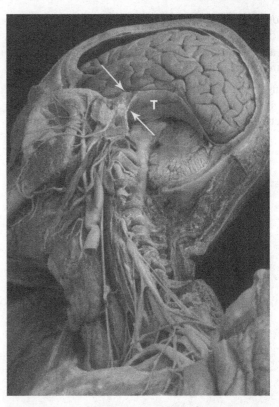

Fig. 2.117 • Posterolateral view. The parietal, temporal and occipital bones have been removed to expose the cortex and petrous portion. The cerebellar hemisphere has been removed to expose the inferior surface of the tentorium (T). The white arrows indicate the superior and inferior layers of the tentorium becoming the periosteum of the petrous portion of the temporal bone.

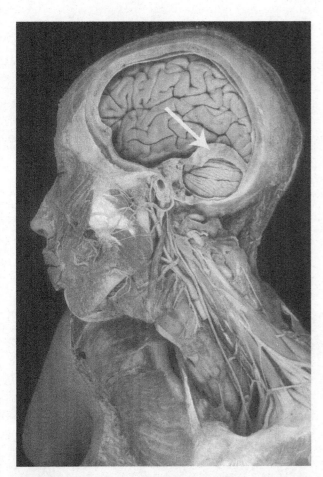

Fig. 2.116 • Lateral view. The parietal, temporal and occipital bones have been removed, as has the dural layer, except for that part forming the external wall of the transverse sinus (white arrow). The cortical and cerebellar hemispheres are exposed.

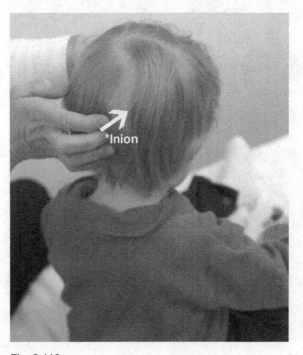

Fig. 2.118

2. The posterior hand introduces a gentle anterior force in the direction of the straight sinus (white arrow). A spreading motion is made with the fingers. This pressure is maintained until a softening is felt.

3. The fingers are repositioned so they lie along the horizontal plane (Fig. 2.119). An anterolateral distracting pressure (white arrows) is directed along the plane of the tentorium in the direction of the sigmoid sinus until a softening is felt.

4. The physician then moves her fingers laterally along the plane of the transverse sinus towards the occipitomastoid articulation, applying the distracting pressure until a change in tissue texture is noted.

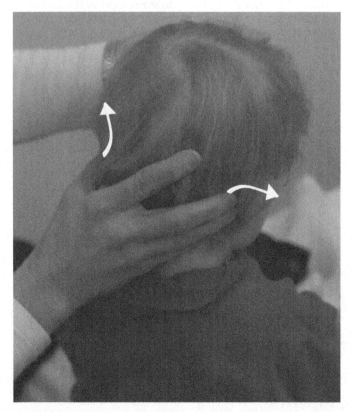

Fig. 2.119

BALANCED MEMBRANOUS TENSION

Temporal Lift

Seated Toddler

The 'temporal bone lift' is used to decompress the occipito-mastoid suture. This procedure is carried out concurrently on both temporal bones. It is an adaptation of the supine technique described earlier.

1. The child is seated on the table or the parent's lap facing away from the physician. The physician stands behind the child (Fig. 2.120). The physician contacts the posterior aspect of the temporal bones bilaterally just anterior to the occipitomastoid suture (OMS) with the thumb and finger of the same hand (Fig. 2.121, asterisk). The other hand stabilizes the child's head.

2. A gentle anterior lateral force is introduced to encourage external rotation of the temporal bones (white arrow).

3. Balanced membranous tension is established within and between the occipitomastoid and petrobasilar articulations bilaterally.

4. The physician maintains this position until there is a change (usually a softening) in the tissue texture at the occipitomastoid junction.

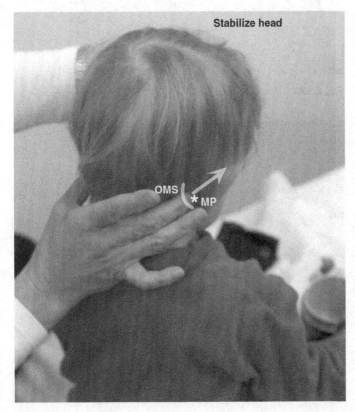

Fig. 2.120

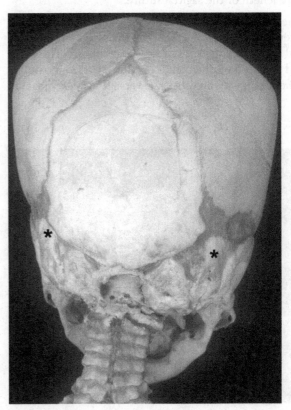

Fig. 2.121

VENOUS SINUS TECHNIQUE

BALANCED MEMBRANOUS TENSION

Falx Cerebri/Sagittal Sinus

Seated Toddler

This technique is intended to improve fluid drainage through the sagittal sinus and address membranous strain in the falx cerebri. These components need to be dealt with simultaneously. The fluid congestion may influence lymphatic and venous drainage. The membranous strain has the potential to influence mechanics in the vault and base (Fig. 2.122).

1. The child is seated. The physician places her hands in a modified vault hold with thumbs crossed and resting on the cranium at the lambdoid (Fig 2.123). The pad of the right thumb should be on the left parietal and the pad of the left thumb on the right parietal (Fig. 2.124).

2. A gentle distracting motion is applied by pushing the right thumb to the left and the left thumb to the right (white arrows, Fig. 2.124) until a subtle change in tissue tension is felt.

3. Maintaining the same hand position, the physician advances her thumbs in small increments over the entire length of the sagittal suture.

4. If the child will not cooperate, an alternative hand placement may be used whereby the physician uses one hand to contact the sagittal suture at lambda. The other hand is placed on the child's head to stabilize it, similar to the first position in the transverse sinus description.

5. A gentle anterolateral distracting pressure is applied over the area of the sagittal suture until a change in tissue texture is noted. Then the fingers are moved anteriorly along the sagittal suture to the next area of restriction.

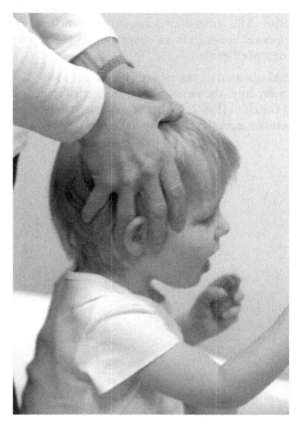

Fig. 2.123

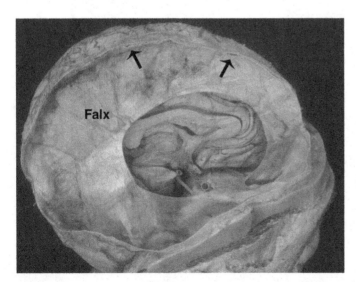

Falx

Fig. 2.122

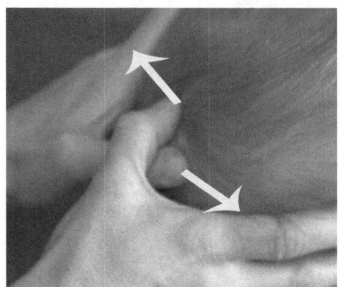

Fig. 2.124

BALANCED MEMBRANOUS TENSION

Petrosphenoid

Seated Toddler

This is a direct approach to establishing balanced membranous tension at the petrosphenoid junction, under which passes the eustachian tube as it exits the temporal bone and enters the posterior pharyngeal tissues (Fig. 2.125).

1. The child is either supine or seated. The physician uses a modified vault hold (Fig. 2.126). The index finger contacts the greater wing of the sphenoid (GW) and the middle finger contacts the anterior squama of the temporal bone (TS) just superior to the pterion (Fig. 2.127). The ring and small fingers monitor the posterior aspect of the temporal squama and the lateral angle of the occiput (LA).

2. A gentle decompression force is introduced into the cranial base (white arrows) with its focus at the petrosphenoid articulation (Fig. 2.125) until balanced membranous tension is felt.

3. The position is maintained until there is a change in tissue texture or an improvement in function.

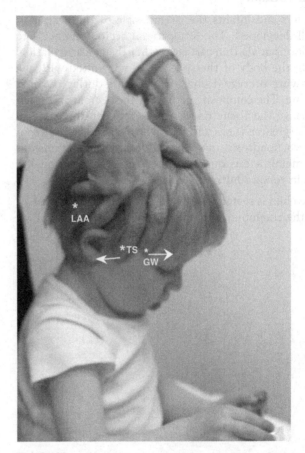

Fig. 2.126

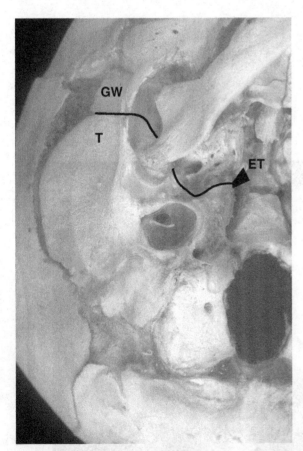

Fig. 2.125 • Inferior view of an infant skull. The petrosphenoid articulation is outlined in black. The location of the eustachian tube is identified (ET) as a black marking. The greater wing of the sphenoid (GW) and the squama of the temporal bone (T) are labeled.

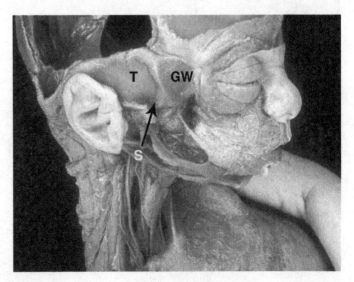

Fig. 2.127

BALANCED MEMBRANOUS TENSION

Sphenobasilar Synchondrosis (SBS)

Seated Toddler

In toddlers and infants the lateral angle of the occiput is not well developed. The intraparietal occiput connects to the basiocciput via thin cartilage rather than an articulation. At birth, the body of the sphenoid is not united with the greater wing–pterygoid units. This occurs during the first year of life. The composite natures of the occiput and sphenoid change the tissue relationships between the external contacts (greater wings and lateral angles) and the sphenobasilar synchondrosis. In young children these relationships have a membranous quality, rather than the bony quality present in young adults.

1. The child is seated. The physician's hands are placed on the cranium in a modified vault hold (Fig. 2.128)

similar to that used in the petrosphenoid technique described above, except in this case the primary contacts are on the greater wing of the sphenoid (GW) and the lateral angle of the occiput (LA), rather than the temporal squama (Fig. 2.129).

2. The SBS pattern is assessed, either through observing passive motion mechanics or through gentle motion testing.

3. The SBS is brought into balanced tension through the contacts on the sphenoid and occiput. Balanced membranous tension is achieved through the reciprocal tension membrane and the SBS, so membranous and osseous mechanics must be addressed.

4. This position is held until there is a change in the quality of motion at the SBS.

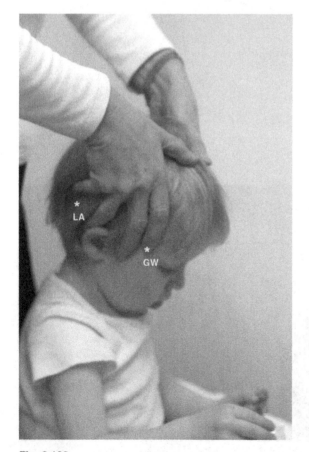

Fig. 2.128

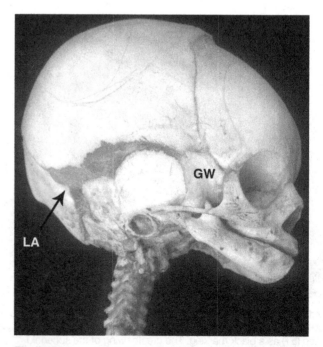

Fig. 2.129

CHRONIC SINUSITIS/CONGESTION

Clinical Notes

Chronic sinusitis may be due to allergic inflammation, persistent or recurrent infection. In young children it will present as cough, stuffiness or congestion with or without nasal discharge. In addition, headaches, facial pain and mild facial edema may be present in adolescents. The cough is often worse at night or when the child is supine, owing to pharyngeal irritation from the postnasal drip. There may be morning nausea or loss of appetite. The child may complain of toothache if the maxillary sinuses are involved, or pain behind the eye if there is frontal, sphenoid or ethmoid involvement. The latter two may also present as headache over the top of the head or behind the eyes.

On physical examination there may be tenderness over the involved sinus. The pharynx may be erythematous, with signs of postnasal drainage. Lymphoid hyperplasia may be visible as a cobblestone appearance of the posterior pharyngeal wall. This effect is produced by lymphadenopathy of the deep pharyngeal nodes draining the sphenoid and ethmoid sinuses. Transillumination of the maxillary and frontal sinuses can be helpful but is often difficult to interpret. Visualization of the nasal passages usually reveals swelling of the nasal turbinates, an erythematous mucosa which may be injected. Thin, stringy mucus suggests allergy, whereas a more purulent discharge implies chronic infection. Having said that, chronic allergic rhinorrhea may appear thickened in the child undergoing long-term treatment with antihistamines, or if the child is slightly dehydrated. Evaluation by X-ray, CT or MRI may be required in complicated or recalcitrant cases. In cases of unresponsive or chronic infection with complications, aspiration of the sinus may be required to obtain definitive identification of the microbe.

Treatment Notes

Chronic sinusitis due to recalcitrant bacterial infection should be treated with appropriate antimicrobials. Prophylactic antibiotics may be necessary. Mechanical obstruction should be dealt with appropriately, usually through surgical intervention. In both infectious and allergic sinusitis, osteopathic treatment to resolve the associated mechanical dysfunctions may help to facilitate mucociliary clearance of the sinuses and promote overall health. Facial mechanics are typically restricted in children with chronic sinusitis. The tissues of the pterygopalatine area are edematous and tender. The space between the pterygoid muscles and the connective tissues of the fossa is often quite narrow and tender on one or both sides. In a cooperative child, use of the maxillary spread and zygoma techniques described below may be helpful in assisting

sinus drainage. Compression at the ethmoid notch is usually present, especially in children with a history of congestion in infancy. There is often restriction of base and vault mechanics. Although it may be difficult to determine the primary dysfunction, normalizing base mechanics prior to addressing the other findings often proves successful. Vault restriction is often secondary to the findings in the cranial base. Dysfunction in the suboccipital muscles may be due to facilitation from pain referred from the sphenoid or ethmoid sinuses via the trigeminal–cervical reflex.

Anterior Cervical Myofascial Release

Supine Child

1. The child is supine and the physician sits at the child's head. With one hand, the physician contacts the occiput and monitors the cranial base. The physician uses the other hand to contact the hyoid and the anterior cervical tissues (Fig. 2.130).

2. The physician assesses the response of the anterior tissues during active motion, when the child swallows, and with passive motion testing of the hyoid.

3. The physician then moves the hyoid through elevation, depression, lateral translation, and rotation to establish balanced tension in its myofascial attachments while monitoring the response in the cranial base.

4. Once balanced tension is achieved the position is maintained until there is a change in tissue texture or an improvement in the strain pattern.

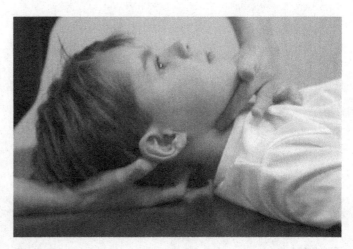

Fig. 2.130

Zygomatic Lift

Child

This is a direct technique that can be used to decompress the maxillary sinus and improve drainage. It is similar in principle and application to a parietal or frontal lift technique. Often after this technique the child's nose will begin to run profusely.

1. The child is supine with the physician seated at his head. The physician contacts both zygomae so that her thumb rests on the superior borders just posterior to the maxillary articulations. The index fingers contact the inferior borders anterior to the zygomatic processes of the temporal bones and posterior to the maxillary articulations (Fig. 2.131).

2. The physician introduces a superolateral motion to 'lift' and 'roll' the zygoma (Fig. 2.131, white arrows) thereby decompressing the articulations with the maxilla (Fig. 2.132, black outline).

3. The physician adjusts the vector of her force to accommodate the resistance in the tissues until balanced tension is achieved.

4. Once balanced tension is established, the physician maintains the position until there a change in tissue texture or an improvement in the strain pattern.

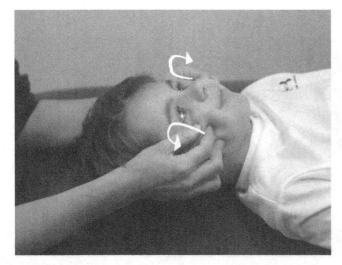

Fig. 2.131

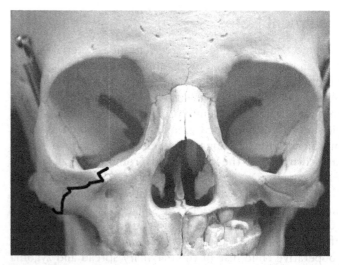

Fig. 2.132

BALANCED LIGAMENTOUS TENSION

Maxillary Spread

Child (Fig. 2.133)

1. The child is supine. The physician sits at the head of the table. One hand is placed under the occiput, with a contact on the suboccipital tissues. The other hand is gloved.

2. The physician places two fingers into the child's mouth just medial to the upper molars, contacting the superior alveolar arches of the maxillae bilaterally. The thumb of the same hand is placed on the glabella.

3. The physician introduces a gentle spreading motion through her fingers, encouraging the maxillae into external rotation while the thumb is used to decompress the glabella area.

4. An anteroinferior traction is introduced (white arrow). The physician maintains this position and monitors the tissue response until there is change in tissue texture, which may be felt as a 'lift and spread' of the maxillae.

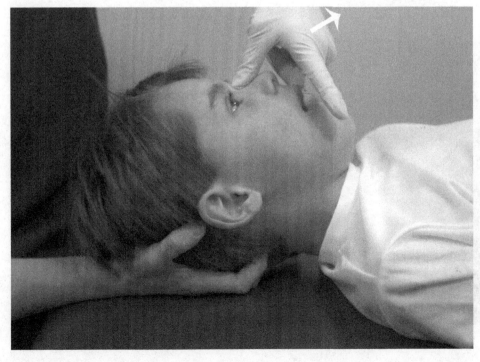

Fig. 2.133 • Anterior view of a child-age skull (note the undescended second teeth). The zygomaticomaxillary articulation is indicated in black.

BALANCED LIGAMENTOUS TENSION

Facial Lift

Child (Fig. 2.134A, B)

1. The child is supine. The physician sits at the head of the table. One hand is placed over the frontal bone contacting the lateral margins. The other hand is gloved.

2. The physician places two fingers into the child's mouth just medial to the upper molars, contacting the superior alveolar arches of the maxillae bilaterally. The thumb of the same hand is placed on the glabella.

3. The physician introduces a gentle spreading motion through her fingers, encouraging the maxillae into external rotation while the thumb is used to decompress the glabella area.

4. The physician internally rotates the frontal bone and introduces an anterosuperior traction (black arrow) while simultaneously introducing an anteroinferior traction through the maxillae (white arrow). The physician maintains this position and monitors the tissue response until there is change in tissue texture, which may be felt as a 'lift and spread' of the tissues.

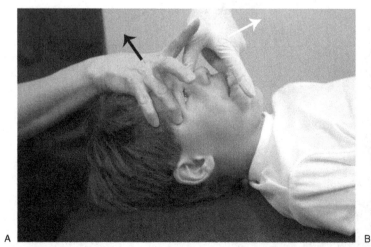

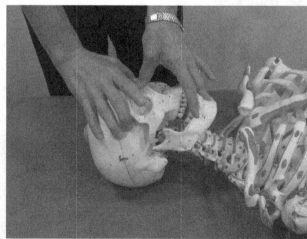

A   B

Fig. 2.134

References

Boersma ER, Offringa PJ, Muskiet FA, et al. Vitamin E, lipid fractions, and fatty acid composition of colostrum, transitional milk, and mature milk: an international comparative study. Am J Clin Nutr 1991; 53: 1197–1204.

Brunetaeu RJ, Mulliken JB. Frontal plagiocephaly: synostotic, compensational, or deformational. Plast Reconstruct Surg 1992; 89: 21–32.

Carreiro JE. An osteopathic approach to children, 2nd edn. Edinburgh: Churchill Livingstone, 2009.

Cheng JC, Au AW. Infantile torticollis: a review of 624 cases. J Pediatr Orthop 1994; 14: 802–808.

Hamanishi C, Tanaka S. Turned head-adducted hip truncal curvature syndrome. Arch Dis Child 1994; 70: 515–519.

Jensen RG, Hagerty MM, McMahon KE. Lipids of human milk and infant formulas: a review. Am J Clin Nutr 1978; 31: 990–1016.

Kane AA, Mitchell LE, Craven KP, Marsh JL. Observations on a recent increase in plagiocephaly without synostosis. Pediatrics 1996; 97: 877–885.

Konishi Y, Mikawa H, Suzuki J. Asymmetrical head turning of preterm infants: some effects on later postural and functional lateralities. Dev Psychobiol 2002; 40: 1–13.

McMaster MJ. Infantile idiopathic scoliosis: can it be prevented? J Bone Joint Surg 1983; 65B: 612–617.

Magoun HIS. Idiopathic adolescent spinal scoliosis. DO 1973; 13–17.

Magoun HIS. Osteopathy in the cranial field, 3rd edn. Kirksville, MO: Journal Printing Company, 1976.

Mills M, Henley C, Barnes L, et al. The use of osteopathic manipulative treament as adjuvant therapy in children with recurrent acute otitis media. Arch Pediatr Adolesc Med 2003; 157: 861–866.

Pang D, Veetai L. Atlantoaxial rotatory fixation: Part 1 Biomechanics of normal rotation at the atlantoaxial joint in children. Neuro-surgery 2004; 55: 614–626.

Philippi H, Faldum A, Jung T, et al. Patterns of postural asymmetry in infants: a standardized video-based analysis. Eur J Pediatr 2006; 165: 158–164.

Ward R. Foundations for osteopathic medicine. St Louis: Lippincott, Williams & Willkins, 2003.

Woodward DR, Rees B, Boon JA. Human milk fat content: within-feed variation. Early Hum Dev 1989; 19: 39–46.

Chapter Three

The spine, rib cage and sacrum

3

OVERVIEW

Anne Wales (personal communication, 1986) often described the human body as a tripod with one leg standing upright. This analogy goes a long way towards describing the precarious nature of posture and balance. The components of the musculoskeletal system interact to provide support, stability and flexibility to the body. The upright leg is a flexible rod with a modified sphere resting atop it. The flexible rod has a serious of sagittal curves that increase the stability of the bipedal system. It is surrounded by a ligamentous stocking that travels from the base of the head to the coccyx. The individual vertebrae are suspended within this stocking, with the cushions of the intervertebral discs sandwiched between them. The entire system works in concert. A force influencing one area of the column influences the entire column.

The rib cage is perched over the middle of the column. This ever-moving structure influences the entire tripod. The diaphragm contracts and the ribs rise and turn at their costovertebral junctions. This influences the vertebrae. As the ribs elevate the tips of their adjacent vertebrae, the thoracic curve flattens slightly. The crurae of the diaphragm increase the tensile load on the anterior longitudinal ligament. This change is transmitted through the fasciae and connective tissues of the ligamentous stocking. The vertebrae and discs lying within it respond. The cervical and lumbar curves decrease slightly. There is activity in the quadratus lumborum and psoas muscles, and that action transmits the influences of respiration into the hips and pelvis. Movements of the ribs and fasciae of the thoracic cage are transmitted to the prevertebral structures and the structures of the posterior thoracic wall, where the sympathetic chain ganglia lie. These movements are slight, but they are repeated throughout the day, throughout the year, throughout life. There are approximately 18 breaths per minute, 60 minutes per hour, 24 hours per day, 365 days per year. That adds up to a lot of motion. Movements at the costovertebral articulations have the potential to influence neural fibers exiting the neural foramina of the thoracic spine (Fig. 3.1).

In the osteopathic structure–function models the mechanical relationships throughout the skeletal system play a key role in the respiratory–circulatory system. From the point of view of the thorax and rib cage this is obvious, but it is often lost in the translation to clinical medicine. In our modern obsession with the minute (cells, chemicals, genes, etc.), medical intervention often neglects the gross structures supporting these marvelous microscopic worlds. Currently, the standard of care for patients with chronic respiratory conditions is pharmacological, and gene therapy is on the not too distant horizon. But patients lose out on the potential benefits of a more global approach, one that addresses the gross work of the respiratory–circulatory system, its energy demands and compensatory mechanisms.

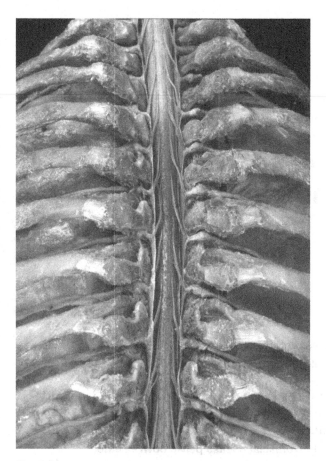

Fig. 3.1

Every aspect of respiratory–circulatory function begins with a breath. The work needed to generate that breath, to sustain it and release it, is based on mechanical functions. These same mechanical processes influence the movement of fluids into and out of tissues. The integrity of the respiratory–circulatory system, especially its low-pressure components, is influenced for better or worse by the mechanical relationships throughout the myofascial system of the body.

THE RESPIRATORY–CIRCULATORY MODEL

Clinical Notes

In the osteopathic concept, unimpeded function of the respiratory circulatory system is fundamental to the maintenance of health and recovery from disease. To further emphasize this, common epitaphs attributed to Still (1899) include: 'The rule of the artery is supreme' and 'By the lymphatics you live or die.' Although these quotations may seem quaint initially, our modern molecular-based medical model cannot dismiss the importance of cellular and tissue health in the prevention and treatment of disease. The delivery of oxygen and nutrients and the removal of waste products are bodily functions that modern medicine has not yet been able to duplicate. Common sense tells us that any patient, regardless of their ailment or state of health, will benefit from optimum function of these systems. Osteopathic manipulative techniques offer a potential tool to assist the body in these processes. Although much research still needs to be done, the potential for benefit and the apparent lack of adverse effects provide a strong motivation to practitioners wishing to help their patients and do no harm.

In older children and adults, ambulation and other voluntary motions assist with the movement of fluids through the peripheral venous and lymphatic channels to the larger collecting channels in the pelvis, abdomen and thorax. Alternating pressures generated through respiration and other involuntary mechanisms assist with fluid movement from these areas back into the circulation. In the osteopathic concept, normal infant functions such as suckling, crying and breathing play an important role in the low-pressure circulatory system, often replacing the influences of more active movement patterns associated with ambulation (Fig. 3.2).

The myofascial and postural relationships throughout the body influence respiratory mechanics (Thach 1979, 1980, Wilson 1980) and lymphatic drainage (Ahlqvist 1985, Agostini and Zocchi 1991, Miller et al. 1992, Aukland and Reed 1993, Negrini et al. 1994). Addressing areas of tissue stress or altered biomechanics may optimize respiratory mechanics and facilitate function of the low-pressure circulatory system. The following sequence of techniques is intended to address the articulatory and myofascial tissues that potentially influence respiratory–circulatory function.

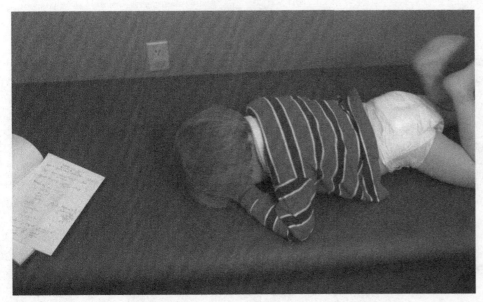

Fig. 3.2 • Two-year-old grandson expressing opinion regarding request that he pose for another batch of photographs. On a positive note, this can be viewed as facilitating fluid movement through the low-pressure circulatory system.

SACRAL–PELVIC BOWL

BALANCED LIGAMENTOUS TECHNIQUE

Supine Infant

This is a general approach to the sacral–pelvic bowl.

1. The infant is supine or held in the parent's arms. The physician sits beside the infant. The physician uses the hand that is closest to the infant's head to contact the posterior aspect of the sacrum along the midline (SBP1). The other hand contacts the anterior superior iliac spines (ASIS) of both innominates (Fig. 3.3A, B). This is a gentle contact.

2. The physician monitors motion and tissue response in the pelvis to breathing. In general, there should be resilience in the sacral–pelvic bowl. This is often described as an expansion during inhalation whereby the innominates flare laterally and the sacrum counternutates. During exhalation, the innominates flare internally and the sacrum nutates.

3. Based on her observations during quiet breathing, the physician will determine whether or not there is a restriction in the normal tissue response.

4. This will be addressed using balanced tension technique. The physician can nutate or counternutate the sacrum by lifting on the superior or inferior aspect. Then the physician uses her contact on the ASIS to rotate and flare or (spread) the innominate, assessing tissue response throughout the sacral–pelvic bowl.

5. Vectors of motion can be fine-tuned to establish balanced tension between the tissues.

6. Once balanced tension is achieved the position is held until the physician feels a change in tissue texture, improvement of involuntary motion or a correction of the strain.

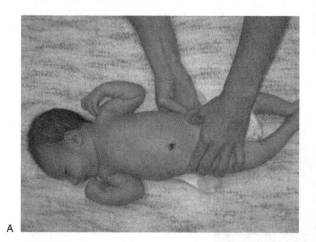
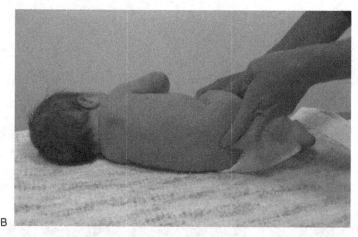

A   B

Fig. 3.3

DIRECT MYOFASCIAL RELEASE

Supine Infant

This is a general fascial approach to the sacral–pelvic bowl. The contact is the same as that used in the balanced ligamentous technique.

1. The infant is supine or held in the parent's arms. The physician sits beside the infant. The physician uses the hand that is closest to the infant's head to contact the posterior aspect of the sacrum along the midline (Fig. 3.4A). The other hand contacts the anterior superior iliac spines (ASIS) of both innominates (Fig. 3.4B). This is a gentle contact.

2. The physician monitors motion and tissue response in the pelvis to breathing. In general there should be resiliency in the sacral–pelvic bowl. This is often described as an expansion during inhalation whereby the innominates flare laterally and the sacrum counternutates. During exhalation, the innominates flare internally and the sacrum nutates.

3. Based on her observations during quiet breathing, the physician will determine whether the restriction exists in inhalation and sacral counternutation, or in exhalation and sacral nutation.

4. The restriction will be addressed using direct myofascial release. As the infant enters the respiratory phase in which the restriction exists, the physician will nutate or counternutate the sacrum (by lifting on the superior or inferior aspect) to load the fascial tissues and engage the restrictive barrier. For example, if the restrictive barrier is in inhalation and sacral counternutation, then as the infant inhales the physician will counternutate the sacrum to engage the restrictive barrier.

5. The physician uses her contact on the ASIS to rotate, and medially or laterally flare the innominates, as is appropriate for the respiratory phase. This further loads the fascial tissues and engages the restrictive barrier.

6. Other vectors of motion, such as compression, decompression and tilt, can be introduced to fine-tune to the restrictive barrier. As the tissue is loaded more precisely, the physician should feel a softening of the restrictive barrier.

7. The physician 'follows' this softening, i.e. further loads the tissue until there is a correction of the barrier.

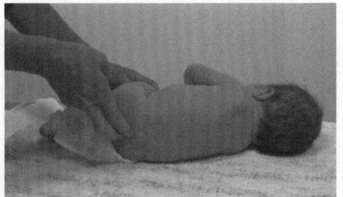

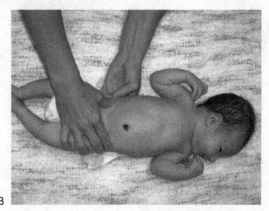

A   B

Fig. 3.4

DIRECT MYOFASCIAL RELEASE

Seated Toddler

This is a general fascial approach to the sacral–pelvic bowl.

1. The toddler is seated. The physician sits beside the child. The physician uses one hand to contact the posterior aspect of the sacral–pelvic bowl, sacrum and iliac crest, and the other to contact the anterior aspect of the innominate (Fig. 3.5).

2. The physician monitors motion and tissue response in the pelvis to breathing. In general there should be resiliency in the sacral–pelvic bowl. This is often described as an expansion during inhalation whereby the innominates flare laterally and the sacrum counternutates. During exhalation, the innominates flare internally and the sacrum nutates.

3. Based on the physician's observation during quiet breathing she will determine within which respiratory phase the restriction exists.

4. The restriction will be addressed using direct myofascial release. As the toddler enters the respiratory phase the physician will use her contacts to introduce compression, decompression, rotation, tilt, flare, nutation and/or counternutation into the myofascial elements to load the fascial tissues and engage the restrictive barrier. For example, if the restrictive barrier is in inhalation the physician will counternutate the sacrum, posteriorly rotate and laterally flare the innominates.

5. As the tissue is loaded more precisely, the physician should feel a softening of the restrictive barrier.

6. The physician 'follows' this softening, i.e. further loads the tissue until there is a correction of the barrier.

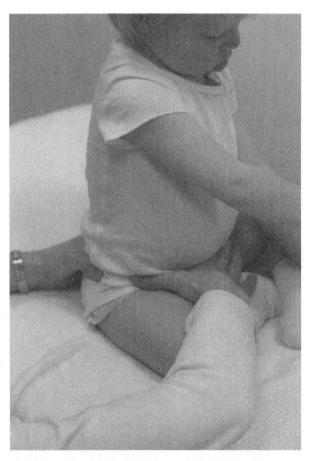

Fig. 3.5

BALANCED LIGAMENTOUS TECHNIQUE

Sacroiliac Joints

Supine Infant

This approach may be performed on a patient of any age. In this example an infant is being treated.

1. The patient is supine or held in the parent's arms. The physician sits beside the patient on the affected side (Fig. 3.6). The physician uses the hand that is closest to the patient's head to contact the posterior aspect of the sacrum as close to the sacroiliac (SI) joint as possible (Figs 3.7 and 3.8). The other hand contacts the anterior superior iliac spine (ASIS) on the same side. This is a gentle contact using either the pad of the fingers or the palm of the hand.

2. The physician lifts the sacrum slightly anteriorly and notes the response of the tissues. The sacrum can also be nutated and counternutated by varying the vector of the anterior lift.

3. Then the physician uses her contact on the ASIS to assess the response of the SI ligaments to rotation and flare of the innominate. The physician determines the position of greater and lesser tissue stress with the innominate in both anterior and posterior rotation and inflare and outflare. These positions will be used to decompress the SI joint in the following step.

4. The physician simultaneously lifts the sacrum anteriorly (white arrow) while moving the innominate in the appropriate direction (black arrows) to decompress the SI joint. Vectors of motion are then introduced into both the sacrum and innominate to fine-tune and establish balanced tension between the tissues.

5. Once balanced tension is established, the position is held until the physician feels a change in tissue texture, improvement of involuntary motion or a correction of the strain.

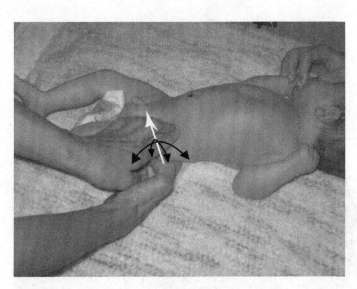

Fig. 3.6

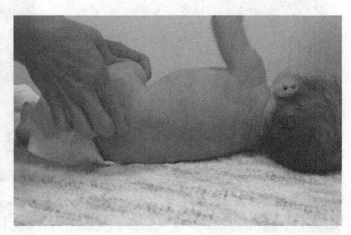

Fig. 3.7   Fig. 3.8

TWELFTH RIB, ARCUATE LIGAMENTS AND DIAPHRAGM

Treatment Notes

The medial arcuate ligament is a tendinous sheath that inserts on the crus of the ipsilateral diaphragm and crosses to the transverse process of L1 (Fig. 3.9A). The psoas passes beneath it. The lateral arcuate ligament is a fascial sheath that inserts onto the transverse process of L1 and the tip of the 12th rib. It extends into the belly of the diaphragm on the ipsilateral side (Fig. 3.9B). The quadratus lumborum muscle passes under the lateral arcuate ligament. Dysfunction of L1, the 12th rib, the psoas or the quadratus lumborum muscles has the potential to affect the mechanics of the diaphragm and the work of respiration. In addition, restrictions in these structures may irritate the lateral cutaneous nerve of the thigh or the iliohypogastric nerve. The former presents with pain and paresthesiae of the anterior thigh, the latter with similar symptoms in the testicle or labia.

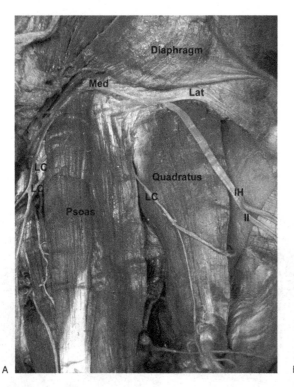
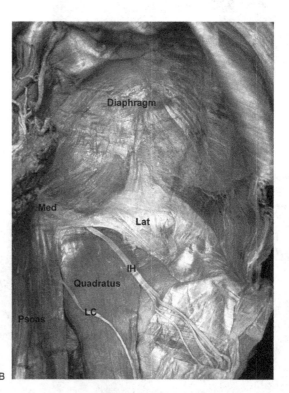

Fig. 3.9 • A,B Anterior view of the left side of the posterior abdominal wall with the abdominal contents, including the peritoneum, removed to expose the deep muscles and the undersurface of the diaphragm. (A) View with the diaphragm lying flat. (B) The diaphragm has been lifted anteriorly to reveal the lateral arcuate ligament extending into the dome of the left diaphragmatic hemisphere. The lateral cutaneous (LC) and iliohypogastric (IH) nerves are labeled.

DIRECT BALANCED LIGAMENTOUS TECHNIQUE

Twelfth Rib, Costal Arches, Diaphragm

Supine Child or Athlete

In older children and athletes, treatment of the 12th rib often requires a direct approach to counterbalance the tissue strain in this area. It is not always easy to locate and contact the 12th rib. This technique employs one hand as a passive hand that uses a plastic contact on the 12th rib, while the other hand plays an active role through the passive hand to establish balanced tension in the tissues (Fig. 3.10). The goal of this approach is to achieve balanced tension between the rib, the arcuate ligaments and their relationship with the diaphragm (Fig. 3.9A). The lateral arcuate ligament forms a modified triangle pointing into the diaphragm (Fig. 3.9B).

1. The child is supine. The physician sits ipsilateral to the side to be treated. The physician places her passive hand beneath the lower rib cage, contacting as much of the 12th rib as possible with the palmar surface of her middle finger (Fig. 3.11). The active hand is placed under the passive hand in a similar plane (Figs 3.10 and 3.12).

2. The physician uses her active hand to lift the middle finger of the passive hand and apply lateral traction along the rib to engage the tissues.

3. The physician then varies the vector of her traction to appropriately counterbalance the forces acting on the rib. Depending on the tissue involved, this may require the inferior, anterior, superior or lateral vectors to be emphasized or de-emphasized to achieve balanced tension. The physician may choose to use a 'stacking' technique to determine the appropriate vectors to employ.

4. Once balanced tension is achieved between the tissues, the physician maintains this position through several respiratory cycles until there is a change in tissue texture, a reduction in tissue stress, or an improvement in respiratory motion of the 12th rib.

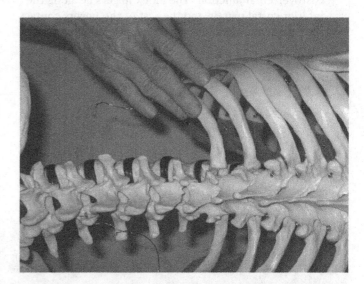

Fig. 3.11

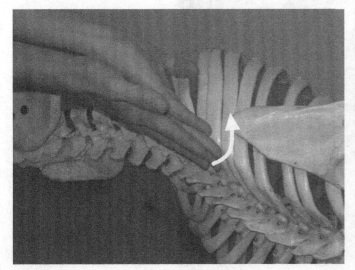

Fig. 3.10

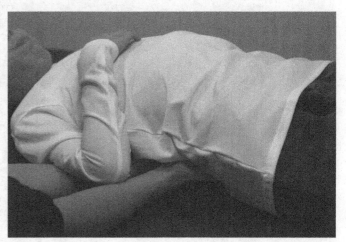

Fig. 3.12

BALANCED LIGAMENTOUS TECHNIQUE

Twelfth Rib, Costal Arches, Diaphragm

Seated Toddler (Fig. 3.13)

The 12th ribs have a caliper-type motion that causes them to spread inferiorly, laterally and posteriorly during inhalation. These ribs play an important role in respiratory mechanics by stabilizing the inferior aspect of the thoracic cage during inhalation. Dysfunction in the pelvis, spine or torso may affect rib motion.

1. The child is seated facing away from the physician. The physician contacts the lower costal margin with both hands so that the thumbs lie along the shaft of the 12th ribs and the tips of the thumbs rest on the costovertebral junction. The index fingers lie along the inferior costal margin and the rest of the fingers contact the myofascial tissues of the superior abdominal wall.

2. The physician assesses rib function during quiet respiration, noting the quality of tissue response.

3. Using the thumbs, the physician introduces a lateral traction in the direction of the shaft of the ribs to decompress the costovertebral junction.

4. Then physician introduces rotation, tilt, translation, depression and elevation into the two ribs, noting the response of the anterior myofascial tissues, the diaphragm and the ribs.

5. The physician uses her contacts to achieve balanced tension through the diaphragm and ribs.

6. Once balanced tension is achieved, this position is maintained until there is a change in tissue texture, an improvement in function or a correction of the dysfunction.

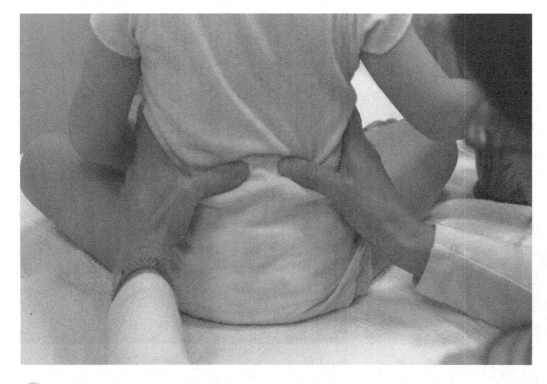

Fig. 3.13

BALANCED LIGAMENTOUS TECHNIQUE

Bilateral 12th Rib, Costal Arches, Diaphragm

Supine Infant

1. The child is supine, seated or on the parent's lap. The physician places one hand around the lower torso and establishes a firm contact on the tip of the 12th rib and the anterior fasciae of the diaphragm. The other hand is placed in a similar position on the other side of the torso (Fig. 3.14A, B).

2. A steady anterolateral traction is placed on the posterior aspect of the rib at a vector of approximately 90° from the spine to establish balanced ligamentous tension between the rib and the vertebra through the arcuate ligaments and the costovertebral ligaments.

3. As this is being done, the physician uses her anterior contact to carry the diaphragm tissues superiorly and either laterally or medially to bring the diaphragm into balanced tension with the position of the 12th ribs.

4. This position is held until the ribs are felt to move more freely with respiration.

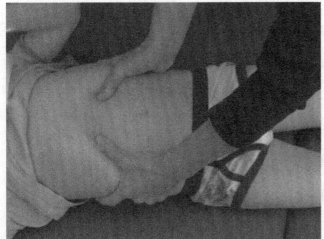

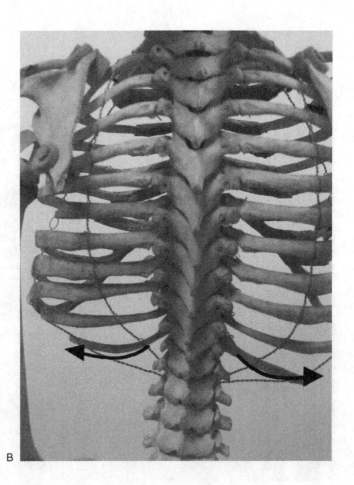

A   B

Fig. 3.14

BALANCED LIGAMENTOUS TECHNIQUE

Thoracic Diaphragm

Supine Infant, Child, Athlete

Although this approach looks similar to the diaphragm-doming technique often used in adults, it is quite different. One should avoid putting any compressive force into the rib cage or diaphragm in infants and young children. One should also avoid anything that causes a marked increase in inhalation volumes, especially if there is concern about an obstructive respiratory condition. Although this approach is described on an infant, it can be used on a patient of any age.

1. The infant is supine. The physician sits beside the infant. The physician contacts the inferior costal margin anteriorly with her thumbs and the thoracic vertebrae posteriorly with her fingers (Fig. 3.15).

2. The physician monitors the response of the lower ribs (9–12), the thoracolumbar vertebrae, and their myofascial components to quiet respiration or, as in this case, active audible respiration.

3. The physician notes tissue resiliency and any areas of restriction.

4. The physician uses her contact on the ribs to decompress the 10th, 11th and 12th ribs at their costovertebral articulations while monitoring the response of the diaphragm.

5. The physician then shifts her force to create balanced tension throughout the dome of the diaphragm. In an infant or young child there should be no compression into the diaphragmatic tissues. In an older child or athlete, compression may be introduced.

6. Once balanced tension is achieved, the position is maintained until there is a change in tissue texture or an improvement in function. The physician releases her contact slowly.

Fig. 3.15

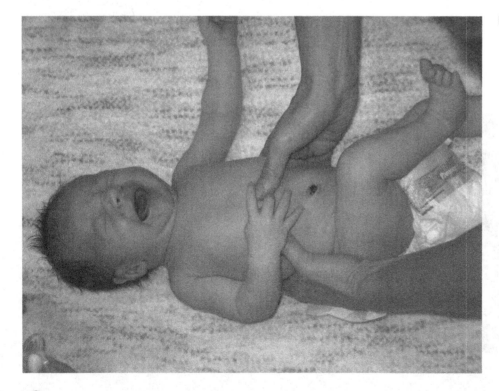

BALANCED LIGAMENTOUS TECHNIQUE

Thoracic Diaphragm

Supine Child or Athlete

This approach is similar to the one previously described, except that each side of the diaphragm and lower rib cage is treated separately. This may be a more effective approach when there has been injury or trauma to one side, such as a seatbelt injury in a motor vehicle accident, when there is postoperative scarring, or in conditions affecting visceral organs that are lateralized, such as the liver, gallbladder, spleen, etc.

1. The patient is supine and the physician sits on the side to be treated. The physician contacts the inferior costal margins of ribs 9 and 10 with the index and middle fingers of one hand. The ring and small fingers of the same hand sink into the anterior abdominal wall under the costal edge. The middle and index fingers of the other hand are placed under the patient, contacting ribs 9 and 10 medially to the rib angle. The thumbs are crossed and contact the lateral margins of ribs 9 and 10 (Fig. 3.16).

2. The physician monitors the response of the lower ribs (9–10), their myofascial components and the ipsilateral side of the diaphragm to quiet respiration.

3. The physician notes tissue resiliency and any areas of restriction.

4. The physician uses her contact on the ribs to decompress the ninth and 10th ribs at their costovertebral articulations by introducing an anterolateral traction through her posterior contacts. The response of the diaphragm and myofascial tissues is noted.

5. The physician then shifts her force to create balanced tension throughout the dome of the diaphragm. This is accomplished by using the anterior contacts to initially lift the tissue cephalad and lateral (black arrow). Depending on the tissue response, the vector may be adjusted by tilting and/or rotating the hands to achieve balanced tension in the tissues.

6. Once balanced tension is achieved, the position is maintained until there is a change in tissue texture or an improvement in function. The physician releases her contact slowly.

Fig. 3.16

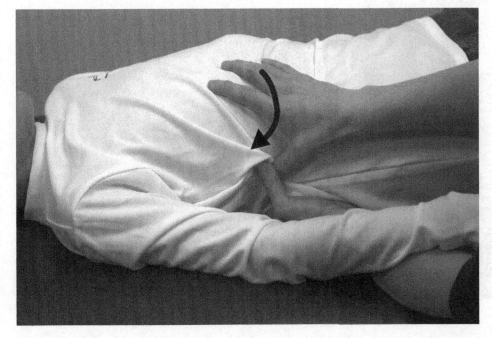

BALANCED LIGAMENTOUS TECHNIQUE

Thoracic Diaphragm

Seated Toddler

In a child less than 3 years old the lower ribs will lie on a more horizontal plane than in a child over 3.

1. The child is seated facing the caregiver, who is responsible for entertainment. The physician sits behind the child. The lower ribs (9 and 10) are contacted bilaterally at the costovertebral junction (Figs 3.17 and 3.18). The fingers are then wrapped around the child's waist along the margin of the ribs (Fig. 3.19). The distal portion of the physician's fingers lies along the margin of the rib cage, contacting the 10th rib as it wraps anteriorly.

2. The physician can use a gentle posterolateral motion such as a caliper opening to engage the tissues of the costovertebral junction. As this is being done, the fingers making contact on the anterior and lateral surfaces of the ribs gently lift the tissues, assessing their response in all planes of motion, including rotation and torsion.

3. The posterior contact takes the ribs laterally, as the lateral and anterior contacts carry the tissues superiorly and in the appropriate direction (see previous step) to achieve balanced tension between the two ribs and the insertion of the diaphragm.

4. Once achieved, balanced tension is maintained until there is a change in tissue texture and sense of increased freedom of motion in the ribs.

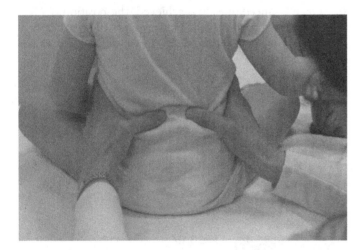

Fig. 3.17

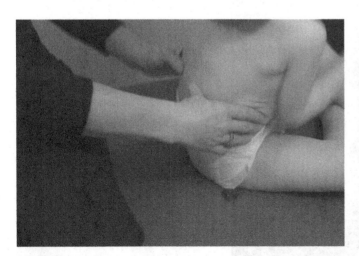

Fig. 3.18

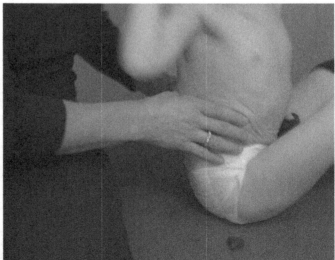

Fig. 3.19

BALANCED LIGAMENTOUS TECHNIQUE

Ribs

Seated Toddler

The ribs have a more horizontal orientation in young children and infants than in adults (Fig. 3.20), and the angles of the ribs are not well developed (Fig. 3.21, black oval).

1. The child is sitting with the affected side towards the physician. The physician contacts the shaft of the rib using the palmar surface of the middle or index finger of one hand anteriorly and one posteriorly (Fig. 3.22).

2. Using the anterior and posterior contacts, the physician tractions the rib laterally adding elevation, depression and/or translation (posterior or anterior) to establish balanced ligamentous tension between the rib and its articular and myofascial connections.

3. Once a point of balance has been reached, the physician holds that position and allows the child to move through a few respiratory cycles. The physician monitors for a change in tissue tension, a correction of the strain or an improvement in function.

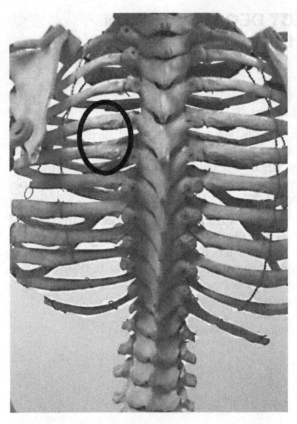

Fig. 3.21

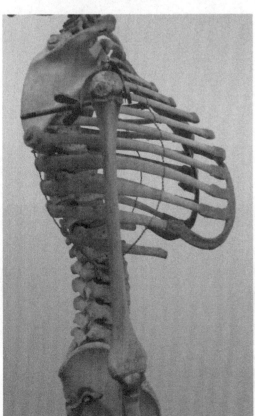

Fig. 3.20 • Lateral view of the skeleton of a 3–4-year-old child. Note the horizontal orientation of the ribs.

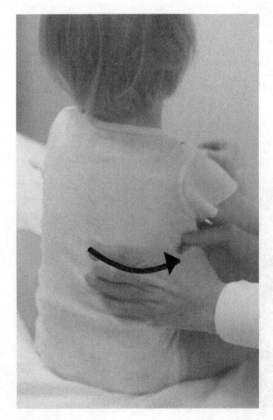

Fig. 3.22

DIRECT DECOMPRESSION TECHNIQUE

Ribs

Supine Infant (Fig. 3.23)

At birth the ribs are very pliable and cartilaginous. This technique can be used to treat a single rib or a group of ribs. Typically in non-ambulating children mid and lower rib dysfunction involves a group of ribs rather than a single rib. Treatment of three ribs is described.

1. The infant is supine or held in the parent's arms. The physician sits beside the infant on the affected side. The physician slides one hand under the infant's back to contact the ribs posteriorly as close to their vertebral articulations as possible (Fig. 3.24). The angles of the ribs are not developed at this age.

2. The other hand is placed over the anterior aspect of the ribs, contacting the costocartilage (Fig. 3.23).

3. The physician observes rib motion during quiet breathing. With her posterior hand the physician lifts the ribs anteriorly while monitoring the tissue response with the other hand. The posterior hand then introduces a lateral traction on the ribs to decompress the costovertebral junction. At the same time, the anterior hand exerts the slightest lateral traction.

4. The vector of motion used by the hands can be individualized to each rib, depending on the tissue response.

5. This position is maintained as the child completes several respiratory cycles until there is a change in tissue resistance or an improvement in function.

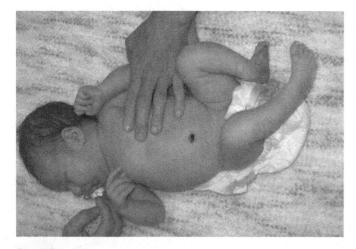

Fig. 3.23

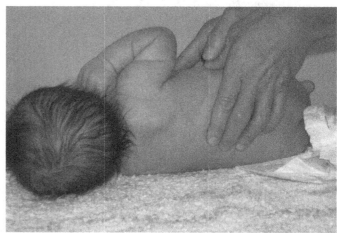

Fig. 3.24

RIB RAISING

Soft Tissue

Supine Child

This technique is appropriate for patients of any age. In this direct technique, the restrictive barrier is engaged but not overcome.

1. The patient is supine. The physician sits ipsilateral to the side to be treated. The physician places both hands under the torso (Fig. 3.25A, B) and uses the pads of the middle, index and ring fingers of both hands to contact several ribs just medial to the rib angle.

2. The physician lifts her fingers into the ribs, carrying each rib anterolaterally in a curvilinear direction to, but not through, the restrictive barrier (curved black arrow). Then the physician releases her forces and allows the tissues to return to their positions. The movement is performed independently of the respiratory cycle.

3. The physician repeats the procedure, lifting her fingers into the ribs and carrying each rib anterolaterally to its restrictive barrier. Then she relaxes her force. This sequence is repeated several times until there is a change in tissue texture.

4. The physician moves her hands superiorly or inferiorly and repeats the sequence on adjacent rib groups.

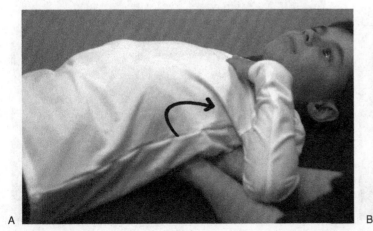 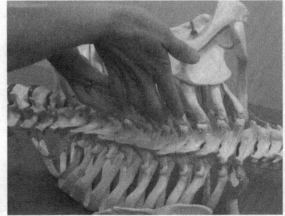

A B

Fig. 3.25

BALANCED LIGAMENTOUS TECHNIQUE

Second and Third Ribs

Supine Infant

The upper ribs are often strained during difficult or prolonged deliveries. The first three ribs play a fundamental role in respiratory mechanics in the thorax and should be treated to optimize respiratory–circulatory function. Treatment of the first rib is described in Chapter 2 (Head and Neck).

1. The infant is supine or held by the parent. The physician sits beside the infant on the affected side (Fig. 3.26A, B).

2. The physician contacts the posterior aspect of the second and third ribs with one hand. Two fingers of the other hand are placed on the anterior aspect of the ribs. The thumbs may be used as a fulcrum in the mid-axillary line.

3. The physician introduces an anterior lift to the posterior aspect of the ribs, monitoring the tissue response.

4. Then the physician simultaneously introduces lateral traction (black arrow) at the anterior and posterior contacts to decompress the costovertebral junction.

5. The physician varies the vector of her forces to achieve balanced tension in the tissues. Once balanced tension is established, the position is maintained until there is a change in tissue texture, a correction of the dysfunction or an improvement in function.

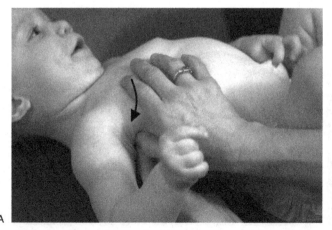

A   B

Fig. 3.26

BALANCED LIGAMENTOUS TECHNIQUE – ALTERNATE TECHNIQUE

Second and Third Ribs

Supine Infant

Rather than introducing forces through the anterior and posterior aspects of the rib, this approach uses a posterolateral contact on the ribs. This approach may be more effective when the upper extremity is involved.

1. The infant is supine or held by the parent. The physician sits beside the infant on the affected side (Fig. 3.27).

2. The physician contacts the posterior aspect of the second and third ribs with one hand. Two fingers of the other hand are placed into the axilla to contact the shafts of the same ribs.

3. The physician introduces an anterior lift to the posterior aspect of the ribs while simultaneously elevating or depressing the shafts of the ribs. Then the physician introduces a lateral traction to decompress the costovertebral junction.

4. The physician uses her two hands to vary the vectors of force as appropriate to achieve balanced tension.

5. Once balanced tension is established, the position is maintained until there is a change in tissue texture, a correction of the dysfunction or an improvement in function.

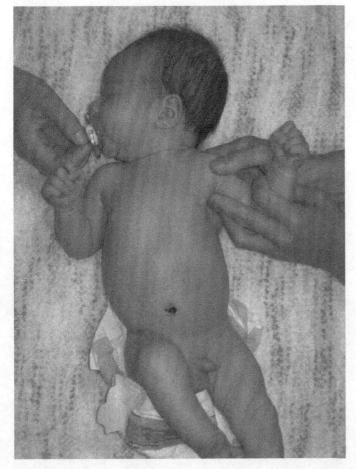

Fig. 3.27

BALANCED LIGAMENTOUS TECHNIQUE

Second and Third Ribs

Seated Toddler

1.   The toddler is seated. The physician sits beside the child on the affected side (Fig. 3.28A, B).

2.   The physician contacts the posterior aspect of the second and third ribs with one hand. Two fingers of the other hand are placed on the anterior aspect of the ribs.

3.   The physician introduces an anterior lift to the posterior aspect of the ribs, monitoring the tissue response anteriorly.

4.   Then the physician simultaneously introduces lateral traction at the anterior and posterior contacts to decompress the costovertebral and costosternal junctions.

5.   The physician varies the vector of her forces to achieve balanced tension in the tissues. Once balanced tension is established, the position is maintained until there is a change in tissue texture, a correction of the dysfunction or an improvement in function.

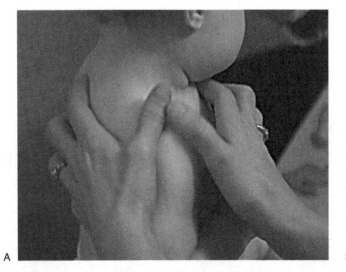
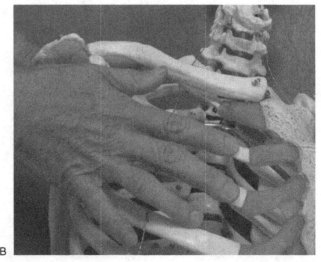

A

B

Fig. 3.28

BALANCED LIGAMENTOUS TECHNIQUE – ALTERNATE TECHNIQUE

Second and Third Ribs

Seated Toddler

The child is seated. The physician sits beside the child on the affected side (Fig. 3.29).

1. The physician contacts the posterior aspect of the second and third ribs with one hand. The thumbs are placed into the axilla, contacting the lateral shaft of the ribs at the mid-axillary line. The pads of two fingers contact the anterior aspect of the same ribs.

2. The physician introduces a slight compression anteriorly with the posterior contacts and posteriorly with the anterior contacts (small black arrows). Then the physician introduces a lateral translation at both contacts to decompress the ribs at their articulations (large black arrow).

3. Using the thumbs as a fulcrum the physician can elevate, depress, translate and rotate the ribs to achieve balanced tension.

4. Once balanced tension is established, the position is maintained until there is a change in tissue texture, a correction of the dysfunction or an improvement in function.

Fig. 3.29

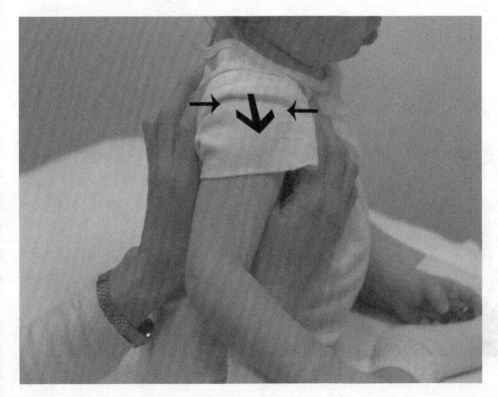

BALANCED LIGAMENTOUS TECHNIQUE

Upper Ribs

Supine Child or Athlete (Fig. 3.30A, B)

By the age of 7, the upper ribs have assumed a more mature shape and pump-handle mechanics. During respiration the anterior aspect rises more than the posterior, and there is a slight rotation at the costovertebral junction during inhalation and exhalation.

1. The child is supine. The physician sits beside the patient on the affected side (Fig. 3.30A).

2. Using the index and middle fingers of one hand, the physician contacts the posterior aspect of two adjacent upper ribs just medial to the rib angle (in this example, ribs 2 and 3 are used). The index and middle fingers of the other hand are placed on the anterior aspect of the same ribs. The thumbs contact the lateral margins of the shafts in the mid-axillary line.

3. The physician introduces an anterior lift and inferior (caudad) traction to the posterior aspect of the ribs, monitoring the tissue response.

4. The physician introduces a superior (cephalad) lift at the anterior contact. Simultaneously, the physician applies lateral traction to the anterior and posterior contacts to decompress the costovertebral junctions.

5. The physician varies the vector of her forces to achieve balanced tension in the tissues. This is done by introducing side-bending, elevation, depression, torsion, compression and decompression into the ribs.

6. Once balanced tension is established, the position is maintained until there is a change in tissue texture, a correction of the dysfunction, or an improvement in function.

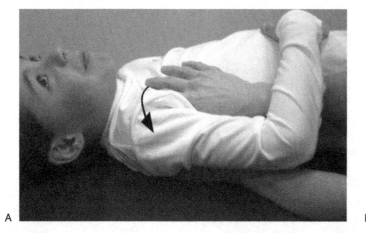

A

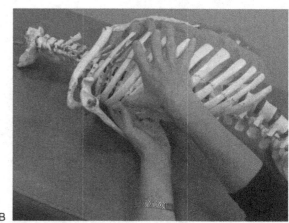

B

Fig. 3.30

BALANCED LIGAMENTOUS TECHNIQUE – ALTERNATE TECHNIQUE

Upper Ribs

Supine Child or Athlete

In this approach the physician uses the upper extremity as a long lever to achieve balanced tension. This may be useful in strains involving the upper ribs and upper extremities. This approach can also be used to treat more than two ribs simultaneously. This contact can also be used to perform a facilitated positional release technique.

1. The child is supine. The physician sits beside the patient on the affected side (Fig. 3.31A).

2. With the index and middle fingers of one hand, the physician contacts the posterior aspect of the ribs to be treated just medial to the rib angle. The other hand is used to abduct the ipsilateral arm. The elbow is flexed and the physician contacts the arm at the elbow.

3. The physician introduces an anterior lift and inferior (caudad) traction to the posterior aspect of the ribs, monitoring the tissue response.

4. The physician then introduces compression through the flexed arm to the level of the ribs (straight white arrow) (Fig. 3.31B).

5. The physician rotates, flexes, extends, abducts and adducts the arm while monitoring the tissue response at the rib and costovertebral junctions.

6. The physician varies the vector of her forces through the arm to achieve balanced tension in the tissues (curved white arrow).

7. Once balanced tension is established, the position is maintained until there is a change in tissue texture, a correction of the dysfunction, or an improvement in function.

TREATMENT

First Rib

These approaches are described in Chapter 2 (Head and Neck).

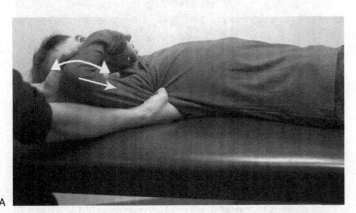

A

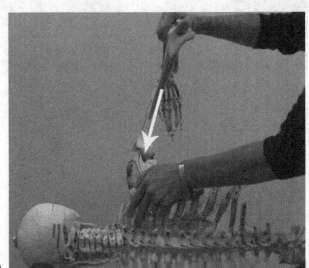

B

Fig. 3.31

CONGENITAL SCOLIOSIS

Clinical Notes

Congenital scoliosis is a malformation of the spine. It may be due to failure of development, failure of segmentation, or a combination of the two (Figs 3.32 and 3.33). Depending on the severity and location of the deformity, congenital scoliosis may not be identified until adolescence. The level of the deformity, the number of segments affected and the extent of neurological involvement will determine whether or not the scoliosis is clinically important. Vertebral deformities can be coupled with tethering of the spinal cord. In mild cases where tethering does not involve motor columns, the child may only present with pain and/or paresthesiae of the distal extremity. Conversely, if a significant portion of the cord is tethered or the tethering affects motor columns, the child may have weakness, paralysis and organ dysfunction. Uncomplicated congenital deformities in the upper thoracic and cervical areas may interfere with the attainment of early motor milestones. The child may present with a torticollis unresponsive to appropriate treatment. Hemivertebrae and fusions in the lower thoracic and lumbar areas may present as an incidental finding on radiography, single curve scoliosis, or as pain exacerbated with activity. Deformities in the very distal lumbar spine may only become symptomatic when the child becomes involved in more demanding activities, such as organized sports (Fig. 3.34).

Treatment Notes

The spinal curves in congenital scoliosis are rigid, so orthotic treatment is of limited value. In most cases conservative management is best. Spinal fusion at the level of the deformity is required when there is instability. Congenital scoliosis can be associated with genitourinary, cardiac and other skeletal abnormalities, such as spina bifida occulta, spinal cord tethers and Klippel–Feil syndrome.

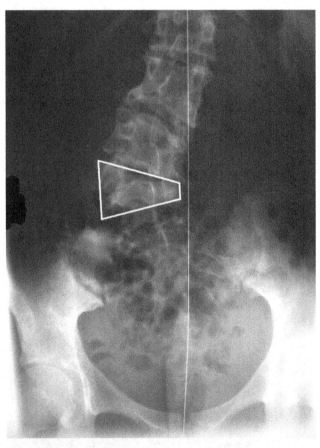

Fig. 3.32 • AP standing X-ray of a 15-year-old girl with low back pain. There is a hemivertebra at L5. This is an example of failure of development.

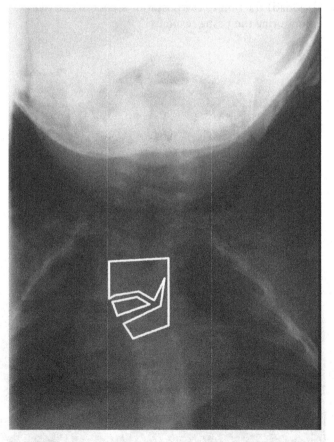

Fig. 3.33 • AP X-ray of a 2-year-old boy with a complex malformation that appears to consist of failure of segmentation of T4, T5, and T6 and failure of development of T5.

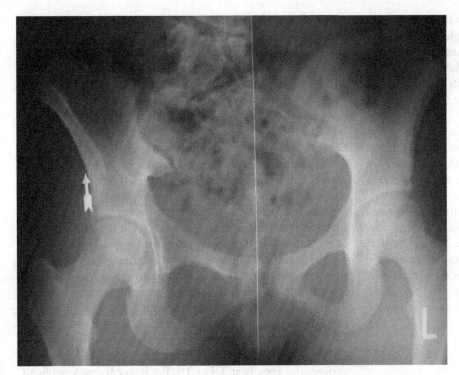

IDIOPATHIC SCOLIOSIS

Clinical Notes

Idiopathic scoliosis is rotational malalignment of one vertebra on another that produces a lateral curvature of the spine. Adolescent idiopathic scoliosis is the most common form, occurring near to or at puberty. There is a structural lateral curvature of the spine of at least 10° for which no cause can be established (Fig. 3.35). Children between 10 and 16 years are at greatest risk for the development and progression of a curve, and girls are almost four times more likely to be affected than boys. Idiopathic scoliosis affects 17 in every 1000 children in western countries.

The most common screening examination is the Adams forward bending test, used to detect asymmetry of the back or the presence of a rib hump. The ribs are rotated posteriorly and are prominent on the convex side of the curve. The positional strain is exacerbated in forward flexion, producing a rib hump. The amount of rib rotation does not always correlate with the scoliosis. Most clinicians can identify a scoliotic curve of 10° using the Adams forward bending test.

A scoliometer or inclinometer can be used to determine the angle of trunk rotation. X-ray evaluation is typically used to establish a precise measurement of the angle. Two views, posteroanterior (PA) and lateral, are obtained for

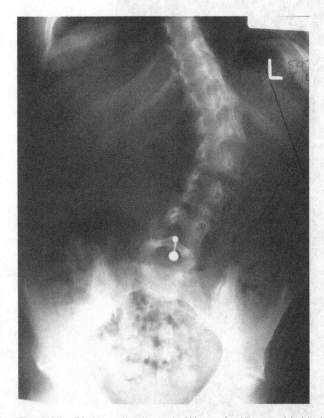

Fig. 3.35 • PA thoracolumbar spinal X-ray of a 17-year-old girl with a 50° left thoracolumbar scoliosis. The patient's belly button ring is clearly visible.

measurement. The degree of curvature is measured from the two end vertebrae (Fig. 3.36). The angle at the line of intersection is Cobb's angle. Curves measuring less than 25° are considered mild. Those measuring between 25° and 40° are considered moderate. Curves greater than 40° are considered severe. The curve is named for the side of the convexity.

Structural curves result from an alteration in the architecture of the vertebrae which distorts the normal spatial relationships of the area. For example, the presence of a hemivertebra will result in side-bending of the vertebra above and below the affected side. Distortion of the shape of the vertebral body from abnormal compressive forces may also produce side-bending of the adjacent vertebrae. Conversely, a functional curve is caused by mechanical and postural forces and will decrease or resolve in certain positions. Functional curves are mechanical adaptations. Passively moving the involved vertebrae in a different plane causes a change in the curve. During the scoliosis screening

examination, the child is asked to bend forward and the back is examined for any evidence of spinal malalignment or rib hump. The area involved is then motion tested by applying a side-bending force and observing the response of the curve. A functional curve will decrease or resolve. Virtually every child with idiopathic scoliosis has some functional component to the curve. This is extremely important, because if left untreated, functional curves will ultimately develop into a structural deformity as the spine grows.

Idiopathic scoliosis is not uncommon. Consequently, it is easy to assume the diagnosis without extensive workup. Knowing the most common presentations of idiopathic scoliosis can help the physician to recognize an adolescent scoliosis that may be due to a more serious pathology. Left-sided thoracic curves and right-sided lumbar curves deserve further investigation, as do thoracic curves that extend into the cervical spine. Scoliosis with pain or significant stiffness is also unusual and may signify something more ominous. Tingling in the extremities or neurological symptoms may represent spinal cord involvement. Scoliosis in the thoracic area is over 90% convexity to the right, with an average of six vertebrae involved. When the upper thorax is concerned, the apex is at T8 or T9. For lower thoracic scoliosis, the apex will be at T11 or T12. Seventy percent of scoliosis in the lumbar spine is convexity to the left. Five vertebrae are generally involved, with the apex at L1 or L2. The upper end of the curve is usually T11 or T12, and the lower end is L3 or L4. Thoracolumbar curves average six to eight vertebrae and are usually convex to the right. The apex is at T11 or T12. Double major curves involve oppositional curves in the thoracic and lumbar areas. Ninety percent of the thoracic curves are convex to the right, with left convexity in the lumbar area. Generally, double major curves involve five thoracic and five lumbar vertebrae, with the respective apices at T7 and L2. Curves that fall outside these parameters merit further investigation.

The progression of scoliosis is due to structural changes that result from the altered biomechanical forces on the vertebrae. Regardless of the etiology, idiopathic scoliosis will eventually cause vertebral asymmetry due to Wolff's law. Growth of the epiphyseal plates on the concave side will be inhibited by the constant increased loading, whereas the epiphyses on the convex side experience relatively accelerated growth. This produces a structural deformity of the vertebral body and articular surfaces. Many children compensate for the curve by exaggerating the lumbar lordosis. This creates increased pressure on the posterior aspect of the vertebral body and reduced pressure anteriorly, with resulting growth differential. These structural and biomechanical forces cause wedging of the intervertebral disc as well as the vertebral body. Researchers have found reduced glycosaminoglycan and increased collagen in the discs of patients with scoliosis. This is probably due to the abnormal stress placed on the disc (Zaleske 1980).

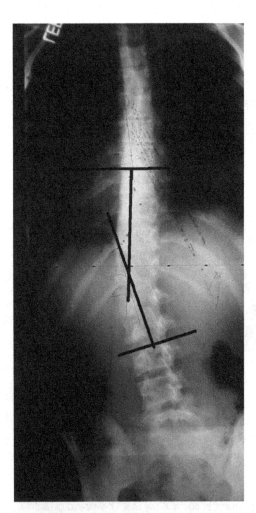

Fig. 3.36 • Full PA thoracic and lumbar spine X-ray with Cobb angle measurements outlined in black.

The child's age at time of diagnosis and the severity of the curve affect the overall progression of the scoliosis. The probability of progression is related directly to the severity of the curve and indirectly to the patient's age at the time of diagnosis. This is probably because progression is most rapid during times of growth. Premenarchal girls with curves over 20° are at the greatest risk for progression. Almost 70% of these children will have worsening of their curves. Double curves appear to progress faster than single curves. The likelihood of progression increases with decreasing age of onset, presumably because the curve has to weather more growth periods. Curves over 20° may be treated conservatively with observation and yearly X-ray. Curves over 40° may require bracing and follow-up X-rays every 6–12 months, depending on the child's age. Once the child passes puberty, progression slows significantly, although curves frequently progress throughout life as a result of the aforementioned biomechanical factors.

The bone age of the child can be used to estimate the risk for progression. Bone age can be measured by X-ray using the Riser scale. A PA view of the pelvis is taken. The iliac crest is then divided into four segments. Ossification of the iliac crest progresses from the anterior iliac spine towards the sacrum. The degree of ossification is measured against the four segments. No ossification is graded 0 and complete fusion of the apophysis is graded 5. This tool allows the radiologist to estimate how much bone growth remains (Fig. 3.37).

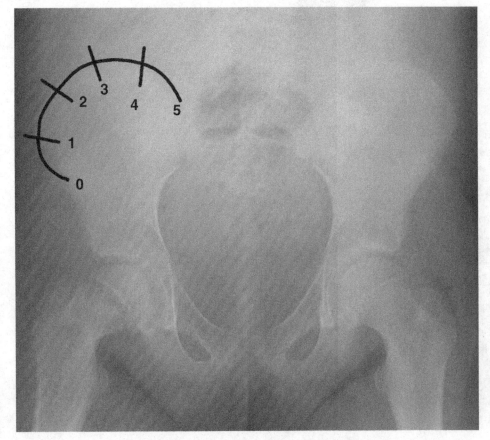

Fig. 3.37 • AP X-ray of female pelvis with Riser scale superimposed in black. Each number equates with a grade. Grade 0 = no ossification, grade 1 = 25% ossification, grade 2 = 26–50% ossification, grade 3 = 51–75% ossification, grade 4 = 76–100% ossification, grade 5 = fusion of the apophysis.

Adams Forward Bending Test

Athlete

The sensitivity and specificity of the Adams forward bending test is greater than 70% for curves less than 10° and more than 90% for curves greater than 20°.

1. The child stands with his feet hip-width apart. The physician stands behind the child. The child is asked to slowly bend forward, allowing his hands to dangle in front of his body (Fig. 3.38).

2. The physician observes the motion of the spine for symmetry during forward bending. If there is rotation of the spine or asymmetry in the appearance of the ribs, the child is instructed to halt his flexion.

3. The physician then introduces side-bending into the curve through the shoulders to test the flexibility of the asymmetry and determine the functional component of the curve.

4. The curve is named for the side of the convexity, which is also the side contralateral to the rib prominence or hump.

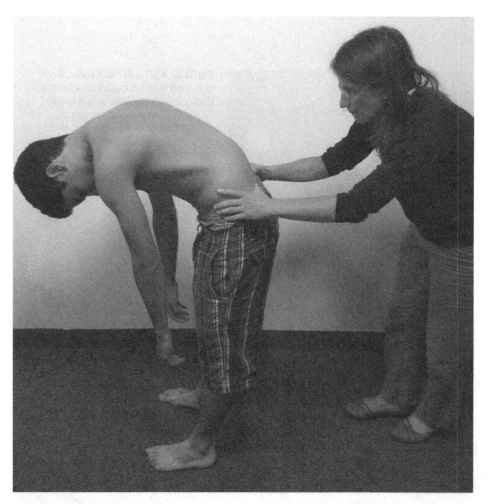

Fig. 3.38 • The Adams forward bending test.

Treatment Notes

Conventional and osteopathic treatment of scoliosis should focus initially on addressing any postural decompensation that has occurred, because of the potential for cardiopulmonary complications. If the curve is greater than 30°, orthotic bracing should be considered. At 40° bracing is highly recommended. Bracing will not correct the curve, but is meant to prevent further progression. Surgery needs to be considered when the curve passes 45°. The procedure consists of internal fixation of the involved vertebrae to prevent further progression. Segmental fixation has been shown to have similar efficacy to regional fixation in many patients. Fusion does not appear to increase the rate of success. Long-term complications of surgery appear to be few and far between. Untreated idiopathic scoliosis increases an individual's mortality by 10%, owing primarily to the cardiopulmonary complications. One-third of patients with scoliosis go on to have constant moderate-to-severe back pain. Approximately 14% have cardiopulmonary symptoms that affect their lifestyle.

Osteopathic manipulative treatment should address all compensatory biomechanical changes resulting from the curve. The functional component should be carefully evaluated, because it is biomechanical and will respond to manipulative treatment, exercise and reconditioning. Frequently, the lumbar component of the double major curve has a strong functional element. In almost every curve there is a functional aspect. In addition to spinal mechanics, rib function on the concave side needs to be addressed. Normal respiratory movement of the ribs is usually restricted on the concave side compared to the convex. It has been shown in experimental animals that the spine will grow away from the side of greater rib motion. Pelvic asymmetries, sacral base unleveling and leg length discrepancies need to be resolved to balance antigravity muscle tone in the pelvis and low back. Dysfunction in the neck and cranium may contribute to the curve through proprioceptive input affecting balance and posture. Lumbar muscle tone is affected by cervical spine mechanics. In the older child, postural rebalancing exercises such as yoga, t'ai chi and even some martial arts can be useful in reconditioning postural muscles. It is paramount that the child and the curve be followed through growth, even if the curve resolves with osteopathic treatment. The growth spurts of puberty will often exacerbate a radiographically resolved curve.

Junctional Areas of the Spine

The junctional areas of the thoracolumbar and lumbosacral areas play an important role in the respiratory–circulatory model of structure and function. Movement of fluids from the lower extremities, pelvis and abdomen is dependent on proper function of the thoracoabdominal cylinder. The effects of the diaphragm and its associated respiratory muscles on the low-pressure circulatory system are impeded by dysfunction in the torso. Because of this, in the respiratory–circulatory model treatment of the junctional areas to facilitate proper arterial, venous and lymphatic movement is essential for health.

Spasm of the quadratus lumborum muscle produces an ipsilateral side-bending of the lumbar spine, an ipsilateral side-bending of the thoracolumbar junction (with a compensatory contralateral rotation), and a contralateral side-bending of the lumbosacral junction (with compensatory ipsilateral rotation). The two following techniques address these components and their compensatory patterns. In the example, the right quadratus lumborum muscle is hypertonic, the lumbar spine is side-bent right, the thoracolumbar junction is side-bent right and rotated left, and the lumbosacral junction is side-bent left and rotated right.

MUSCLE ENERGY ISOMETRIC

Lumbosacral Junction

Supine Athlete

1. The patient lies in a lateral recumbent position on the side contralateral to the lumbosacral side-bending, in this example the right side (Fig. 3.39). The white line indicates the position of the lumbosacral junction, side-bent left (inferior on the left side).

2. The physician rests her forearm on the patient's hip, posterior and inferior to the ischial tuberosity. With her hand, she monitors the lumbosacral junction.

3. The other hand contacts the patient's shoulder and rotates the patient's thoracic and lumbar spines towards the ceiling until the lumbosacral junction is engaged.

4. The physician rotates the patient's sacrum and pelvis towards the floor and in a superior direction

(white arrow) to engage the lumbosacral junction. The torsional forces generated from the pelvic rotation meet the torsional forces descending from the thorax and lumbar spine.

5. The physician instructs the patient to push her hip against the physician's forearm (black arrow). The physician opposes this motion with an equal and opposite force. The physician should feel the lumbosacral muscles engage. This isometric contraction is maintained for 4–5 seconds.

6. The physician instructs the patient to relax as she simultaneously relaxes her counterforce. There is a 4–5-second pause.

7. The physician moves the lumbosacral junction to the new barrier by rotating the sacrum and pelvis towards the floor.

8. The sequence is repeated twice more.

Fig. 3.39

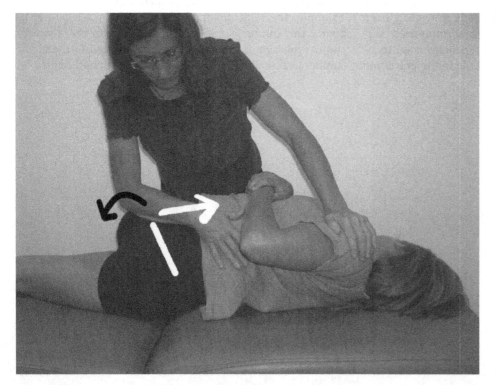

MUSCLE ENERGY ISOMETRIC

Thoracolumbar Junction and Quadratus Lumborum Muscle

Supine Athlete

1. The patient lies in a lateral recumbent position on the side contralateral to the thoracolumbar side-bending, in this example the left side (Fig. 3.40). The white curved line indicates the convexity of the lumbar spine, side-bent right (convex on the left side).

2. The physician rests her forearm on the patient's hip, superior to the femoral head, along the blade of the ilia. With her hand, she monitors the quadratus lumborum muscle or the thoracolumbar junction.

3. The other hand contacts the patient's shoulder and rotates the patient's thoracic spine towards the ceiling until the thoracolumbar junction is engaged.

4. The physician rotates the patient's lumbar spine and pelvis towards the floor in an inferior direction

(black arrow) to engage the thoracolumbar junction. The torsional forces generated from the lumbar and pelvic rotation meet the torsional forces descending from the thorax.

5. The physician instructs the patient to push her hip against the physician's forearm (white arrow). The physician opposes this motion with an equal and opposite force. The physician should feel the lumbosacral muscles engage. This isometric contraction is maintained for 4–5 seconds.

6. The physician instructs the patient to relax as she simultaneously relaxes her counterforce. There is a 4–5-second pause.

7. The physician moves the thoracolumbar junction to the new barrier by rotating the lumbar spine and pelvis towards the floor.

8. The sequence is repeated twice more.

Fig. 3.40

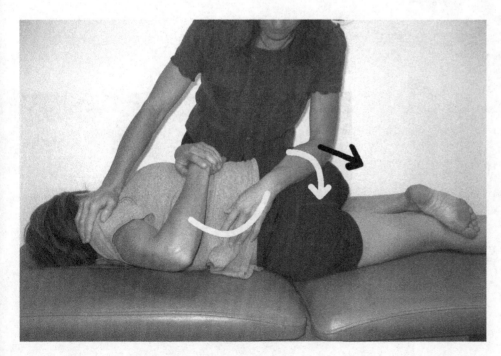

BALANCED LIGAMENTOUS TECHNIQUE

Lumbar or Thoracic Spine

Seated Toddler (Figs 3.41 and 3.42)

This approach can be used to treat the lumbar or thoracic spine.

1. The child is seated. The physician sits on the affected side. The physician uses one hand to stabilize the torso anteriorly. The other hand contacts the spinous processes of three adjacent vertebrae. The middle finger should contact the segment of primary dysfunction (Fig. 3.41).

2. The physician uses the spinous processes and the anterior hand to influence the position of the vertebrae. Introducing an anterior vector to the inferior surface of the spinous processes produces extension. Rotation is accomplished by introducing the appropriate lateral force (white arrows). Flexion can be achieved by lifting cephalad on the inferior aspect of the spinous process (black arrow) and using the appropriate level of contact on the torso as a fulcrum.

3. The physician uses her hand contacts to introduce the appropriate force vectors into the three vertebrae until balanced ligamentous tension is achieved. Force vectors may be introduced simultaneously into all three vertebrae, or sequentially in a stacking method.

4. The involuntary motions associated with respiration are incorporated into the positioning of the vertebrae.

5. Once balanced tension is achieved, the positions are maintained until there is a change in tissue texture, a correction of the dysfunction or an improvement in function.

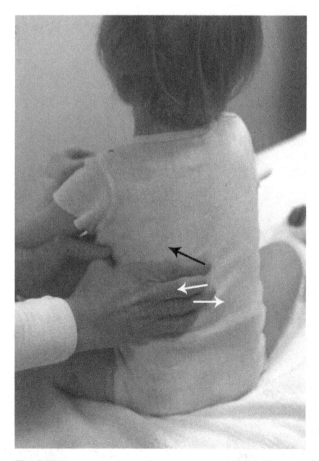

Fig. 3.41

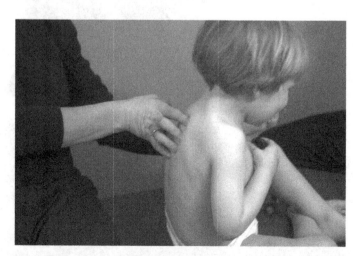

Fig. 3.42

BALANCED LIGAMENTOUS TECHNIQUE

Lumbar and Thoracic Spine

Supine Infant

1. The infant is supine. The physician sits beside the infant. The physician places one hand under the lumbar spine, contacting the spinous processes of three adjacent vertebrae with her index, middle and ring fingers (Fig. 3.43). The other hand monitors the anterior tissues and keeps the infant from rolling (Fig. 3.44).

2. With her hands on the spinous processes the physician assesses involuntary vertebral motion during breathing (and crying perhaps).

3. The physician uses the spinous processes to assess motion restriction (Fig. 3.43). Introducing an anterior vector to the inferior surface of the spinous processes produces translation and extension. Rotation is accomplished by introducing the appropriate lateral force (small white arrows). Flexion can be achieved by lifting cephalad on the inferior aspect of the spinous process (black arrow).

4. The physician uses her hand contacts to introduce the appropriate force vectors into the three vertebrae to evaluate tissue response and the presence of restrictive barriers. After assessing one group of vertebrae the physician 'walks' her fingers to the next group (Fig. 3.45). This can be done along the lumbar and thoracic spine to determine the area of greatest restriction and the group to be treated.

5. Once the physician has ascertained the area to be treated, she contacts the vertebrae with the greatest restriction with the pad of her middle finger and the two adjacent vertebrae with her index and ring fingers.

6. Using her finger pads to introduce the appropriate force vectors the physician establishes balanced ligamentous tension between the three vertebrae. Force vectors may be introduced simultaneously into all three vertebrae, or sequentially in a stacking method.

7. The involuntary motions associated with respiration are incorporated into the positioning of the vertebrae.

8. Once balanced tension is achieved, the positions are maintained until there is a change in tissue texture, a correction of the dysfunction or an improvement in function.

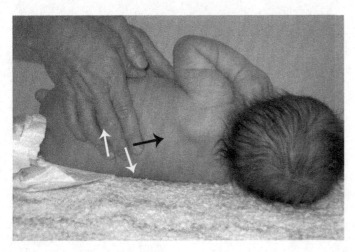

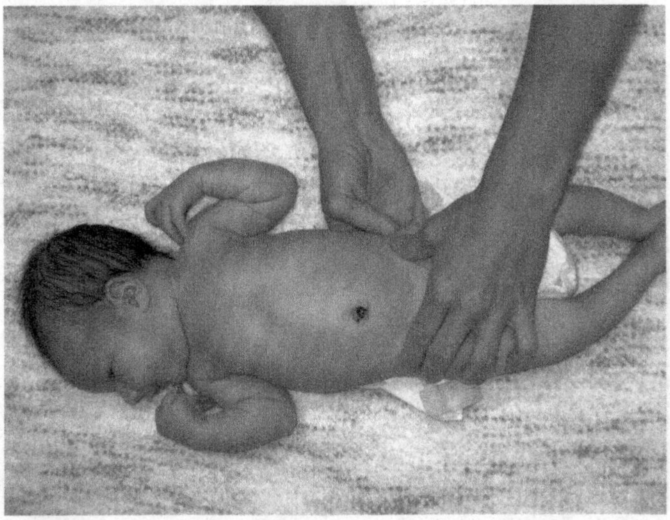

Fig. 3.43

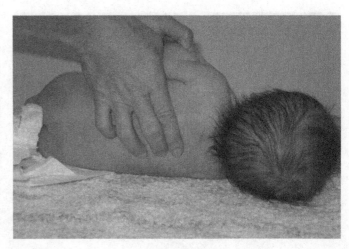

Fig. 3.44

Fig. 3.45

COSTOVERTEBRAL JUNCTION

Treatment Notes

Somatic dysfunction in the thoracic spine typically creates compensatory changes in the biomechanics of the associated ribs, and vice versa. Often resolution of the primary dysfunction is followed by changes in the compensatory adaptations. Sometimes the vertebral and rib dysfunctions must be treated separately. Periodically, the primary dysfunction is at the costovertebral junction. This is often the case in ligamentous strains and chronic dysfunctions. Treatment can be carried out with the patient seated or supine.

BALANCED LIGAMENTOUS TECHNIQUE

Costovertebral Junction

Seated Toddler

1. The child is seated with the physician sitting on the affected side. One hand is placed on the back, contacting the rib to be treated and its two articulating vertebrae (Fig. 3.46 labeled V, R,V). The other hand is placed on the torso in the same plane.

2. The rib is gently tractioned anterolaterally (Fig. 3.47, black arrow) while the physician uses the spinous processes to rotate the two vertebrae towards or away from the rib (white arrows) to establish balance within the vertebrae–rib unit (the vertebrae–rib unit includes the rib and both involved vertebra.). The entire unit needs to be brought to a point of balance.

3. Once found, the position of balance is held through a series of respiratory cycles until a change in tension is felt.

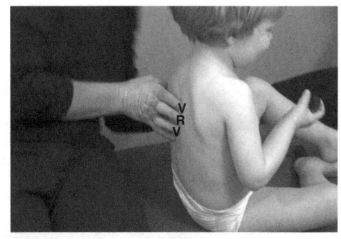

Fig. 3.46

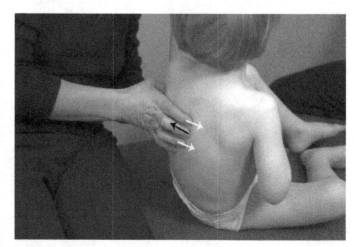

Fig. 3.47

BALANCED LIGAMENTOUS TECHNIQUE

Costovertebral Junction

Supine Athlete/Child

In this technique, the physician uses one hand to contact the vertebrae and the other to contact the rib (Fig. 3.48).

1. The child is supine and the physician sits ipsilateral to the rib to be treated. The physician contacts the rib with the middle or index finger of one hand. With the other hand, the physician contacts the spinous processes of the two adjacent vertebrae (Fig. 3.49).

2. In all typical ribs the costotransverse articulation is between the rib and the transverse process of the associated vertebra (Fig. 3.50). The costovertebral articulation occurs between the head of the rib and the demifacets located on the vertebral bodies of the vertebra above and the associated vertebra (Fig. 3.51).

3. The physician introduces a lateral traction through the rib in a curvilinear direction (black arrow). The fingers of her other hand are used to rotate the vertebrae either away from or towards the rib. (The direction will depend on the dysfunction in the rib and each vertebra.)

4. The physician uses her contacts to introduce the appropriate vectors into the tissues of the costovertebral unit until there is balanced tension. This position is maintained through several respiratory cycles until there is a change in tissue texture, an improvement in motion or a correction of the strain.

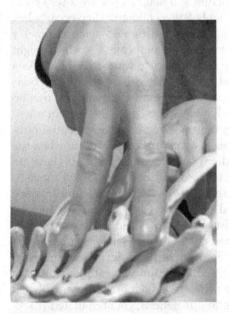

Fig. 3.48

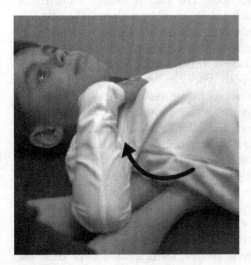

Fig. 3.49

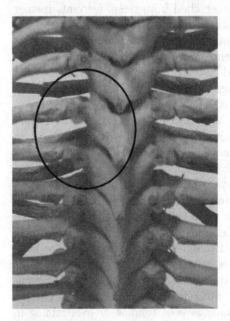

Fig. 3.50

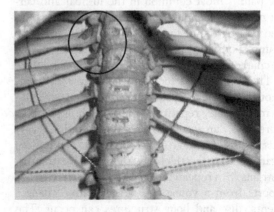

Fig. 3.51

BACK PAIN

Clinical Notes

Back pain in children was once thought to be rare and only due to malignant organic pathology. Today most healthcare professionals recognize that back pain is not an uncommon complaint in children. The differential diagnosis of back pain in children must include mechanical, inflammatory/infectious, neoplastic, developmental and psychosomatic etiologies. Spondylolysis and spondylolisthesis are the most common developmental pathologies seen with back pain. They may be congenital or traumatic, and are most common in the lower lumbar spine, L5 and L4. Spondylolysis and spondylolisthesis need to be ruled out in athletes using repetitive extension and rotation motions. Congenital deformities such as hemivertebrae and spinal fusions are rare.

Pain that persists regardless of activity level or position, or pain that awakens the child from sleep, warrants further investigation to rule out an inflammatory condition, neoplasia or infection. Back pain associated with incontinence suggests spinal cord compromise and requires urgent intervention. Pain that is aggravated by certain movements or positions and relieved with rest suggests a mechanical etiology. However, ascertaining the actual etiology of the pain and finding a method to alleviate the patient's symptoms is often a challenge. Mechanical back pain may present with radiculopathy: pain, burning, weakness, reflex changes and/or numbness along the anatomic distribution of the nerve root. Progressive signs of nerve root involvement include depressed reflexes, muscular weakness and muscular atrophy. Back strain is a more common condition in children and relates to injury to the paraspinal muscles and ligaments. It is associated with spasm of the involved muscles. Neurological signs are lacking. The clinical presentation consists primarily of pain, stiffness and tightness in the affected area. Back strain may occur as a result of trauma, although it is often related to a chronic or repetitive stress such as poor training or overtraining in athletes, poor posture or awkward sleeping habits.

Discogenic pain is most common in the lumbar and cervical areas. It may be secondary to trauma or chronic strain and should be part of the differential diagnosis in any back or neck pain unresponsive to conservative management. The condition is characterized by changes in the architecture of the disc. There is often a localized inflammatory component. Although discogenic pain is typically considered a condition of middle age, repetitive injury, such as neck or lumbar compression, can accelerate disc degeneration.

Spondylosis is less common in the pediatric population, although it can be seen in athletes with repetitive trauma, such as equestrians with repeated falls, or athletes who engage in contact sports from a young age. Degenerative changes of the ligaments, disc and bony structures can occur. The pain is typically localized to a broad area around the spinal segments, although there can be radiation into an extremity if the dorsal ramus is involved. There is a reduced range of motion and muscular tightness on physical examination. The neurological evaluation is normal. Degenerative processes result in a decreased ability to effectively distribute pressures between disc, vertebral endplates and facet joints, and may predispose the adolescent to further problems in adulthood.

Facet syndrome usually occurs after an extension or backward bending injury. In the neck it is associated with headaches; in the spine with localized axial pain. The diagnosis may be confirmed by fluoroscopic injection of an anesthetic agent which provides temporary symptomatic relief.

In children, as in adults, the sacral area is a common pain generator. Sacral dysfunctions may occur between the sacrum and L5 or between the sacrum and ileum. Sacral torsions are strains between the sacrum and ileum. They are a very common strain pattern in ambulating children. They occur when one sacroiliac joint is loaded, the lumbar spine is quickly rotated and the sacrum cannot compensate, such as might happen when running and turning to hit a tennis ball. As a result, the sacrum and L5 are rotated in opposite directions and thus unable to move in synchrony. Under normal motion mechanics, when the lumbar spine flexes the sacrum counternutates, and during lumbar extension or in a neutral position the sacrum nutates. A sacral torsion may occur when the sacrum is in a nutated or counternutated position. These are called forward sacral torsions and backward sacral torsions, respectively. The former happens when the lumbar spine is upright or extended, the latter when the lumbar spine is flexed. The strain exists between L5 and the sacral base. If the sacrum was nutated at the time of injury, symptoms are typically worse when the patient has a flexed lumbar spine, as in bending forward. If the sacrum was counternutated at the time of injury the patient will be more symptomatic in a standing or prone position. In general, counternutated (backward) sacral torsions are more symptomatic than nutated (forward) sacral torsions. The pain is usually a deep ache across the lower back accompanied by stiffness. The pain may radiate into the buttock or posterior thigh. Forward sacral torsions are better with rest. Children with backward sacral torsions typically have a difficult time finding a comfortable sleeping position. Both types can be treated effectively with balanced ligamentous techniques as well as muscle energy.

Sacroiliac strains are another common source of back pain. The pain is unilateral and extends into the buttocks and posterior thigh. It may be accompanied by mild paraesthesiae without other neurological signs. Sacroiliac dysfunctions can occur concomitantly with lumbosacral strains. In chronic conditions, one may be compensatory for the other: the dysfunction may predominantly involve the sacrum, or an innominate dysfunction may be the primary dysfunction. The seated and standing flexion tests can differentiate between the two. The balanced ligamentous techniques described later treat the strain in the sacrum and innominate simultaneously.

POSITIONAL DIAGNOSIS

Sacrum

Athlete/Child (Table 3.1)

The following assessment tools can be used with variable accuracy in older children. They are most appropriate for adolescents and young adults, in whom the necessary anatomical landmarks are better developed. There are four pieces of information needed to determine the diagnosis in most sacral dysfunctions: the laterality of the seated flexion test, the sacral response to lumbar motion, the inferior or posterior inferior lateral angle (ILA) of the sacrum, and the deep sacral sulcus.

Seated Flexion Test

The seated flexion test identifies the side of the sacrum that is restricted. This test is most accurate in older adolescents and young adults, when the posterior superior iliac spine has developed more prominence.

1. The child is seated with his knees flexed. The physician kneels behind the patient with her eyes at the level of the pelvis and her thumbs contacting the posterior superior iliac spines (PSIS) (Fig. 3.52).

2. The child is asked to bend forward slowly. The physician observes the anterosuperior movement of the PSIS.

3. The side that moves initially or demonstrates the greater excursion is the side of sacroiliac restriction. This is the positive side. In the figure, the right side has greater superior excursion.

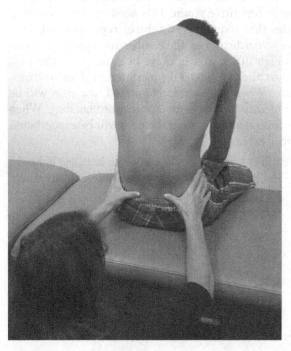

Fig. 3.52

Table 3.1 Comparison of osteopathic structural examination findings for diagnosis of sacral dysfunction				
Diagnosis	**Positive seated flexion test**	**Sacral sulcus**	**Inferior lateral angle**	**Resists**
Right unilateral nutation	Right	Deep right	Posterior inferior right	Counternutation on the right
Left unilateral nutation	Left	Deep left	Posterior inferior left	Counternutation on the left
Right unilateral counternutation	Right	Shallow right	Anterior superior right	Nutation on the left
Left unilateral counternutation	Left	Shallow left	Anterior superior left	Nutation on the right
Bilateral nutation	Bilateral	Deep bilaterally	Posterior inferior bilaterally	Counternutation
Bilateral counternutation	Bilateral	Shallow bilaterally	Anterior superior bilaterally	Nutation
Left on left torsion	Right	Deep right	Posterior inferior left	
Right on right torsion	Left	Deep left	Posterior inferior right	
Left on right torsion	Left	Deep right	Posterior inferior left	
Right on left torsion	Right	Deep left	Posterior inferior right	

Seated Sacral Nutation and Counternutation
(Figs 3.53 and 3.54)
During lumbar flexion the sacral base should counternutate, i.e. move posteriorly. During lumbar extension the sacral base should nutate, i.e. move anteriorly. The ability of the sacrum to nutate and counternutate in response to lumbar mechanics can be compromised in athletes as a result of trauma or repetitive strain. This needs to be considered in activities that require persistent or repetitive hyperextension or hyperflexion of the lumbar spine, such as gymnastics, weightlifting and hockey. In either case the pain is located at the lumbosacral junction and does not usually radiate. When the sacrum is nutated, the pain will be exacerbated with lumbar flexion or forward bending. When the sacrum is counternutated, the pain will be exacerbated with lumbar extension.

1. The child is seated with the physician kneeling behind him. The physician contacts the sacral sulci bilaterally.

2. The child is instructed to drop his head and slowly bend forward (see Fig. 3.53). The physician observes the flexion of the lumbar spine and notes the timing and symmetry of sacral counternutation. The child then resumes the seated position.

3. The child is asked to look up at the ceiling and slowly extend or arch his back (Fig. 3.54). The physician observes the extension of the lumbar spine and notes the timing and symmetry of sacral nutation. The child resumes the seated position.

4. The sulci should move symmetrically through nutation and counternutation. Resistance of motion indicates a restrictive barrier. The restrictive barrier may be unilateral or bilateral. The dysfunction is named for its position of ease. Unilateral dysfunctions are often called 'sacral shears.' Restrictive barriers that prevent the sacrum from nutating are the most symptomatic.

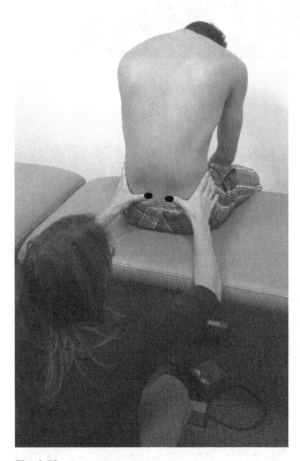

Fig. 3.53

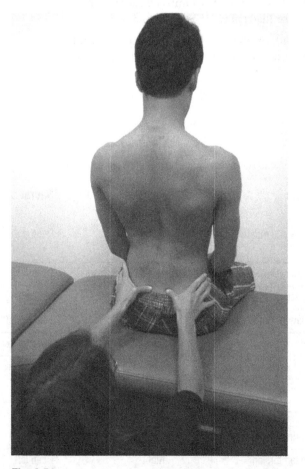

Fig. 3.54

Sacral Sulcus

In infants and toddlers, the posterior superior iliac spines are rather flat and the sacral sulci are not well developed.

Once the sacrum begins to assume its convex shape and the PSIS develop, the sacral sulci become more apparent.

1. The child is supine. The physician stands beside the child and contacts the posterior superior iliac spines with her thumbs.

2. The physician then slides her thumbs medially off the PSIS and drops them into the sacral sulci (Fig. 3.55).

3. The depths of the sulci are compared. If the deeper sulcus is ipsilateral to the positive seated flexion test, then the sacrum has nutated on the opposite oblique axis. If the deep sacral sulcus is contralateral to the positive seated flexion test, then the sacrum has counternutated on the ipsilateral oblique axis. This is confirmed by the presence of a prominent inferior lateral angle contralateral to the deep sacral sulcus.

Inferior Lateral Angles

The inferior lateral angles are absent in infants and toddlers and not well developed in younger children. In adolescents and young adults they are fairly easy to locate.

1. The child is supine. The physician stands beside the child and palpates the sacral sulci with her thumbs.

2. The physician then walks her thumbs inferiorly along the sacrum to the inferior lateral angles (Fig. 3.56).

3. The ILAs are compared to assess which one is more superior or more posterior.

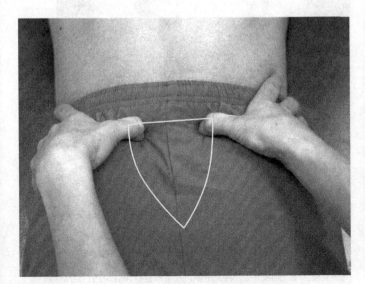

Fig. 3.55

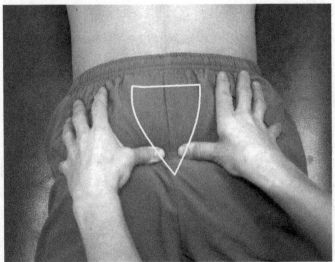

Fig. 3.56

ASSESSING MOTION CHARACTERISTICS

Lumbosacral Spine

Supine Athlete/Child/Toddler

1. The child is supine. The physician sits beside the child near the pelvis. The physician places her hands beneath the child so that her most superior hand contacts the transverse processes of L5, while the inferior hand contacts the spines of the sacrum (Fig. 3.57). In children the unossified sacrum is in five segments. The physician should have contacts on at least the superior three segments (Fig. 3.58, black circles).

2. Through her contacts the physician can assess the inherent and passive motion characteristics of L5 and the sacral segments simultaneously. Interosseous strains may present as areas of compression or torsion between the sacral segments.

3. The physician observes the involuntary motion characteristics of the area. This is done with the child breathing quietly. As with the rest of the spine, the strain pattern is often exaggerated during the inhalation phase.

4. After assessing involuntary motion characteristics, the physician assesses passive motion of the sacrum on the two oblique axes and the horizontal axis. The response of L5 is noted. The physician then tests L5 mechanics through all planes of motion while observing the response of the sacrum.

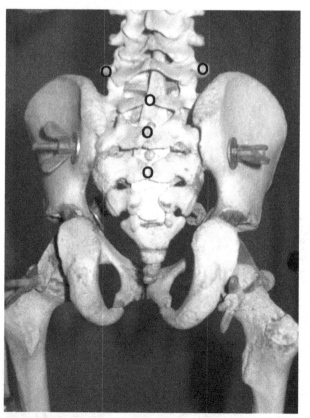

Fig. 3.58 • Posterior view of a pediatric skeleton, approximately 5 years old, showing the sacrum, lower lumbar spine and pelvis. This child had spina bifida and the midline fusion of the neural arch is defective. Nevertheless, the segmentation between the sacral parts is visible.

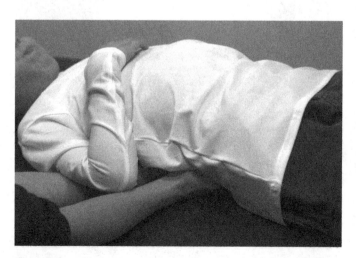

Fig. 3.57

BALANCED LIGAMENTOUS TECHNIQUE

Lumbosacral Junction

Supine Athlete/Child/Toddler

1. The physician uses the contacts described previously for this technique, the only difference being that she sits ipsilateral to the shallow sacral sulcus, or on the counternutated side of the sacrum (Fig. 3.59A, B).

2. Through her contacts, the physician can simultaneously introduce motion into L5 and the sacral segments. The physician observes the involuntary motion characteristics of the area as she does this.

3. The physician uses her contacts on the transverse processes of L5 to rotate, side-bend, translate, flex and extend the vertebra. Her fingers contacting the sacral segments can introduce rotation, compression or decompression. The physician uses these vectors to establish balanced ligamentous tension between L5 and the sacral segments.

4. Once balanced ligamentous tension is established, the position is maintained until there is a change in tissue texture, improvement in involuntary motion or a correction of the strain.

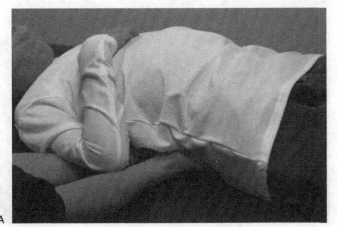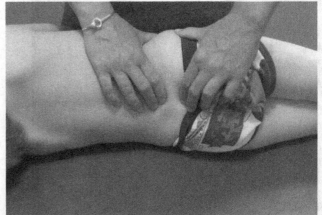

A   B

Fig. 3.59

ASSESSING MOTION CHARACTERISTICS

Sacrum and Ileum/Sacroiliac Joint

Supine Athlete/Child/Toddler

1. The child is supine. The physician sits beside the child near the pelvis. The physician places the hand closest to the child's head beneath the pelvis such that she contacts the lateral aspect of the upper three sacral segments as close to the joint as possible (Figs 3.60, 3.61, black circles). Depending on the age of the patient, the sacroiliac joint may be a composite joint of the ileum with two or three sacral segments, rather than a single sacral bone. The other hand is placed over the anterior superior iliac spine (Fig. 3.62).

2. Through her contacts, the physician can assess the inherent and passive motion characteristics of the ileum and the sacral segments simultaneously. Interosseous strains may present as areas of compression or torsion between the sacral segments.

3. The physician observes the involuntary motion characteristics of the sacroiliac area. This is done with the child breathing quietly. The strain pattern is often exaggerated during the inhalation phase.

4. After assessing involuntary motion characteristics, the physician assesses passive motion between the sacral segments and the ileum. This is accomplished by compressing the ileum towards the sacrum while stabilizing the sacrum (Fig. 3.62, straight black arrow). This disengages the SI joint. Rotation (curved black arrow) and flare (curved white arrow) are then introduced into the innominate. The sacrum can be rotated, nutated and counternutated with the posterior contacting hand. The response of the sacroiliac ligaments and fasciae is observed.

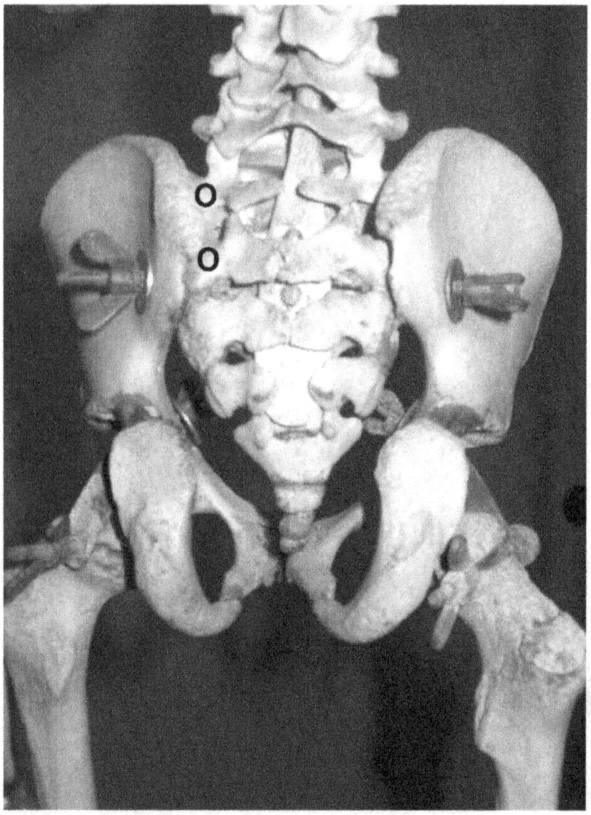

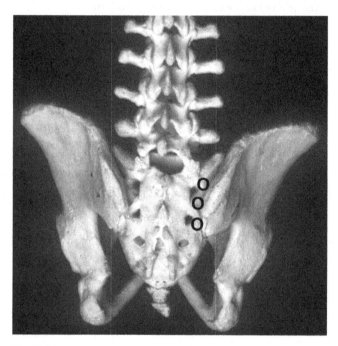

Fig. 3.61

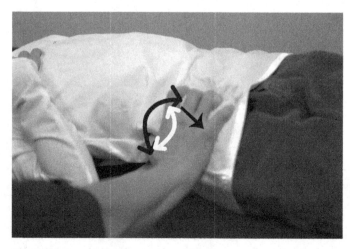

Fig. 3.62

Fig. 3.60

BALANCED LIGAMENTOUS TECHNIQUE

Sacrum and Ileum/Sacroiliac Joint

Supine Athlete/Child/Toddler

This approach is similar to the sacroiliac balanced ligamentous technique described for newborns. However, in an ambulating child the orientation of the sacroiliac joint is more oblique and the force used to disengage the articulation typically needs to be stronger and more medially directed.

1. The physician uses the contacts described above for this technique. The physician treats the restricted side first, but regardless of the side of the dysfunction both sacroiliac joints are treated (Fig. 3.62). The physician contacts the lateral aspect of the upper three sacral segments as close to the SI joint as possible. She curls her finger pads up into the joint space, creating a fulcrum between the sacrum and the innominate.

2. The physician uses her contact on the ileum to compress (straight black arrow), decompress, rotate (curved black arrow) and flare (curved white arrow) the ileum on the sacrum.

3. The fingers contacting the sacral segments can introduce rotation, compression, or decompression to the segments.

4. The physician modifies her forces and vectors to bring balanced tension between the posterior (Fig. 3.63) and anterior (Fig. 3.64) sacroiliac ligament complexes, the ileum and the associated sacral segments. Both the anterior and posterior sacroiliac ligaments need to be brought into balanced tension.

5. Once balanced tension is reached, the positions are maintained until there is a change in tissue texture, an improvement in involuntary motion or a correction of the strain.

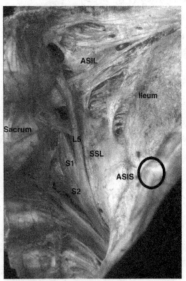

A

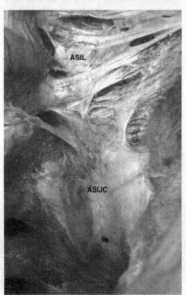

B

Fig. 3.64 • A,B Anterior view of the right sacroiliac joint. The deep pelvic muscles, fasciae and organs have been removed. The L5, S1 and S2 nerves are labeled. The anterior superior iliac spine (ASIS) is indicated by the black circle. The anterior sacroiliac ligament (ASIL) extends from the crest of the iliac blade over the anterior surface of the sacroiliac joint. In many specimens it is continuous with the iliolumbar ligament. The sacrospinous ligament (SSL) is visible in dissection 1. (B) A slightly different perspective and close-up view of the same anterior sacroiliac ligament with the nerves removed and the sacrospinous ligament cut. The anterior surface of the articular capsule (ASIJC) is labeled.

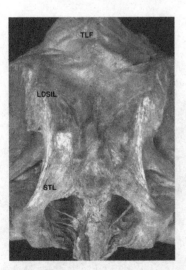

Fig. 3.63 • Posterior view of the sacrum and pelvis with the lumbar spine flexed. All the muscles have been removed. The gluteal–multifidus raphe has been cut. The inferior aspect of the thoracolumbar fascia (TLF) is intact. The sacrotuberous ligament (STL) and long dorsal sacroiliac ligament (LDSIL) are labeled.

Sacral Diagnosis

Seated Toddler

1. The toddler is seated facing away from the physician. The physician contacts the sacrum and pelvis bilaterally such that her thumbs rest on the sacrum just medial to the SI joint and her fingers contact the iliac crest and anterior superior iliac spines (Fig. 3.65).

2. The physician stabilizes the innominate and sacrum on one side as she carries the opposite innominate into anterior and posterior rotation, nutating and counternutating the sacrum. This is repeated on the opposite side.

3. The tissue response and quality of motion at the sacroiliac joints are compared to determine the side and characteristics of the restriction.

4. Once the side of the restriction is identified the physician contacts the sacral segments with the pads of her fingers along the SI joint (Fig. 3.66, left side is assessed). The other hand contacts the ipsilateral innominate.

5. The physician motion tests the innominate, noting the location of the tissue restriction.

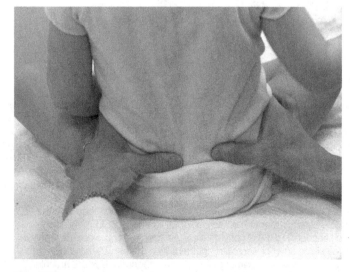

Fig. 3.65

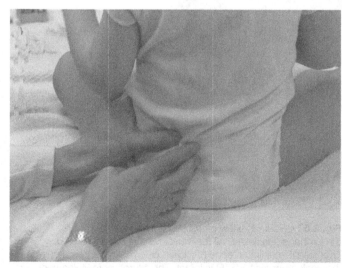

Fig. 3.66

PRIMARY SACRAL OR SACROILIAC DYSFUNCTION

Intraosseous Sacral Dysfunction

Seated Toddler

In younger children and toddlers, the sacral segments are not fused. Intraosseous strains may develop between the composite parts of the sacrum and alter the shape of the sacrum or its articular surface at the iliosacral joint. This influences sacroiliac mechanics and may result in compensatory changes in the biomechanical position of the innominate.

1. The child is seated facing the parent or some toys. The physician sits behind the child. One hand contacts the first three or four sacral segments on the sacral spines.

2. The other hand contacts the innominate on the involved side with the thumb on the posterior superior iliac spine, the hand along the ileum and the finger on the anterior superior iliac spine (Fig. 3.67).

3. The innominate is taken into anterior and posterior rotation with inflare and outflare as the intraosseous sacrum is monitored.

4. Balanced tension is achieved between the segments of the sacrum and the ileum. If the dysfunction involves the ligamentous connection with the ischial tuberosity, the technique may need to be performed with the child supine and the hip extended to reduce tension from the hamstring group.

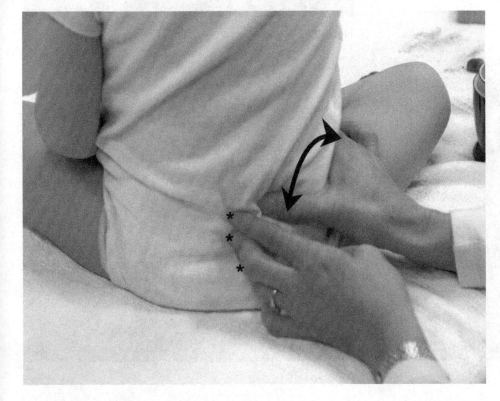

Fig. 3.67

ARTICULATORY TECHNIQUE

Sacroiliac Joint

Prone Athlete

This is a general mobilization technique which can be used to address restriction at the sacroiliac joint.

1. The patient is placed in a lateral Sim's position with the affected sacroiliac joint superior and the thorax and lumbar spine rotated away from the affected joint (turned towards the table). The physician stands on the opposite side of the patient (Fig. 3.68). In the example, the left sacroiliac is being treated. The physician places the hypothenar eminence of her contralateral hand (in this case right) on the sacrum just medial to the sacroiliac joint (Fig. 3.69).

2. The patient flexes her ipsilateral hip and knee (left). The physician grasps the leg under the knee.

3. The physician further flexes the patient's hip until motion is felt at the sacroiliac joint. The physician then abducts thigh until a slight resistance is felt at the sacroiliac joint (Fig. 3.70).

4. The patient is instructed to take in a deep breath and hold it. The physician circumducts the thigh by abducting and extending the hip (white arrow). At the end of extension the patient is told to exhale.

5. The procedure is repeated with the patient lying on the other side to treat the opposite sacroiliac articulation.

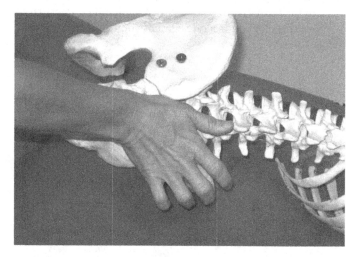

Fig. 3.69

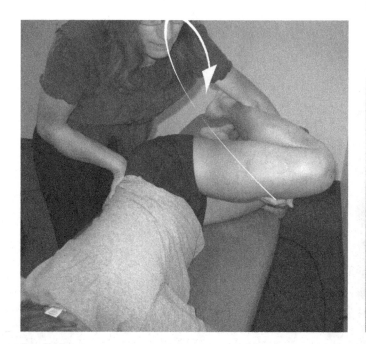

Fig. 3.68

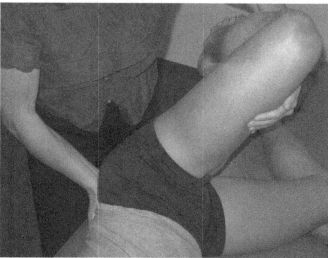

Fig. 3.70

ARTICULATORY TECHNIQUE/ SACRAL WOBBLE

Sacroiliac Joint

Prone Child

This is a general mobilization technique for the sacroiliac joint which uses an opposing force on the sacrum and ileum to spring the joint. Both sides are treated.

1. The patient is supine (Fig. 3.71A, B). The physician stands facing the child, ipsilateral to the SI joint to be treated. The hypothenar eminence of one hand is placed over the PSIS and along the iliac portion of the SI joint, as close to the joint as possible but not on the sacrum. The hypothenar eminence of the other hand contacts the superior aspect of the sacrum near the sacral sulcus.

2. The hand contacting the sacrum applies an anteriorly directed force to engage the restrictive barrier at the sacrum. The force may be directly anterior or anterocephalad. The hand contacting the innominate applies an anteriorly directed force to engage the restrictive barrier at the ileum.

3. The physician applies a short, quick impulse simultaneously to the restrictive barriers at the sacrum and ileum. The impulse is used to spring or 'wobble' the sacrum and ileum on their articular axes.

4. The other SI joint is treated in the same manner.

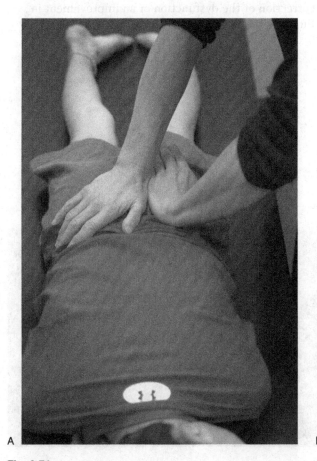
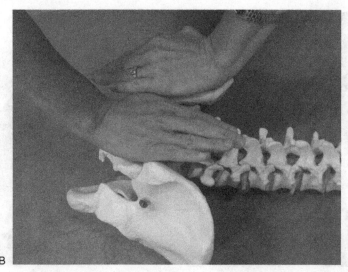

Fig. 3.71

BALANCED LIGAMENTOUS TECHNIQUE

Lumbar and Thoracic Spines

Supine Child/Athlete

This approach can be used in any age group. It is an alternative to the technique described for the infant. Both hands are used simultaneously, with the two index fingers contacting two adjacent vertebrae, or contacting several vertebrae with multiple fingers (Fig. 3.72).

1. The child is supine. The physician sits beside the child. The physician places both hands under the spine, contacting the spinous processes of two or more adjacent vertebrae with the appropriate fingers. In this example, four adjacent vertebrae are being contacted (Fig. 3.73).

2. With her hands on the spinous processes, the physician assesses involuntary vertebral motion during breathing.

3. The physician uses the spinous processes to assess motion restriction. Introducing an anterior vector to the inferior surface of the spinous process produces translation and extension. Rotation is accomplished by introducing the appropriate lateral force (Fig. 3.72, black arrows). Flexion can be achieved by lifting cephalad on the inferior aspect of the spinous process (larger black arrow).

4. The physician uses her hand contacts to introduce the appropriate force vectors into the vertebrae to evaluate tissue response and the presence of restrictive barriers. After assessing one group of vertebrae, the physician 'walks' her fingers to the next group. This can be done along the lumbar and thoracic spines to determine the area of greatest restriction and the group to be treated.

5. Once the physician has ascertained the area to be treated she contacts the spinous process of the vertebra with the greatest restriction using the pad of her middle finger and the spinous processes of the two adjacent vertebrae using her index and middle fingers.

6. Using her finger pads to introduce the appropriate force vectors the physician establishes balanced ligamentous tension between the three vertebrae. Force vectors may be introduced into all three vertebrae, either simultaneously or sequentially in a stacking method.

7. The involuntary motions associated with respiration are incorporated into the positioning of the vertebrae.

8. Once balanced tension is established, the positions are maintained until there is a change in tissue texture, a correction of the dysfunction or an improvement in function.

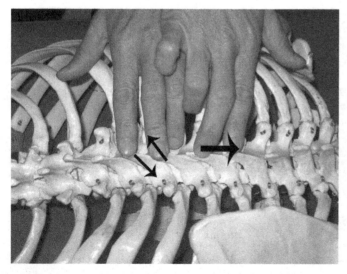

Fig. 3.72

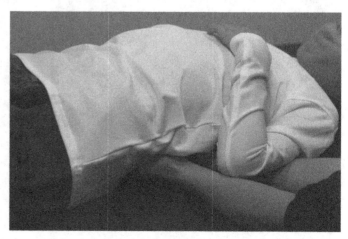

Fig. 3.73

SCHEUERMANN'S DISEASE

Clinical Notes

Scheuermann's disease is a less common developmental condition affecting the thoracic spine. The child develops an exaggerated kyphosis that is rigid. It most often occurs in the thoracic spine, but can also occur at the thoracolumbar junction and in the lumbar spine. There may be an associated mild scoliosis. Children complain of back pain, stiffness and fatigue. Symptoms are usually exacerbated with activity or as the day progresses. Pain is more severe when the thoracolumbar or lumbar areas are affected. The severity of the curve will also influence the pain level. Typical pain patterns may be subscapular, infrascapular or above the iliac crest, depending on the location of the apex of the kyphosis. In general, Scheuermann's kyphosis does not predispose the child to progressive disability or respiratory compromise as an adult (Murray 1993).

Diagnosis is by X-ray or MRI. There is anterior wedging of the vertebrae and endplate deformity. Scheuermann's disease is more common in boys and usually presents between the ages of 10 and 12 years. Although the pathophysiology is unclear, the mechanical loading of the anterior aspect of the vertebrae is thought to contribute to the wedging as well as the increased tension in the anterior longitudinal ligament. Bracing has been shown to reduce the progression of the wedging in some patients. The hallmark of Scheuermann's kyphosis is the rigidity of the curve. Compensatory changes include increased tension in the hamstrings and thoracolumbar fascia, and shortening of the pectoral muscles and fasciae.

Treatment Notes

In most cases, stretching, strengthening and appropriate exercise are the treatments of choice for children with Scheuermann's disease. Isotonic and isometric muscle energy techniques may be useful to strengthen and stretch the costal muscles. The child should also be encouraged to undertake exercises that encourage spinal extension, such as swimming, volleyball and equestrian sports. Unrelenting pain, a rapid increase in the curve or the extent of the wedging warrants consideration for bracing or surgery. Signs of respiratory or spinal cord compromise deserve surgical consultation.

Braces are initially used all day long. They influence the mechanical loading of the vertebral endplate. Manipulation, physical therapy and bracing can be used together in most patients. Casts are used in some children and worn for two consecutive 45-day periods. With both casts and braces there is often an initial improvement, but the duration of the effects depends on the severity of the curve, the age of the child and patient compliance. Surgical correction and stabilization are necessary in approximately 5% of patients.

MUSCLE ENERGY ISOMETRIC

First Rib

Supine Athlete

The first rib moves with a type of pump-handle motion: the anterior aspect moves caudad as the posterior aspect moves cephalad. The first rib is most often elevated posteriorly by the scalene muscles. This is a common finding in neck injuries, chronic postural adaptations and shoulder conditions. This technique uses isometric contraction of the scalene muscles.

1. The patient is supine. The physician stands beside the patient on the affected side. The patient places her hand palm up over her forehead (Fig. 3.74).

2. The physician grasps the posterior surface of the rib to be treated and depresses it to the restrictive barrier (Fig. 3.75). The physician places her other hand over the patient's supinated palm. The patient's head should be turned 5–10° away from the dysfunctional rib to engage the anterior and middle scalene muscles.

3. The patient is instructed to lift her head against the physician's hand (white arrow, Fig. 3.74). This engages the scalene muscles (Fig. 3.76). The physician resists this movement with an equal and opposite force for 4–5 seconds to create an isometric contraction of the scalene muscles.

4. The patient is asked to relax. The physician waits 3–4 seconds and then depresses the posterior aspect of the first rib to the new restrictive barrier.

5. The sequence is performed a total of three times. Respiratory motion is reassessed.

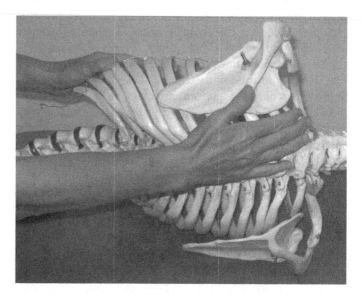

Fig. 3.75

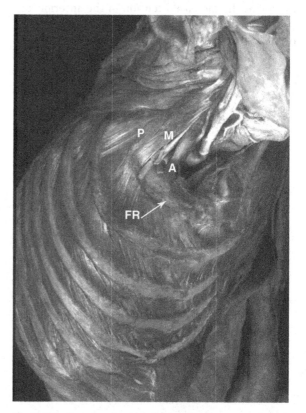

Fig. 3.76 • Anterior superior view of the upper thorax with the shoulder complex removed. The anterior (A), middle (M), and posterior (P) scalene muscles are labeled, as is the first rib (FR).

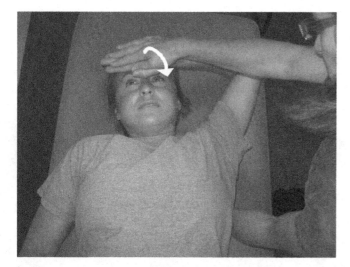

Fig. 3.74

MUSCLE ENERGY – ISOTONIC

Mid Ribs – Depressed

Supine Athlete

Ribs 2–5 have pump-handle motions similar to the first rib. This technique uses the pectoral muscles to lift the anterior aspect of the rib.

1. The patient is supine. The physician stands beside the patient on the affected side. The patient places the dorsum of her hand alongside her cheek (Fig. 3.77).

2. The physician grasps the posterior surface of the rib to be treated and depresses it to the restrictive barrier (Fig. 3.78). The physician places her other hand over the patient's elbow.

3. The patient is instructed to bring her elbow towards her opposite hip (white arrow). The physician resists this movement with an equal and opposite force to engage the pectoral group.

4. As the tension in the pectoralis muscles increases the physician increases her caudal force on the posterior aspect of the rib, pulling it inferiorly and creating an isotonic contraction of the pectoral muscles. This is maintained for 4–5 seconds.

5. The patient is told to relax, and as she does, the physician depresses the posterior aspect of the rib to the new restrictive barrier.

6. This sequence is performed a total of three times. The respiratory motion is rechecked.

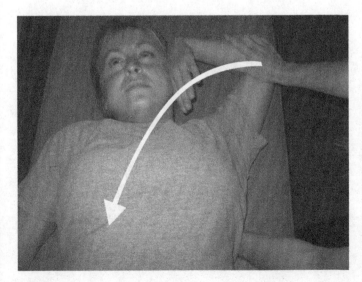

Fig. 3.77

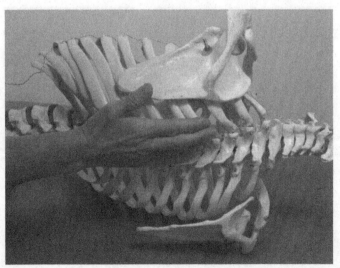

Fig. 3.78

MUSCLE ENERGY – ISOTONIC

Lower Ribs – Depressed

Supine Athlete

Ribs 6–9 move with a bucket-handle type of motion. The lateral edge rises as the anterior and posterior aspects are depressed. This technique uses the serratus anterior muscle to raise the lateral border.

1. The patient is supine. The physician stands beside the patient on the affected side. The patient flexes, abducts and externally rotates her arm so it lies beside her head (Fig. 3.79).

2. The physician grasps the posterior surface of the rib to be treated and depresses it to the restrictive barrier (Fig. 3.80). The physician places her other hand over the patient's elbow.

3. The patient is instructed to bring her elbow towards the ceiling (Fig. 3.79, white arrow). The physician resists this movement at the elbow while simultaneously pulling the restricted rib inferiorly to create an isotonic contraction of the serratus anterior muscle. This is maintained for 4–5 seconds.

4. The patient is told to relax. As she does so, the physician depresses the posterior aspect of the rib to the new restrictive barrier.

5. This sequence is performed a total of three times. The respiratory motion is rechecked.

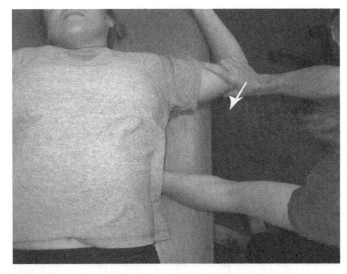

Fig. 3.79

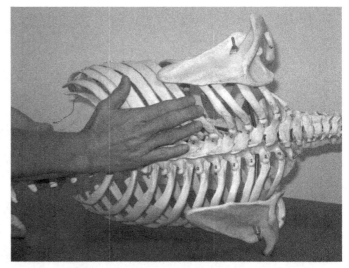

Fig. 3.80

MUSCLE ENERGY – ISOMETRIC

Lowest Ribs – Depressed

Supine Athlete

Ribs 10–12 are described as moving with a caliper motion. This technique employs the latissimus dorsi muscle.

1. The patient is supine. The physician stands beside the patient on the affected side. The patient flexes, abducts and externally rotates her arm so it lies beside her (Fig. 3.81).

2. The physician grasps the posterior surface of the rib to be treated (ribs 10–12) and depresses it to the restrictive barrier (Fig. 3.82). The physician places her other hand over the patient's elbow.

3. The patient is instructed to bring her elbow towards her ipsilateral hip (Fig. 3.81, white arrow). The physician resists the movement of the elbow with an equal and opposite force to create an isometric contraction of the latissimus dorsi muscle. This is maintained for 4–5 seconds.

4. The patient is told to relax. The physician waits 3–5 seconds for the post-isometric relaxation phase. Then physician depresses the posterior aspect of the rib to the new restrictive barrier.

5. This sequence is performed a total of three times. The respiratory motion is rechecked.

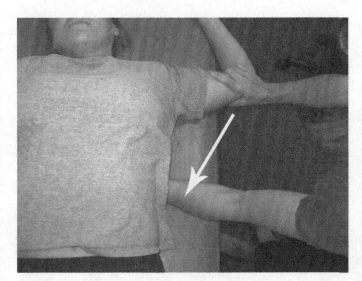

Fig. 3.81

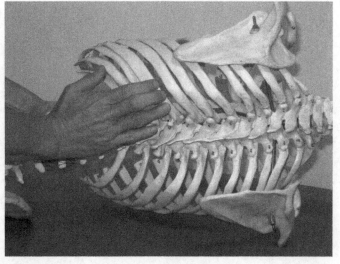

Fig. 3.82

MUSCLE ENERGY

Lower Ribs – Elevated

Supine Athlete

Respiratory mechanics are engaged in this technique.

1. The patient is supine. The physician stands at the head of the table towards the affected side. The physician places her thenar eminence along the shaft of the involved rib in the mid-axillary line (Fig. 3.83).

2. The physician places her other hand under the patient's head and neck (Fig. 3.84). The physician flexes and side-bends the patient towards the affected rib until the restrictive barrier at the rib is felt.

3. The patient is instructed to inhale and exhale deeply.

4. With each inhalation the physician resists the elevation of the rib. As the patient exhales, the physician follows the depression of the rib and exaggerates the flexion and side-bending.

5. This sequence is repeated a total of three times. The physician maintains the position of the rib as she lowers the patient's head.

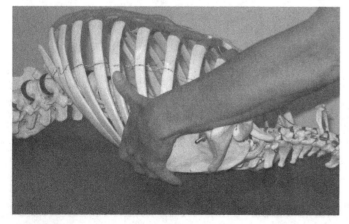

Fig. 3.83

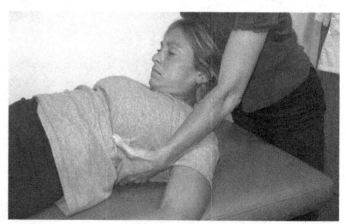

Fig. 3.84

References

Agostoni E, Zocchi L. Starling forces and lymphatic drainage in pleural liquid and protein exchanges. Respir Physiol 1991; 86: 271–281.

Ahlqvist J. On the structural and physiological basis of the influence of exercise, movement and immobilization in inflammatory joint diseases. Ann Chir Gynaecol 1985; 198: 10–18.

Aukland K, Reed RK. Interstitial–lymphatic mechanisms in the control of extracellular fluid volume. Physiol Rev 1993; 73: 1–78.

Miller AJ, DeBoer A, Palmer A. The role of the lymphatic system in coronary atherosclerosis. Med Hypotheses 1992; 37: 31–36.

Murray PM, Weinstein SL, Spratt KF. The natural history and long-term follow-up of Scheuermann kyphosis. J Bone Joint Surg Am 1993; 75: 236–248.

Negrini D, Ballard ST, Benoit JN. Contribution of lymphatic myogenic activity and respiratory movements to pleural lymph flow. J Appl Physiol 1994; 76: 2267–2274.

Still A. Philosophy of osteopathy. Kirksville, MO: AT Still, 1899.

Thach BT, Thach BT, Abroms IF. Intercostal muscle reflexes and sleep breathing patterns in the human infant. J Appl Physiol 1980; 48: 139–146.

Thach BT, Stark AR. Spontaneous neck flexion and airway obstruction during apneic spells in preterm infants. J Pediatr 1979; 94: 275–281.

Wilson SL, Thach BT, Brouillette RT, Abu-Osba YK. Upper airway patency in the human infant: influence of airway pressure and posture. J Appl Physiol 1980; 48: 500–504.

Zaleske DJ, Ehrlich MG, Hall JE. Association of glycosaminoglycan depletion and degradative enzyme activity in scoliosis. Clin Orthop Relat Res 1980: 148: 177–181.

Chapter Four

The shoulder complex

CHAPTER CONTENTS

OVERVIEW

The shoulder complex comprises three articular units: the glenohumeral joint, the sternoclavicular joint, and the scapulothoracic joint. Typically when one thinks about 'shoulder problems' it is the rotator cuff that is actually being considered. However, the functional mechanics of the shoulder complex are dependent upon proper performance of all three articular units. Normal movements of the upper extremity require some involvement of these three articular components, and disorders of the arm are almost never isolated to one joint mechanism. Slight variations in mechanics at the shoulder complex can influence movements at the elbow and wrist. Furthermore, dysfunction affecting any one area of the arm will affect other areas, just as dysfunction in any one articular component of the shoulder complex will ultimately influence the other components.

The tissues of the shoulder are particularly susceptible to repetitive microtrauma or overuse syndrome. Microtrauma occurs primarily through three mechanisms: acceleration or explosive force, sustained force, and static or isometric force (Hill 1983). Acceleration force best describes the mechanism of injury in racquet and pitching sports, where the athlete uses optimum load to generate force. In racquet sports the resistance of the racquet connecting with the ball increases the load on the muscle. Dynamic force describes the action of the shoulder muscles during sports such as swimming, where the arm is moving against the sustained resistance of the water. Static force describes the action of the shoulder muscles when they are held in a constant position with isometric contraction, such as may occur in a dancer or gymnast.

Sports involving repetitive, accelerated overhead movements are particularly hazardous for the shoulder. In throwing and tennis the arm is often abducted to 90°, externally rotated and extended. The anterior articular capsule and anterior glenohumeral ligament are maximally tightened and stressed. The tendon of the subscapularis, which typically provides some anterior stability, is positioned superiorly, compromising its role. Virtually all the muscles of the rotator cuff, as well as the deltoid, are active in this position. For the arm to accelerate forwards to throw the ball or move the racquet, the anterior muscles – the pectoralis and subscapularis – must rapidly internally rotate the humerus. This is the shortest but most stressful movement for the glenohumeral joint and rotator cuff muscles because it places excessive loads in multiple planes across the ligaments, tendons and articular capsule. Once the ball has been released the arm continues through flexion, internal rotation and adduction carried by its own momentum. Although the surrounding muscles make an effort to decelerate the arm, the fascial and ligamentous tissues will absorb much of this load. At the very end of follow-through the posterior articular capsule will be maximally loaded. Because of the loads placed on these tissues, all are vulnerable to overtraining or inappropriate use. The resulting repetitive microtrauma will lead to inflammation, ischemia, and in some cases degeneration.

Swimmers are another group of athletes at risk for shoulder injuries, owing primarily to the extraordinarily high rate of repetitive motion required in the sport. Although specific variations exist for particular strokes, there are two distinct phases of shoulder motion involved with the typical stroke: the pull phase and the recovery phase. During the pull phase the athlete generates the force to pull herself through the water. This can be likened to the acceleration phase of throwing or racquet sports, although the load on the tissues is greater in swimming because of the resistance of the water. As in throwing and racquet sports, the pectoralis major provides much of the force during the pull phase, while the subscapularis acts to stabilize the humeral head.

In most shoulder injuries the relationship between the deltoid and rotator cuff is uncoupled. Typically these two components counterbalance each other to stabilize the humeral head and disperse forces into the soft tissue and away from the articular and epiphyseal surfaces. When inadequately opposed, the actions of the large muscles of the shoulder complex – the latissimus dorsi, pectoralis and deltoid – will displace the humeral head, leading to impingement and subluxation.

IMPINGEMENT SYNDROME

Clinical Notes

Impingement syndrome in young athletes usually involves compression of the supraspinatus and biceps tendons. The subacromial bursa may be involved in older patients (Micheli 1983, Cofield 1985). Impingement syndrome represents a continuum of worsening microtrauma, inflammation, and eventually compression of the soft tissue structures. Because of the inherent laxity of the pediatric shoulder joint, the rotator cuff muscles in young athletes are under greater demand to provide dynamic stability than those of an adult (Tibone 1983, Curtis 1994). Elite athletes place an even higher demand on these muscles when they use overhead motions. The subacromial bursa, long bicipital and supraspinatus tendons are compressed into a relatively small space surrounded by the walls of the acromion, coracoid and coracoacromial ligament. Additionally, the compact arrangement of structures provides little room for adaptation to biomechanical changes at the scapulothoracic or sternoclavicular areas. For example, overdevelopment of the pectoral and deltoid muscles in weightlifters may contribute to impingement syndrome. Athletes using repetitive overhead motions, such as swimmers, pitchers and tennis players, are more susceptible to injuries in these tissues (Rupp et al. 1995, Yanai et al. 2000). Overuse results in repetitive contact between the tendons and the coracoacromial arch. Initially, the repetitive contact results in inflammation and swelling. Over time, repetitive microtrauma causes scarring that alters the structure of the articular capsule, tendons and ligaments. Pain inhibits muscle firing, which leads to muscle weakness. Deltoid tone is no longer counterbalanced by rotator cuff activity. As a result, during adduction or early flexion the humerus is elevated, compressing the soft tissue structures between the humeral head and the coracoacromial arch. This exacerbates the inflammatory changes that can weaken the structure of the tendon, predisposing the patient to partial and complete tears.

Assessment

The young athlete with impingement syndrome usually complains of anterior shoulder pain with overhead motion, flexion or internal rotation. As inflammatory changes progress the pain may persist at rest. There may be reduced strength in abduction and internal rotation against resistance. Symptoms of supraspinatus impingement are exacerbated by abduction of the humerus. Supination and flexion will elicit pain if the bicipital tendon is inflamed. Full flexion of the arm (Neer test) or 90° flexion with internal rotation (Hawkins test) reproduces the symptoms of impingement.

When signs of impingement are present the shoulder also needs to be assessed for laxity and instability. The drop arm test is performed to evaluate the rotator cuff for full-thickness tears. The athlete is instructed to abduct the arm and then slowly lower it. Inability to do so is indicative of a full-thickness tear. Exacerbation or worsening of pain with lowering suggest a partial-thickness tear. The drawer test can be used to evaluate laxity of the rotator cuff. The anterior apprehension test can be used to rule out anterior subluxation. Plain X-rays are normal in patients with impingement syndrome. MRI may demonstrate increased signal in patients with full-thickness tears. However, full-thickness tears are rare in children. The differential diagnosis of impingement syndrome includes stress fracture, adhesive capsulitis, and thoracic outlet syndrome.

There are several classification systems used to describe impingement syndrome (Jobe and Jobe 1983, Curtis 1994). Most refer to the presence or absence of instability and the degree of chronic inflammatory change.

Treatment Notes

In the treatment of impingement syndrome, normalization of shoulder complex biomechanics is imperative to reduce or eliminate the irritation to the supraspinatus and biceps tendons. The mechanics of the clavicle and scapula should be addressed first, because these structures form the foundation for the mechanics at the glenohumeral joint.

The physician can use the child's symptoms to guide decision-making about continued participation in the sport. In general, if pain only occurs with activity, treatment may proceed in conjunction with training as long as improper training practices are addressed. If the pain persists after the activity is completed, then training should stop until there is no pain at rest.

If there is pain at rest, passive indirect and passive balancing techniques can be used. These may also be used prudently in cases of suspected tears or instability. In patients without a suspected tear or instability, active direct techniques such as isotonic concentric muscle energy can be employed as part of a strengthening and retraining program, along with band therapy and free weights. Isometric muscle energy techniques can be used to regain range of motion and flexibility. The patient should be pain free at rest before passive direct techniques are employed. Passive direct techniques should be avoided in patients with joint instability. Re-evaluation and adjustment of the athlete's training program is essential to prevent further injury.

In general, children respond well to conservative treatment of shoulder problems. Patients with either persistent pain at rest following 4 weeks of appropriate treatment, or pain with activity following 12 weeks of treatment, may require further diagnostic work-up or intra-articular injection.

Apprehension Test (Fig. 4.1)

This test should be performed gently and with caution.

1. The patient is seated. The physician places one hand on the posterior aspect of the glenohumeral joint. The other hand grasps the patient's forearm.

2. The affected arm is abducted to 90° and the elbow is flexed. The physician applies a steady anterior force to the back of the glenohumeral joint while gently attempting to externally rotating the humerus.

3. Pain or voluntary resistance to motion is indicative of anterior instability.

Fig. 4.1

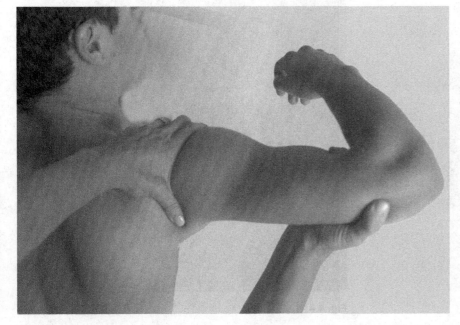

BALANCED LIGAMENTOUS TECHNIQUE

Clavicle

Seated Athlete

The function of the clavicle is assessed by palpating its motion during active circumduction of the shoulder and passive respiration. The positions of the two clavicles are compared at the sternoclavicular joints. The inferior clavicle is treated first. The fulcrum for superoinferior movement of the clavicle is the costoclavicular ligament, located approximately 1 inch lateral to the sternoclavicular joint. This technique addresses clavicle restrictions prior to the BLT scapulothoracic technique described next.

1. The patient is seated facing the physician (Fig. 4.2). The physician contacts the distal end of the clavicle with one hand, resting his fingers across the acromioclavicular joint and the pad of his thumb under the distal clavicle. The other thumb is placed inferior to the proximal end of the clavicle, just lateral to the sternoclavicular joint (Fig. 4.3).

2. The patient is asked to lean forward onto the operator's thumbs (Fig. 4.4, white arrow). The operator applies a gentle pressure to the shoulder at the acromion (black arrow) until a subtle engagement is felt at the acromioclavicular (AC) joint.

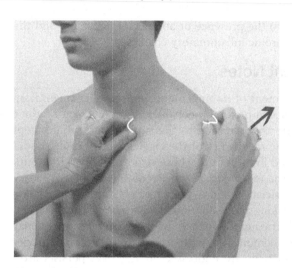

Fig. 4.3

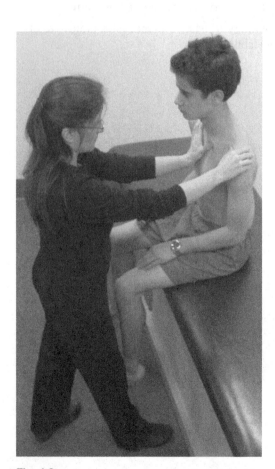

Fig. 4.2

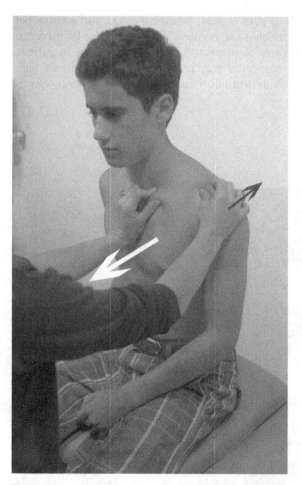

Fig. 4.4

3. The patient is then asked to carry the contralateral shoulder posteriorly (Fig. 4.3, black arrow), thereby engaging the sternal end of the clavicle. These two movements are performed to establish a balance in the ligaments at the articulations (Fig. 4.5).

4. The claviopectoral fascia (CPF, Fig. 4.6) and the subclavius (SubC) muscle can be described as fulcrums for motion of the clavicle. According to Sutherland's model, the claviopectoral fascia has a similar role to the interosseous membranes of the forearm and lower leg, in that it guides and limits movement of the bone.

5. The clavicle is taken through various planes of motion until balanced tension is achieved between the clavicle and the surrounding tissues. This position is held as the patient breathes, until a slight 'shift' in the clavicle is felt and it moves freely with the respiratory movement of the first rib.

6. The patient is then asked to slowly carry his contralateral shoulder forward, and then to sit upright. The operator maintains contact with the clavicle until the patient is upright and all weight is removed from the thumbs.

7. The sequence is repeated on the other clavicle.

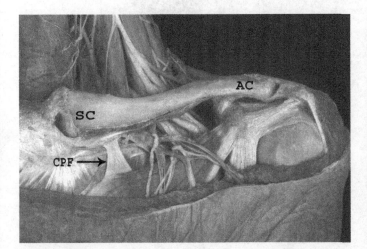

Fig. 4.5 • An anterior view of the left side of the thoracic outlet. The skin, superficial fasciae and sternocleidomastoid muscle have been removed. The claviopectoral fascia (CPF) extends from the inferior margin of the proximal clavicle to the superior margin of the pectoralis muscle.

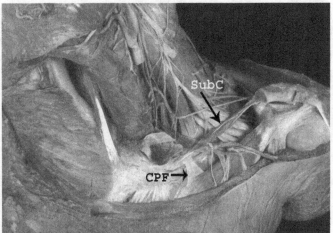

Fig. 4.6 • A slightly superior anterior view of the left thoracic outlet with the clavicle removed. The insertion of the claviopectoral fascia (CPF) into the subclavius muscle (SubC) is identified. The subclavius inserts along the inferior margin of the clavicle. In infants and young children it assists in respiration.

BALANCED LIGAMENTOUS TECHNIQUE

Scapulothoracic Joint

Seated Athlete

1. The patient is seated on the edge of the table. The table is positioned so that the patient's shoulder is at the same height as the physician's. The physician stands at the patient's side and slightly behind him. Treatment of the left shoulder will be described.

2. The physician uses her thumb as a fulcrum beneath the scapula. The physician places her left hand so that her fingers are on the anterior chest wall and the thumb is in the axilla on the side to be treated.

3. The palmar surface of the thumb is placed on the lateral surface of the second or third rib with the tip facing posteriorly (Fig. 4.7). The thumb should be anterior to the latissimus dorsi muscle (Fig. 4.8).

4. The physician gently slides her thumb posteriorly along the surface of the rib until it rests between the scapula and the rib. The thumb will act as a fulcrum for treatment of the scapulothoracic joint. The dorsal surface of the thumb contacts the subscapularis muscle, while the plantar surface contacts the serratus anterior (Fig. 4.9).

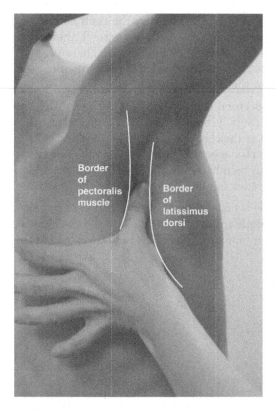

Border of pectoralis muscle

Border of latissimus dorsi

Fig. 4.8

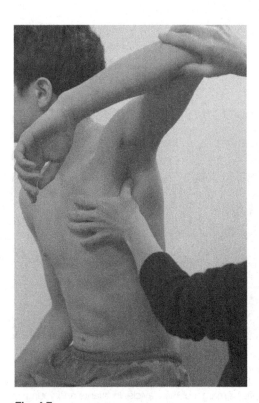

Fig. 4.7

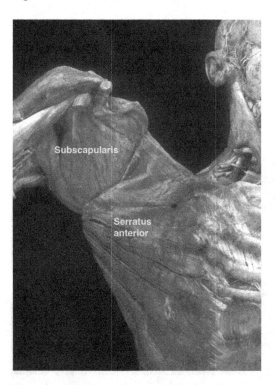

Subscapularis

Serratus anterior

Fig. 4.9 • Anterior view into the axilla. The clavicle, pectoralis muscles and posterior stabilizers of the scapula have been removed. The shoulder and arm have been pulled laterally away from the torso to reveal the insertion of the serratus anterior onto the medial border of the inferior surface of the scapula.

5. The physician places the other hand over the posterior aspect of the scapula. The base of the hand is on the apex of the scapula. The fingers grasp the spine of the scapula (Fig. 4.10).

6. The physician uses the posterior hand to protract, retract, adduct, abduct, elevate and depress the

scapula to achieve balanced tension in all the tissues attached to it.

7. The physician uses both hands to balance the entire shoulder girdle complex (anterior and posterior attachments) to the thorax (Fig. 4.11).

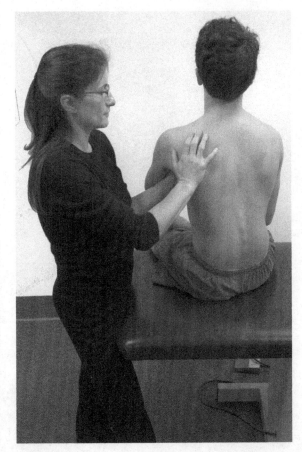

Fig. 4.10

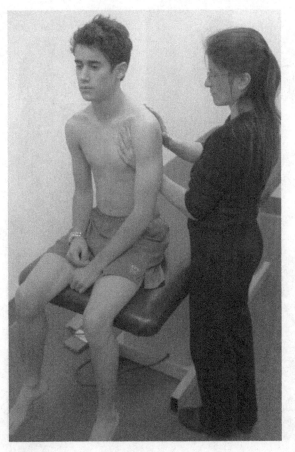

Fig. 4.11

BALANCED LIGAMENTOUS TECHNIQUE

Humerus/Rotator Cuff

Seated Athlete

This approach may be used in an acute or painful shoulder as a way to address the pain and splinting. In this approach the physician directs her attention to the muscles and fasciae of the rotator cuff complex. This technique can also be used in conjunction with the Spencer muscle energy techniques in the treatment of rotator cuff dysfunction.

1. The patient is seated on the edge of the table. The table is positioned so the patient's shoulder is at the same height as the physician's shoulder. The physician stands beside and slightly behind the patient on the side to be treated (Fig. 4.12).

2. The physician grasps the humeral shaft with both hands. The thumbs are placed together over the lateral surface. The fingers interlock on the medial surface of the humerus. Care is taken not to compress the neurovascular bundle.

3. The physician pushes with both hypothenar eminences against the humeral shaft. Her index finger and thumbs act as a fulcrum so that the humeral head is abducted as the humerus is adducted. The patient is instructed to place his ipsilateral hand on the opposite side of his chest. This internally rotates the adducted humeral head.

4. The patient is instructed to move his elbow forward (thereby internally rotating the humerus) and then backward (externally rotating the humerus). The physician determines which direction enhances balanced tension. The patient is instructed to maintain his arm in the position of maximum balanced tension.

5. The physician fine-tunes the tensions at the glenohumeral joint to achieve balanced tension. Once balanced tension is achieved, the physician maintains that position until a correction in the mechanical strain or improvement in tissue function is noted.

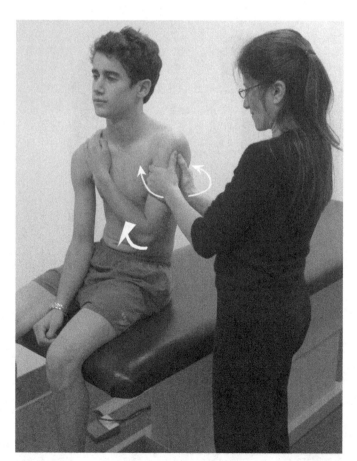

Fig. 4.12

ROTATOR CUFF DISORDERS

Clinical Notes

The glenohumeral joint probably has the greatest range of motion of any joint in the body. To some extent stability is sacrificed to achieve this multiplanar range of motion. The muscles of the rotator cuff act as dynamic stabilizers of the glenohumeral joint. The subscapularis, supraspinatus, infraspinatus and teres minor muscles act in concert to compress the humeral head into the glenoid fossa, counterbalancing the translational forces of larger muscles acting on the joint. For example, when the arm is lifted to throw a ball, the deltoid and the rotator cuff muscles act in concert to stabilize and move the arm. The deltoid attaches to the spine of the scapula, the acromioclavicular area and the clavicle. When the deltoid contracts, the counterforce of the rotator cuff muscles stabilizes the head of the humerus and prevents it from translating cephalad. The combined forces result in abduction of the humerus. The subscapularis is the anterior stabilizer and under the greatest strain when the arm is lifted over the head. The supraspinatus, infraspinatus and teres minor act as posterior and superior stabilizers. Together, the muscles of the rotator cuff also play a role in actions of the latissimus dorsi and pectoralis major muscles.

Whereas the muscles of the rotator cuff stabilize and execute actions at the glenohumeral joint, the scapulothoracic and sternoclavicular muscles are silent partners whose involvement is necessary for both stabilization and motion. If this is lacking, inappropriate forces are transferred to the muscles of the rotator cuff. Scapular motion in particular plays an important role in rotator cuff function. Restrictions in scapular flare or elevation will change the contractile force, tension, length and eccentric contractile loads placed on the muscles of the rotator cuff. In many cases it is the pain or injury to the muscles of the rotator cuff that brings the patient in for evaluation. However, a rotator cuff problem often represents an accumulation of dysfunction and strain in other components of the shoulder complex.

Problems of the rotator cuff can be described as a continuum of increasing levels of inflammation and trauma, progressing from chronic microtrauma to complete tears.

Rotator cuff disorders are classified into four categories representing increasing degrees of injury similar to those described for impingement syndrome. Stage 1 injury occurs when there is microtrauma with inflammation. Stage 2 describes tendonitis with fibrotic changes. Stage 3 refers to degeneration of the tendon called a partial-thickness tear. Stage 4 is a full-thickness tear in the tendon. Fortunately, in young athletes stage 4 is rare.

Treatment Notes

Stage 1 and 2 injuries respond to conservative management addressing biomechanical dysfunction, muscle spasm and improper training practices. Removal from play should be considered, depending on the persistence of symptoms. There is some evidence that ultrasound and massage aid in treatment (Hill 1983). Muscle retraining may be necessary. Stage 3 requires complete removal from play. Steroid injections may be warranted, and gentle resistance exercises are added to the aforementioned. Stage 4 requires surgical consultation.

Prior to treatment of the rotator cuff, dysfunctions in the scapulothoracic and acromioclavicular areas need to be dealt with as previously described. Normalizing mechanics in these areas will facilitate appropriate retraining of the rotator cuff muscles.

ISOMETRIC MUSCLE ENERGY TECHNIQUE

Spencer Sequence

Side-lying Athlete

The Spencer sequence or 'stages of Spencer' employs a muscle energy approach to address dysfunction in the rotator cuff and surrounding muscles. Various authors describe seven or eight stages in the sequence. These techniques address all of the muscles of the shoulder girdle, using the arm as a long lever. The sequence should be carried out in the order described below because of the increasing complexity of movements required of the patient with each stage. Patients should be progressed through the sequence as tolerated. Pain is an indication that progression should be stopped until the next visit. In all of the stages the physician should support the acromioclavicular joint, monitor tensions in the muscles and stabilize the shoulder joint.

During all stages the patient will be in the lateral recumbent position, with the shoulder to be treated uppermost (Fig. 4.13).The physician may stand either in front of or behind the patient. This approach may be used with caution in patients with chronic shoulder dislocation. In all patients pain, apprehension or abnormal guarding are signs to discontinue the sequence.

Stage 1: Extension
Normal extension is approximately 90°.

1. Isometric contraction is used to lengthen the pectoralis major, pectoralis minor and anterior deltoid muscles. The scapula is stabilized. The arm is flexed at the elbow and the shoulder is slowly carried to its barrier in extension (Fig. 4.14).

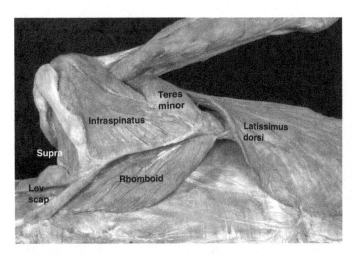

Fig. 4.13

2. The athlete is instructed to move his arm forward (flex his shoulder, black arrow). The physician resists this movement with an equal and opposite counterforce (white arrow) to the extent that the pectoralis major, pectoralis minor and anterior deltoid are engaged (Figs 4.15 and 4.16).

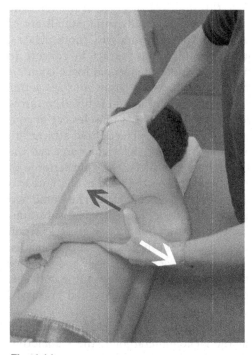

Fig. 4.14

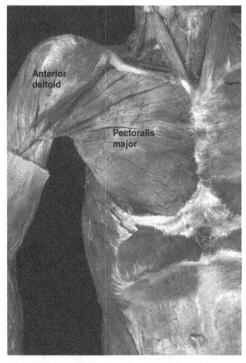

Fig. 4.15

3. This isometric contraction is maintained for 4–5 seconds. The athlete is asked to cease contraction while the physician simultaneously reduces her counterforce.

4. The physician maintains contact and waits for tissue relaxation (approximately 4–5 seconds).

5. The physician then extends the shoulder to the new restrictive barrier. The sequence is repeated twice.

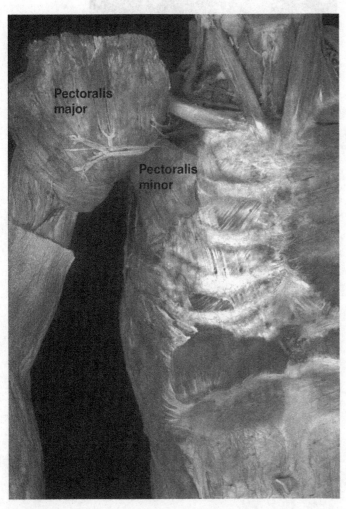

Pectoralis major

Pectoralis minor

Fig. 4.16

Stage 2: Flexion

Normal flexion is approximately 180°.

1. Isometric contraction is used to lengthen the latissimus dorsi, teres major and minor, and posterior deltoid muscles. The scapula is stabilized. The elbow is flexed and the shoulder is slowly carried to its barrier in flexion (Fig. 4.17).

2. The athlete is instructed to move his arm backwards (extend his shoulder, black arrow). The physician resists this movement with an equal and opposite counterforce (white arrow) to the extent that the latissimus dorsi, teres major and minor, and posterior deltoid muscles are engaged (Fig. 4.18).

3. This isometric contraction is maintained for 4–5 seconds, and then the athlete is asked to cease contraction while the physician simultaneously reduces her counterforce.

4. The physician maintains contact and waits for tissue relaxation (approximately 4–5 seconds).

5. The physician then flexes the shoulder to the new restrictive barrier. The sequence is repeated twice.

Stage 3: Circumduction without Traction

This is a passive range of motion stretch.

1. The arm is flexed at the elbow. The scapula is stabilized and abducted to 90°. The shoulder is circumducted from the midline in small concentric circles in a clockwise direction with a gradual increase in the radius of the circle (Fig. 4.19).

2. If the arc flattens over any portion of the circle the range of motion in that direction is gently increased to tolerance. The same technique is carried out in a counter-clockwise direction.

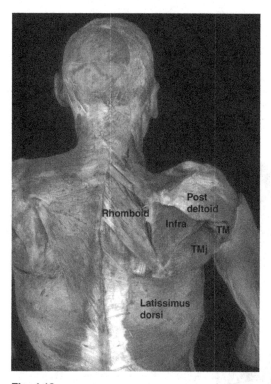

Fig. 4.18

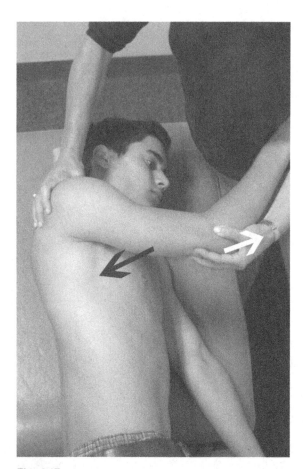

Fig. 4.17

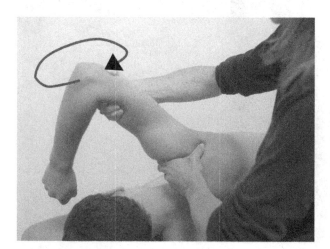

Fig. 4.19

Stage 4: Circumduction with Traction

This is passive range of motion stretch.

1. The elbow is flexed. The arm is grasped proximal to the elbow and approximately 5–10 lb of traction is applied to the shoulder (large black arrow). The scapula is stabilized and the arm abducted to 90° (Fig. 4.20).

2. The shoulder is circumducted, as in stage 3 (small black arrow), in both clockwise and counter-clockwise directions, with maintenance of traction.

Stage 5: Abduction

Normal abduction is approximately 135° (this is the motion limited in impingement syndrome and inflammation of the subacromial bursa).

1. The arm is flexed at the elbow and the scapula stabilized. The shoulder is carried to its limit in abduction (Fig. 4.21). The athlete is asked to bring his arm towards his body (adduct the arm, black arrow).

2. The physician resists this movement (white arrow) with an equal and opposite counterforce to the extent that the pectoralis minor, teres minor and infraspinatus muscles are engaged (Fig. 4.22).

3. This isometric contraction is maintained for 4–5 seconds, then the patient is asked to cease contraction while the physician simultaneously reduces her counterforce.

4. The physician maintains contact and waits for tissue relaxation (approximately 4–5 seconds).

5. The physician abducts the arm to the new restrictive barrier. The sequence is repeated twice.

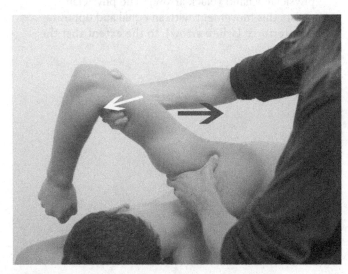

Fig. 4.21

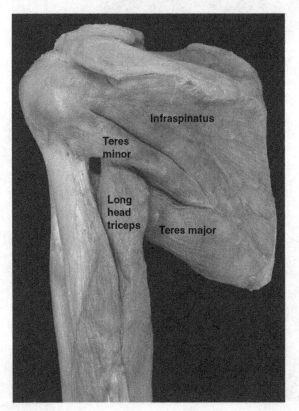

Fig. 4.22

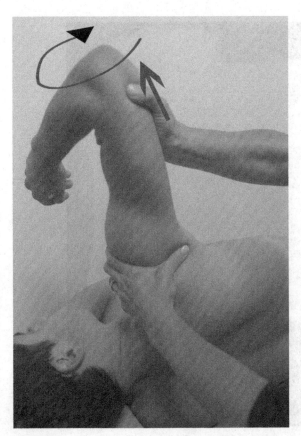

Fig. 4.20

Stage 6: Adduction

1. The physician stands facing the athlete. The physician's arm stabilizes the scapula. The patient's arm is rested on the physician's forearm (Fig. 4.23). The physician's other hand is used to move the patient's elbow medially (white arrow), thereby introducing adduction as well as external rotation at the shoulder.

2. The patient is asked to lift the elbow against the physician's hand (black arrow). The physician resists this movement with an equal and opposite counterforce (white arrow), to the extent that the subscapularis and teres major muscles are engaged (Fig. 4.24).

3. This isometric contraction is maintained for 4–5 seconds, and then the patient is asked to cease contraction while the physician simultaneously reduces her counterforce.

4. The physician maintains contact and waits for tissue relaxation (approximately 4–5 seconds).

5. The physician moves the elbow medially to the new restrictive barrier. The sequence is repeated twice.

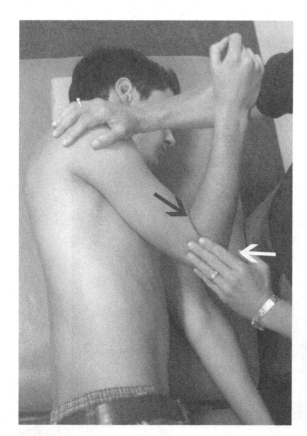

Fig. 4.23

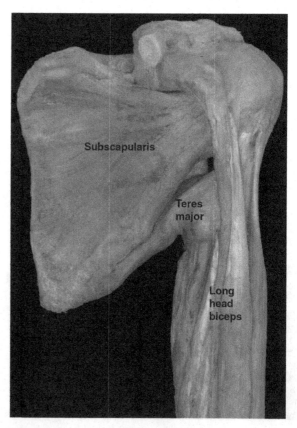

Subscapularis

Teres major

Long head biceps

Fig. 4.24

Stage 7: Internal Rotation

This is one of the most difficult stages and should be used with great care. It is contraindicated in patients with shoulder instability.

1. The arm is flexed at the elbow. The scapula is stabilized and the arm is carried to its barrier in internal rotation. The palm is facing posteriorly and the hand may be placed behind the patient (Fig. 4.25). The physician places her hand on the patient's elbow.

2. The patient is instructed to push the elbow backwards into the physician's hand (externally rotate the humerus, black arrow).

3. The physician resists this movement (white arrow) with an equal and opposite counterforce, to the extent that the supraspinatus and infraspinatus muscles are engaged (Fig. 4.26).

4. This isometric contraction is maintained for 4–5 seconds. The patient is then asked to cease contraction while the physician simultaneously reduces her counterforce.

5. The physician maintains contact and waits for tissue relaxation (approximately 4–5 seconds).

6. The physician internally rotates the humerus to the new restrictive barrier. This can be done by moving the elbow anteriorly. The sequence is repeated twice.

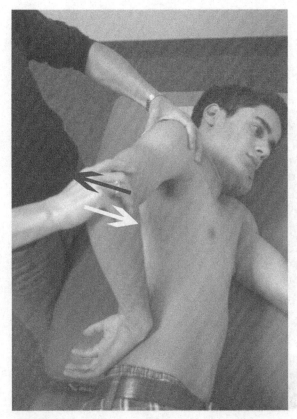

Fig. 4.25

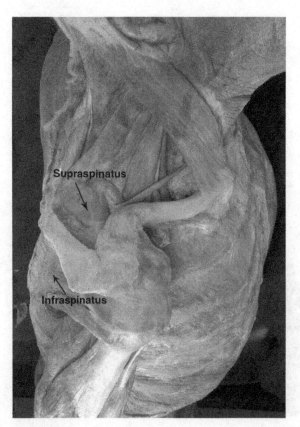

Supraspinatus

Infraspinatus

Fig. 4.26

Stage 8: Abduction with Resisted Traction

This stage is contraindicated in patients with shoulder instability.

1. The arm is abducted and elevated. The physician clasps his hands around the deltoid muscle and the distal humerus and adds 3–4 lb of traction to the shoulder (Fig. 4.27, white arrow).

2. The physician carries the shoulder to its barrier in abduction while maintaining traction (Fig. 4.28, white arrow).

3. From this stretched position the patient is instructed to pull his arm towards his shoulder joint and body (adduction, black arrow)

4. The physician resists this movement with an equal and opposite counterforce.

5. This isometric contraction is maintained for 4–5 seconds. Then the patient is asked to cease contraction while the physician simultaneously reduces her counterforce.

6. The physician maintains contact and waits for tissue relaxation (approximately 4–5 seconds).

7. The physician increases the traction on the shoulder to the new restrictive barrier. The sequence is repeated twice.

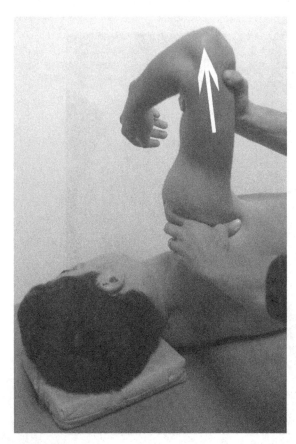

Fig. 4.27

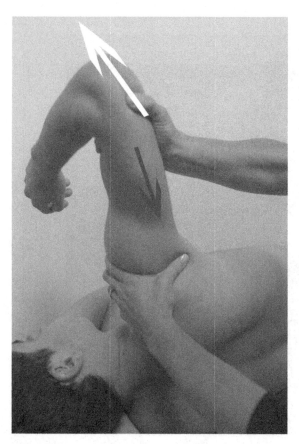

Fig. 4.28

ACROMIOCLAVICULAR SPRAIN/ STRAIN/DISLOCATION

Clinical Notes (Figs 4.29 and 4.30)

An acromioclavicular sprain, strain or dislocation is usually a traumatic injury that occurs secondary to a fall or in contact sports. Ligamentous sprain and strain may result from impacts that drive the scapula inferiorly and stretch the capsular tissues and ligaments. Injuries may also result from repetitive forceful adduction that strains the stabilizing ligaments. Normal joint glide during arm movement is essential at the AC joint. Abnormal muscle balance, biomechanical dysfunction, and altered tissue loading of the scapula, clavicle or associated tissues may interfere with normal glide of the articular surfaces during arm movement, resulting in repetitive microtrauma. Because the acromioclavicular ligament and capsule are the major stabilizers of the AC joint, they are most vulnerable to repetitive strain.

When there is displacement of the joint, a tender step-off or bump is present. Passive motion may be more painful than active motion, especially adduction of the arm across the body. Mild injury or strain involves the acromioclavicular capsule and ligament, causing mild swelling and tenderness to palpation. Moderate injury stretches the capsule and ligament, and also involves the coracoclavicular ligament. This results in an increased movement at the joint with translation. Severe injury disrupts both ligaments and presents clinically as pronounced instability.

Treatment Notes

Strain and mild to moderate injuries of the acromioclavicular joint respond to conservative treatment. Moderate injuries may benefit from short-term immobilization to promote proper scarring. However, immobilization carries the risk of developing adhesions. Direct techniques can be used in acute injury without instability. In other cases, balancing, deep tissue techniques and passive range of motion may be applied.

Mechanics at the clavicle and scapula need to be considered during treatment, including the anterior cervical and thoracic muscles and fasciae and the scapula.

In young children or those with dislocation it is preferable to treat the clavicles using balancing techniques with the patient in the supine position rather than seated. Direct techniques may be used prudently if ligamentous disruption has been ruled out.

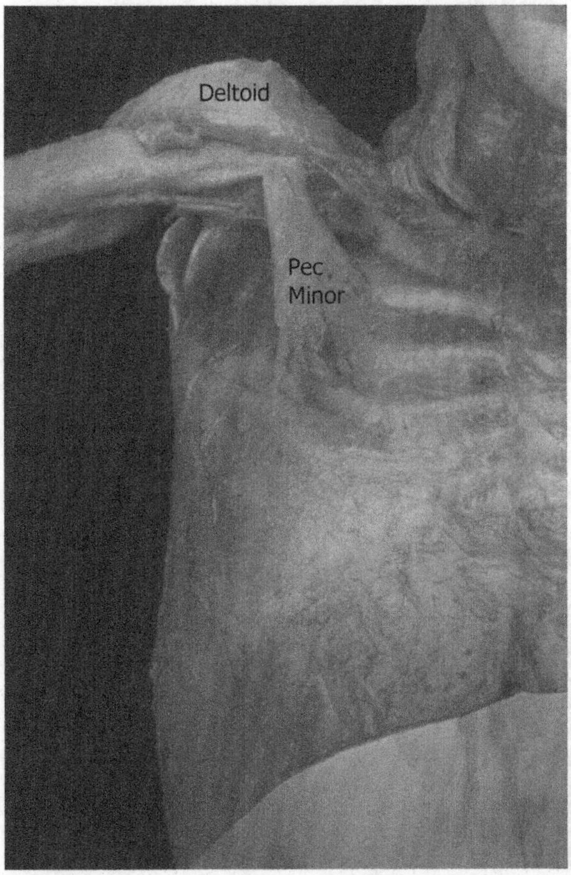

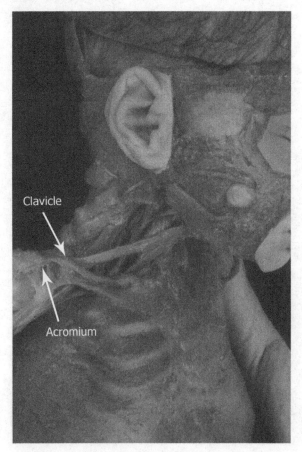

Fig. 4.29

Fig. 4.30

DIRECT MYOFASCIAL RELEASE TECHNIQUE

Anterior Cervical Fascia

Seated Athlete

1. The patient is seated facing the physician. The physician places her thumbs along the superior margin of the clavicles, just distal to the sternocleidomastoid insertion (Fig. 4.31).

2. The patient drapes his arms over the physician's and flexes the head and neck. This allows the physician's fingers to sink into the supraclavicular space (Fig. 4.32).

3. The patient is instructed to breathe deeply. During inhalation, the physician resists the superior movement of the supraclavicular fasciae. During exhalation, the patient exaggerates the flexed posture of the head and neck and the physician follows the tissues as they descend into the thoracic inlet.

4. This is repeated three to four times. Then the patient is instructed to take a deep breath and sit up straight, as the physician maintains resistance on the supraclavicular tissues.

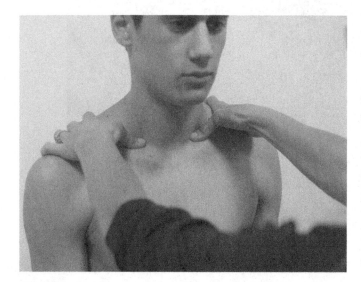

Fig. 4.31

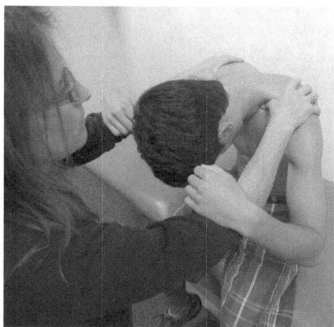

Fig. 4.32

MYOFASCIAL RELEASE TECHNIQUE

Anterior Cervical Fascia

Seated Toddler

This may also be done in the supine position on infants.

1. The child is seated. The physician uses the thumb and index finger of one hand to contact the supraclavicular tissues along the margin of the clavicle lateral to the sternocleidomastoid. The thumb and index finger of the other hand contact the posterior aspects of the first ribs bilaterally (Fig. 4.33).

2. Using the posterior contact, the physician applies a gentle force to the ribs in a direct or indirect manner (as described below), while monitoring the response of the anterior myofascial tissues. The anterior hand monitors the change in tissue tensions with respiration.

   a. Direct technique: During exhalation the fingers contacting the posterior ribs sink into the tissues following the motion of the ribs. During inhalation the fingers gently resist the movement of the tissues. The vectors of force are adjusted to accommodate the tissue response anteriorly.

   b. Indirect technique: During inhalation the fingers exaggerate the tissue tensions in the direction of ease. The vectors of force are adjusted to accommodate the tissue response anteriorly. During exhalation the physician relaxes her pressure and allows the tissue to rebalance.

Fig. 4.33

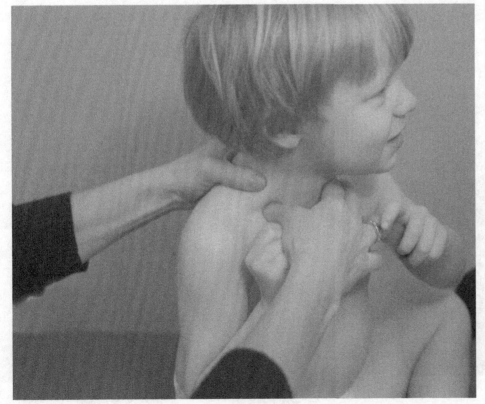

BALANCED LIGAMENTOUS TECHNIQUE

Clavicle

Supine Athlete

1. The patient is supine with the physician standing ipsilateral to the clavicle to be treated. The physician contacts the clavicle at the inferior aspect of the sternoclavicular and acromioclavicular articulations (Fig. 4.34).

2. A slow, steady, posterior and cephalad force (black arrows) is introduced at each of the points of contact until there is a slight change in tissue texture.

3. Compression, rotation, abduction, adduction, flexion and extension are introduced at each end until balanced tension is felt between the clavicle and its adjacent tissues. This position is held until there is a change in tissue texture and the clavicle moves freely with respiration.

4. The technique is repeated with the other clavicle.

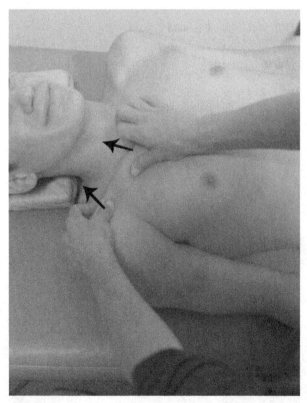

Fig. 4.34

ARTICULATORY TECHNIQUE

Acromioclavicular Joint

Seated Athlete

The arm is used as a short lever to move the scapula on the clavicle (Fig. 4.35).

1. The patient is seated. The physician stands behind the patient, with her thumb contacting the clavicle at the distal end. The motion at the acromioclavicular joint is monitored with the thumb superiorly and the middle finger inferiorly.

2. The physician grasps the patient's elbow with the other hand. The patient's humerus is abducted and the elbow flexed (Fig. 4.36).

3. The acromioclavicular joint is used as a fulcrum. The restrictive barrier of the AC joint is engaged by using a small amount of either compression or traction along the long axis of the arm into the joint (large white arrow).

4. The patient's arm is then circumducted in both clockwise and counterclockwise directions (circular white arrow) while the physician engages the restrictive barrier until the acromion moves freely on the clavicle.

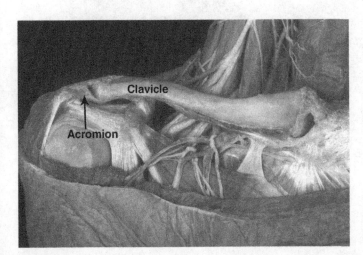

Fig. 4.35

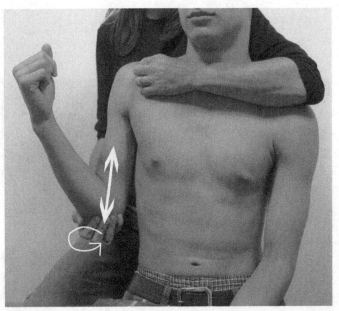

Fig. 4.36

ARTICULATORY TECHNIQUE

Sternoclavicular Joint

Seated Athlete

The arm is used as a long lever to move the clavicle on the sternum (Fig. 4.37).

1. The patient is seated. The physician stands behind the patient with her thumb contacting the jugular notch. The motion at the sternoclavicular end of the clavicle is monitored with the index finger superiorly and the middle finger inferiorly.

2. The physician grasps the patient's elbow with the other hand. The patient's humerus is abducted and the elbow flexed (Fig. 4.38).

3. The restrictive barrier of the sternoclavicular joint is engaged by using a small amount of either compression or traction (large white arrow) along the long axis of the arm into the clavicle.

4. The patient's elbow is then flexed across the chest and the arm is circumducted superiorly and then posteriorly (circular arrow) while the physician engages the restrictive barrier until the clavicle moves freely at the sternum. This may also be done in the opposite direction.

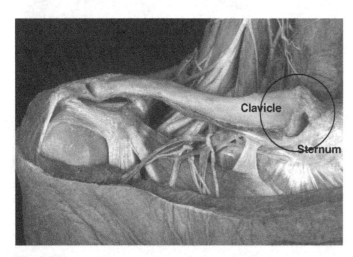

Fig. 4.37

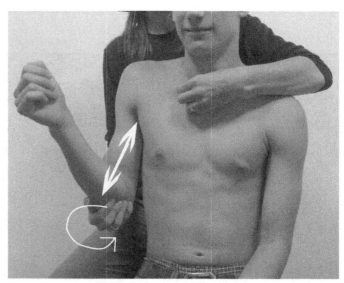

Fig. 4.38

DIRECT MYOFASCIAL TECHNIQUE

Scapula

Supine Athlete

This technique may improve circulation to the muscles of the shoulder complex, and may reduce muscle splinting (Fig. 4.39).

1. The patient lies on the unaffected side. The physician stands in front of the patient. The patient's affected arm is internally rotated and placed behind his back.

2. The physician's contacts the medial border of the scapula with one hand. The other hand is placed over the superior aspect of the scapula and shoulder (Fig. 4.40). The hand on the scapula and shoulder applies an inferior force (white arrow) to move the scapula into the physician's other hand. At the same time the other hand is used to lift the scapula away from the thoracic cage.

3. The physician uses the two hands to engage the restrictive barrier. The physician introduces rotation, flaring, elevation and/or depression into the scapula.

4. Once the restrictive barrier is engaged, the physician holds this position until there is a release in tissue texture, improved range of motion and relaxation of muscle spasm.

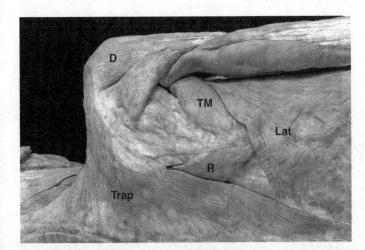

Fig. 4.39 • Posterior view of the muscles of the upper back and shoulder. Trapezius (Trap), deltoid (D), rhomboid (R), latissimus dorsi (Lat), teres major (TM).

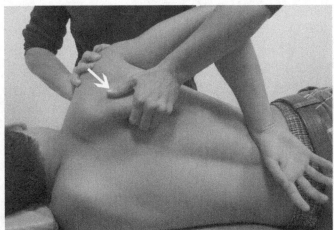

Fig. 4.40

SHOULDER (GLENOHUMERAL) DISLOCATION/INSTABILITY

Clinical Notes

The glenohumeral joint is inherently unstable owing to the disproportionate sizes of the glenoid fossa and humeral head. The glenoid labrum, fibrous capsule and glenohumeral ligaments all act to reinforce this articulation. Anterior dislocation results from forced extension, adduction and external rotation. Posterior dislocation arises from forced flexion, adduction and internal rotation. Both can occur during a fall or a blow to the shoulder. Anterior dislocation is most common and is named for the position of the humeral head anterior to the fossa. For example subcoracoid dislocation occurs when the humeral head is positioned anterior to the fossa and inferior to the coracoid process. When the humeral head is anterior and inferior to the glenoid fossa, it is classified as a subglenoid dislocation. Rarely, the humeral head may be dislocated inferior to the clavicle (subclavicular) or between the ribs (intrathoracic). Posterior dislocations are rare in children and have similar nomenclature, although the humeral head is positioned posterior to the fossa.

The patient with acute shoulder dislocation presents with pain, a limited range of motion and muscle spasm. The humeral head may be palpable in an anterior dislocation. Prominence of the coracoid process and flattening of the anterior shoulder contour suggest a posterior dislocation. Differential diagnosis includes fracture. In adolescents damage to the humeral epiphysis may occur concomitantly with the dislocation. Compression fractures of the humeral head, called Hill–Sachs lesions, can occur with shoulder dislocation.

Recurrent anterior dislocation is common in young athletes. In the immediate post-reduction period immobilization should be considered. With repeated dislocation the anterior articular capsule and ligaments become stretched or torn and are unable to stabilize the humeral head during external rotation. Hill–Sachs lesions alter the biomechanics at the glenoid fossa, thereby contributing to the instability. With recurrent dislocation the area of the compression fracture may be re-injured, leading to chronic degenerative changes in the joint. Recurrent dislocation also leads to scarring and edema of the capsule and ligaments, further compromising the stability of the joint.

Treatment Notes

Dislocations can be reduced by various methods that employ traction with abduction, flexion, and external rotation. Post-reduction treatment focuses on correcting biomechanical dysfunction associated with the injury, strengthening and retraining of stabilizing muscles, and addressing secondary dysfunction in the neck and thorax. Spencer's techniques for the shoulder may be beneficial in restoring muscle balance and range of motion.

BALANCED LIGAMENTOUS TECHNIQUE

Humerus/Rotator Cuff

Supine Athlete/Child

This approach may be used in an acute or painful shoulder as a way to address the pain and splinting. In this approach the physician directs her attention to the muscles and fasciae of the rotator cuff complex. This is a short lever technique.

1. The patient is supine with the arm resting in a comfortable position. The physician sits beside and slightly behind the patient on the side to be treated.

2. The physician places one hand over the top of the shoulder, contacting the scapula and clavicle (Fig. 4.41). The other hand grasps the humerus close to the glenohumeral joint. Care is taken not to compress the neurovascular bundle.

3. While stabilizing the scapula the physician uses a stacking technique to gently take the humerus through various planes of a motion, moving it only a few degrees into each plane to test the tissue response in order to achieve balanced tension (Fig. 4.42).

4. Once balanced tension is achieved, the physician maintains that position until a correction in the mechanical strain, a reduction in pain and muscle splinting, or improvement in tissue function is noted.

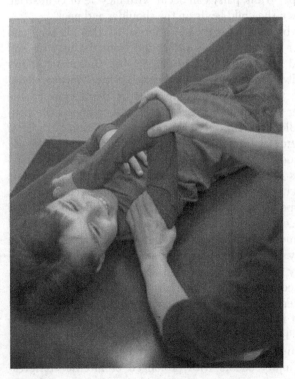

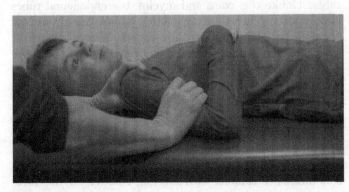

Fig. 4.41

Fig. 4.42

BRACHIAL PLEXUS INJURY/ERB'S PALSY

Clinical Notes

Injury to the brachial plexus may occur as a result of excessive stretching or compression of the nerve roots or peripheral nerves of the brachial plexus. Erb's palsy, a partial brachial nerve plexus palsy involving damage to C5 and C6 nerves, classically occurs in large neonates during vaginal delivery. The injury to the upper brachial trunk (levels C5 and C6) is thought to be due to traction and side-bending (lateral flexion) of the head and neck during delivery. Other risk factors include mid-forceps delivery and vacuum assistance. Erb's palsy may be associated with facial nerve palsy, ipsilateral fractured clavicle, ipsilateral Horner's syndrome, and congenital torticollis, all of which are thought to result from the traumatic delivery. Erb's palsy is named for 'Erb's point,' the junction where the fifth and sixth cervical nerves come together. Pressure at this site superior to the clavicle and posterior to the sternocleidomastoid muscle produces the characteristic paresis of Erb's palsy. When injury extends to the lower brachial trunk (C5–T1) it is called Erb–Duchenne–Klumpke's palsy. This may occur with traction of the arm during delivery. In older children and adults brachial plexus palsy may occur due to trauma in the thoracic outlet (Fig. 4.43). Lower trunk palsy typically results from forceful traction and abduction of the upper extremity. Upper trunk palsy can occur with bicycle or equestrian falls when the child lands on the shoulder and neck.

The brachial plexus lies inferior to the clavicle and shoulder complex and is suspended from the first rib and coracoid process by fasciae (Fig. 4.44). Traumatic injury is usually due to one of two possible mechanisms. Side-bending of the neck accompanied by depression of the shoulder will simultaneously stretch and compress the neural bundle. Forceful traction and hyperabduction of the arm can stretch the brachial plexus, or in extreme cases avulse nerve roots or rupture the axons. There are four classifications of nerve injury. First-degree injury is the mildest and occurs as a result of short-term nerve compression. This type of injury may result from swelling and edema of adjacent tissues. There is degeneration of myelin and impediment of depolarization, but no disruption of axonal anatomy. Once the compression is relieved, functional recovery is complete. Second-degree injury occurs with prolonged compression. There is obstruction of neural veins and arteries, resulting in interruption of axoplasmic and nutrient flow. Degeneration of the myelin sheath and axons occurs. The axons and myelin are capable of regenerating, and complete recovery may take weeks to months. Third-degree injury occurs with prolonged or intense compression. There is venous congestion, obstruction of axoplasmic

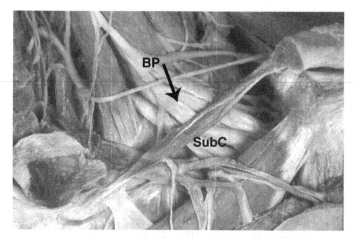

Fig. 4.43 • Anterior view of the left thoracic outlet. The clavicle and superficial muscles and faciae have been removed. Note the close proximity of the brachial plexus (BP) to the subclavius muscle.

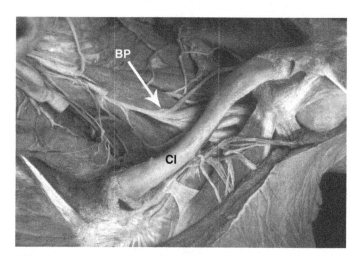

Fig. 4.44 • A superior view of the left side of the thoracic outlet. The skin, superficial fascia and sternocleidomastoid muscle have been removed. The brachial plexus (BP) can be seen passing inferior to the midpoint of the clavicle (Cl).

flow, myelin degeneration and disruption of the endoneural tubes. Unlike the axons and myelin, the endoneural tubes have poor regenerative capabilities. Consequently, recovery may be incomplete in third-degree injuries. Partial or complete transaction of the nerve or avulsion of the nerve root disrupts the perineurium and requires surgical repair. Recovery is poor. In general, axonal regeneration is said to occur at a rate of approximately 1 mm/day and is more likely to occur if the endoneural tubes are intact.

Classic upper brachial plexus injuries (Erb's palsy) involve C5 and C6 nerve roots. The typical posture of the infant with Erb's palsy is a flaccid shoulder that is adducted and internally rotated with internal rotation of the forearm. Upper brachial plexus injury affects the elevators and abductors of the scapula, the elbow flexors and the forearm supinators. Wrist and finger flexion are usually intact and have greater tone than extensor muscles, resulting in a posterior facing, and flexed wrist and hand. Ipsilateral palmar grasp reflex may be present but weak. The Moro reflex is asymmetrical. When C4 is involved there is hemidiaphragm paralysis (phrenic nerve), which may present as cyanosis, tachypnea, and in severe cases respiratory distress. There is sensory loss in the C5 and C6 dermatomes. The prognosis for Erb's palsy is good. Although the neural injury may repair in less than 6 months, functional recovery may be prolonged owing to the development of compensatory motor patterns and movement strategies.

Lower brachial plexus injuries involve the C7–T1 nerve roots. More often than not upper and lower injuries occur together. Isolated lower plexus injuries are uncommon. Function of the upper arm and shoulder is not affected in a pure lower plexus palsy. The motor deficit affects the elbow extensors, wrist extensors, finger flexors and extensors, and intrinsic muscles. The ipsilateral grasp reflex is absent in newborns. If the sympathetic fibers at T1 are involved the child will have Horner's syndrome. In lower plexus palsy there is sensory loss over the C7 dermatome and the distribution of the ulnar nerve. In combined upper and lower palsy there is complete sensory loss and paresis in the limb. This is called flail arm. The extent of the sensory loss predisposes the child to repetitive hand injury. The prognosis for Erb–Duchenne–Klumpke's palsy is significantly more guarded than for Erb's palsy (Eng et al. 1978, Eng et al. 1996). If recovery does occur, it may take 2 or more years.

In children with Erb's palsy the shoulder adductors and internal rotators (the latissimus dorsi, subscapularis and teres minor muscles) become shortened as a result of unopposed tone from the weakened serratus anterior and rhomboid muscles. Over time, contractures develop in the shortened muscles, whereas the muscles affected by the palsy atrophy. In addition, the unopposed contraction of the rotator cuff changes the arc of movement of the humerus during flexion and abduction. The infant compensates by elevating the shoulder, abducting the humerus and flexing the elbow when spontaneously attempting to reach out. In the infant, muscle contractures and imbalances can affect the development of muscle firing patterns. During this early developmental phase, this compensatory adaptation becomes learned as a dominant movement pattern. This is called Erb's engram. Unfortunately, once in place, the abnormal patterning may persist even after neural recovery. Contractures develop in some of the rotator cuff muscles, placing the humerus in an internally rotated position. The anterior portion of the joint capsule tightens and the posterior aspect stretches. This predisposes the child to posterior humeral subluxation. Over time the clavicle, glenoid fossa, humeral head, acromion and coracoid processes may be deformed by the abnormal tensions in the shoulder complex.

The development of hand function and hand–eye coordination can also be affected owing to learned compensatory motor patterning and abnormal positioning. The forearm typically assumes a pronated posture over time due to shortening of the elbow flexors. The adaptive posturing of the arm causes shortening of the anterior joint capsule and stretching posteriorly, which contributes to instability and functional loss. These secondary consequences complicate recovery even after nerve healing. What is more, mechanical dysfunction in the shoulder complex can influence the low-pressure circulatory system, prolonging tissue edema and congestion and delaying healing.

Severe pain is a primary component of brachial plexus injuries in adults and older children. This is especially true with avulsion of the nerve or nerve root. The pain may be constant, or sudden and intense. It is often described as crushing and burning. Nerve root compression injuries in adults and older children typically present with a radiating pain pattern that is described as electrical, burning, or a deep ache. Although the characteristics and localization of the pain may differ from that in an older child or adult owing to the immaturity of cortical mapping, one must assume the presence of nociceptive activity in infants with brachial plexus injuries. Transcutaneous electric stimulation can be used to manage pain in older children, but is contraindicated in infants.

Treatment Notes

In general, manipulative treatment needs to be directed at normalizing muscle resting lengths, preventing contractures, facilitating normal biomechanical motions, reducing pain, supporting normal movement strategies, and improving lymphatic and vascular flow. The rationale for manipulative treatment includes the respiratory–circulatory, the nociceptive, and the biomechanical/postural models. Motor patterning, stretching, muscle training and hand–eye coordination all need to be part of the rehabilitation strategy. Gentle passive range of motion movements can be taught to parents to encourage lengthening of the affected muscles. Active range of motion should be employed to reinforce normal movement patterns and inhibit compensatory strategies. Initially, movements should be attempted in a gravity-neutral position and then progressed to movement against gravity. Gravity-neutral positioning can be achieved by the child lying supine or held in the caregiver's arms. The affected arm is supported as the child reaches. Alternatively, the child can be placed on the unaffected side with the head supported in a neutral position (no lateral flexion) and the affected arm allowed to drop across the body midline. Laying the child on the affected side should be avoided in the acute phase. Because of the abnormal tone the child will adapt compensatory patterns of movement. These strategies must be discouraged and inhibited, whereas normal strategies are repeated. For example, compensatory elevation of the shoulder during reaching can be discouraged by stabilizing the scapula. Although the child may not be able to reach as far, normal patterning within that range of motion is maintained and reinforced. During active movement, normal muscle patterning is more important than range of motion. Passive exercises can be used to maintain appropriate range of motion without compromising patterning. Properly trained caregivers can perform passive and active exercises with the child throughout the day. Some children with Erb's palsy may develop an associated oropharyngeal dysfunction that is usually related to speech articulation. Strains in the myofascial tissues of the anterior neck may play a role in the oropharyngeal dysfunction.

In severe cases of paralysis where the forearm is fixed in supination and there is limited elbow flexion, hand function is severely affected. Osteotomy with rotational correction may be necessary to optimize function.

BALANCED LIGAMENTOUS TECHNIQUE

Scapulothoracic Joint

Seated Toddler or Infant

Balanced ligamentous treatment of the scapulothoracic joint can be used to address the resting length and function of the serratus anterior, subscapularis, rhomboid, latissimus dorsi and lower trapezius muscles (Fig. 4.45).

1. The child is seated. The physician sits beside the child on the side to be treated.

2. The physician places one hand over the posterior surface of the scapula, contacting the spine of the scapula with her fingers (Fig. 4.46). The thumb of the same hand is positioned high in the axilla, with a contact on the medial inferior surface of the humerus. Care is taken to not compress the neurovascular bundle.

3. The other hand is placed over the anterior chest wall, contacting the clavicle and upper ribs with the fingers. The thumb of this hand is positioned in the axilla, contacting the lateral margin of the uppermost ribs (Fig. 4.47). The physician gently slides the thumb posteriorly until it is deep to the anterior surface of the scapula. The two thumbs are now crossed in the axilla.

4. The tensions in the surrounding myofascial attachments of the scapula are brought into balanced tension and the scapula is balanced on the thorax. The physician maintains this position until a correction in the mechanical strain or improvement in tissue function is noted.

5. This technique may also be performed with the child supine (Figs 4.48 and 4.49).

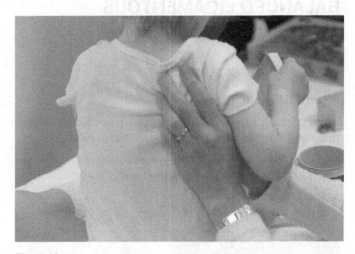

Fig. 4.46

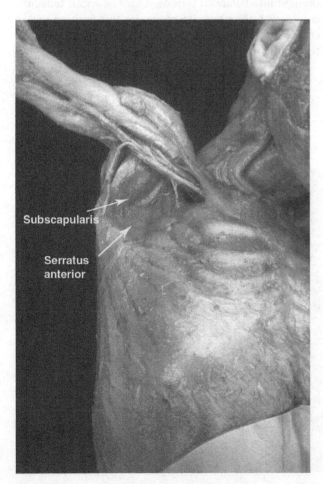

Subscapularis

Serratus anterior

Fig. 4.45

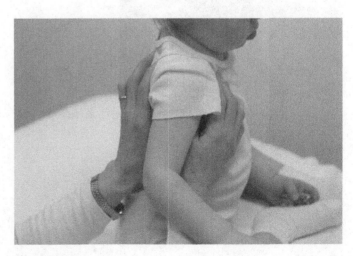

Fig. 4.47

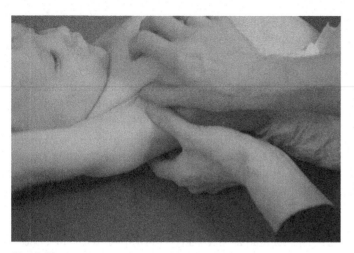

Fig. 4.48

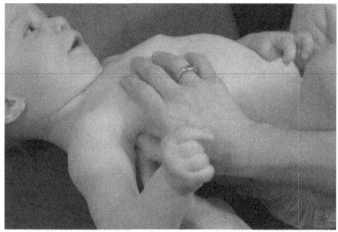

Fig. 4.49

BALANCED LIGAMENTOUS TECHNIQUE

Scapulothoracic Joint

Alternate Technique

This approach may be used if muscle spasm prevents positioning of the thumb in the scapulothoracic space.

1. The physician contacts the scapula posteriorly with one hand (Fig. 4.50). The opposite hand is used to contact the anterior surface of the scapula (Fig. 4.51). The index, middle or small finger (as appropriate) can be used as the fulcrum for positioning the scapula.

2. The fascial and muscular attachments of the scapula are brought into balanced tension. Once balanced tension is achieved, the physician maintains this position until a correction in the mechanical strain or improvement in tissue function is noted.

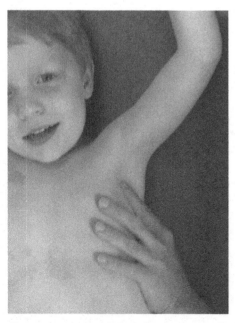

Fig. 4.50

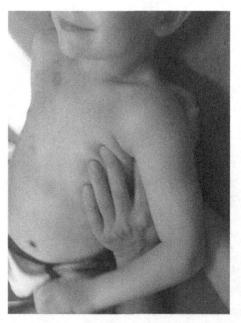

Fig. 4.51

BALANCED LIGAMENTOUS TECHNIQUE

Clavicle–First Rib

Seated Toddler

Treating the clavicle and first rib may improve lymphatic and vascular flow through the thoracic inlet and to the extremity. This approach addresses the thoracic inlet as a complex comprising the bilateral clavicles and first ribs. The image of a flexible ring may be used to describe the relationship between the structures.

1. The toddler is seated on the table or the physician's lap facing away from the physician (Fig. 4.52).

2. The physician contacts the clavicles bilaterally so that the index fingers are at the sternoclavicular articulation and the ring fingers are at the acromial portion of the clavicle. The middle fingers contact the anterior margin of the first rib.

3. The thumbs are placed on the superoposterior margin of the first ribs bilaterally.

4. The physician uses the contact of the thumbs on the ribs as a fulcrum to introduce a gentle posterior lateral motion into both clavicles simultaneously to 'open' the sternoclavicular junction (white curved arrow).

5. The bilateral clavicle–first rib complex is treated as a single functional unit. The physician introduces side-bending, rotation, translation, depression and elevation to establish balanced tension in the costoclavicular complex and its associated myofascial tissues.

6. Once balanced tension is achieved, the physician maintains that position until a correction in the mechanical strain or improvement in tissue function is noted.

ALTERNATIVE TECHNIQUE

Using the same contact as described above, the tissues are brought into the position of ease rather than balanced tension and held until a release in tissue tension is felt.

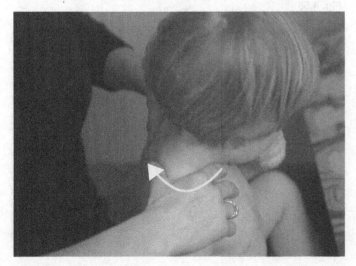

Fig. 4.52

BALANCED LIGAMENTOUS TECHNIQUE

Thoracic Inlet – Complete

Toddler, Infant

Indications for treatment of the thoracic inlet include improving lymphatic and vascular flow through the inlet, and addressing mechanical strains in the thoracic inlet complex. This particular approach addresses the thoracic inlet by contacting the ribs, sternum and T1 vertebra. The hand position described below is used to contact the T1 vertebra, sternum, first rib and clavicle simultaneously and bring the entire thoracic inlet into balance. The image of a caliper may be used to describe the relationship between the structures, with T1 as the center of the caliper and each rib as one of the arms (Fig. 4.53). This approach may be effective when there is sternal or anterior chest wall involvement.

1. The child is supine, seated or held in a parent's arms. The physician sits to the side and slightly above the child's shoulder. The physician uses one hand to contact the first ribs anteriorly. The middle finger and thumb of the same hand are placed on either side of the sternum just inferior to the clavicle and lateral to the costosternal junction on the anterior surface of each first rib. The index finger monitors the manubrium (Fig. 4.54).

2. The other hand is placed posteriorly, with a contact on each first rib and the spinous process of T1. The precise position of the fingers will vary depending on the size of the child and the size of the physician's hands (Fig. 4.55).

3. The anterior hand is used to introduce a lateral traction to the sternal end of each first rib until the posterior hand contacting that same rib feels a release (Figs 4.56 and 4.57, white arrows). The manubrium is monitored.

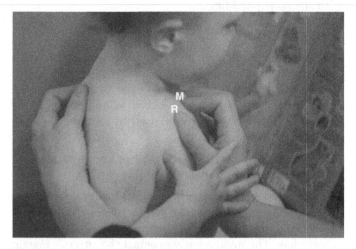

Fig. 4.54

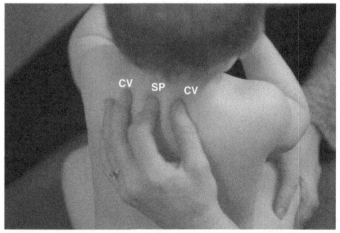

Fig. 4.55

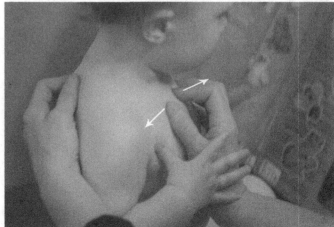

Fig. 4.56

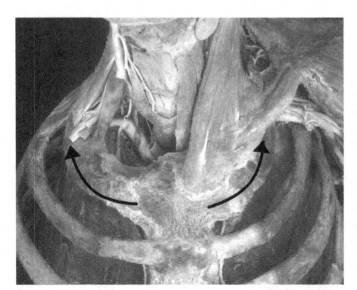

Fig. 4.53

(The parts of the sternum do not begin to unite until mid-puberty, and the manubriosternal joint is present throughout life in most people.)

4. The physician then uses both hands to induce rotation, side-bending, translation, and compression to bring the entire first rib–T1–sternal complex and its associated tissues into balanced tension.

5. Once balanced tension is achieved, the physician maintains that position until a correction in the mechanical strain or improvement in tissue function is noted.

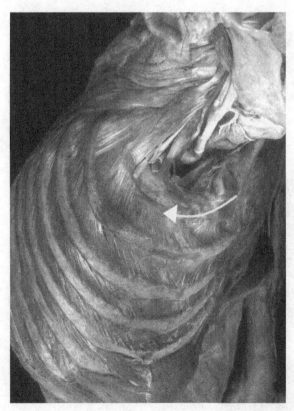

Fig. 4.57

BALANCED LIGAMENTOUS TECHNIQUE

Clavicle

Seated Infant

This may be performed with the infant supine, seated, or held in the parent's arms. This technique is contraindicated in acute clavicle fractures. The alternative technique may also be used in this age group when the tissue does not respond to compression.

1. The infant is seated, supine, or lying in the caregiver's arms. The physician is seated ipsilateral to the side to be treated. The clavicle is contacted at the sternoclavicular and acromioclavicular ends. The physician evaluates passive motion with respiration (Fig. 4.58).

2. A gentle compression is applied along the long axis of the bone (black arrows). The vector of the compression is changed depending on the response of the tissue. The presence of torsional forces is counterbalanced in the direction of the restrictive barrier without engaging the restrictive barrier.

3. The clavicle is then balanced along its axis and its attachments to the clavipectoral fascia and the subclavius muscle. These are then balanced in relation to the movements of the first rib.

4. Balanced tension is maintained until a change in tissue texture, correction in the mechanical strain or improvement in tissue function is noted.

ALTERNATIVE TECHNIQUE

The position and hand contacts are the same as described above; however, traction rather than compression is employed along the long axis of the clavicle.

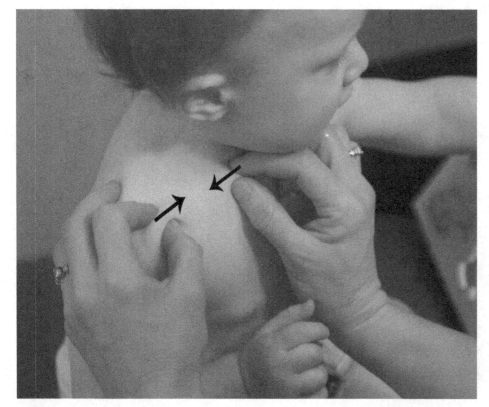

Fig. 4.58

BALANCED LIGAMENTOUS TECHNIQUE

Glenohumeral Joint

Seated Toddler

This is a long lever technique and may also be performed in the supine position. The scapulothoracic area and clavicle should be treated before applying this technique.

1. The child is seated. The physician sits beside or behind the child. With one hand the physician contacts the scapula and clavicle on the side to be treated. The other hand holds the distal end of the humerus (Fig. 4.59).

2. The physician stabilizes the scapula and clavicle. Compression, distraction, rotation, abduction and adduction are introduced into the glenohumeral tissues through the long lever of the humerus until balanced tension is achieved.

3. Once the glenohumeral tissues are positioned in balanced tension, the position is maintained until a correction in the mechanical strain or an improvement in tissue function is noted.

4. In the picture balanced tension was achieved with the humerus in extension, adduction and internal rotation (Fig. 4.60).

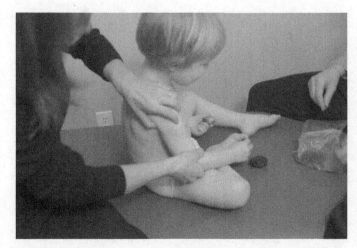

Fig. 4.59

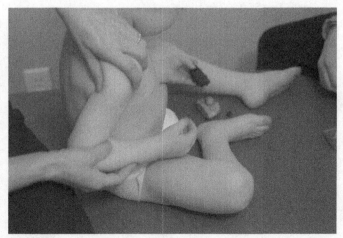

Fig. 4.60

STINGER/ACUTE NERVE INJURY

Acute injury to the nerves of the upper extremity typically occurs from a blow to the shoulder such as might occur in a contact sport. The athlete complains of burning numbness in the shoulder that may radiate into the hand. The specific nerves involved depend on the direction of the impact and the position of the shoulder at the time of contact. Nerve damage may be due to stretching or compression. In the vast majority of cases the neuropathy is temporary. Rebalancing and indirect techniques can be used to address secondary somatic dysfunction that may impede venous and lymphatic drainage and contribute to discomfort.

DISORDERS AFFECTING UPPER EXTREMITY STABILIZATION

Clinical Notes

In the infant and toddler the development of motor patterns for precisely coordinated arm and hand movement depends on proper biomechanical relationships throughout the arm. The child must be able to stabilize the shoulder to execute reaching, writing, lifting, and all the other activities requiring precision interaction with a target. Abnormalities in shoulder mechanics due to birth injury or abnormal muscle tone will affect the appropriate development of these skills. This becomes especially important in the long-term management of children with congenital conditions affecting the upper extremity. Normalizing mechanics at the scapulothoracic and glenohumeral joints will improve the child's ability to perform strengthening, motor planning and motor patterning rehabilitation.

Older children with spasticity experience difficulties with motor patterning. This affects agonist–antagonist relationships and the coordination of movements in those with even mild involvement. One of the goals of osteopathic treatment in these children should be the normalization of baseline levels of tone and the correction of dysfunction due to abnormal compensation patterns.

Children with primary muscle disease or hypotonia of other origin have difficulty in maintaining posture. Postural and antigravity muscles respond by shortening. Many flexors become deconditioned and stretched. Myofascial contractions in the tissues of the anterior torso and the neck are common. This produces the classic posture of internally rotated shoulders, a straightened cervical lordosis, extended and anteriorly translated occiput and a forward-leading chin. In these children the anterior myofascial and cervical tissues need to be addressed prior to treatment of the shoulder complex.

BALANCED LIGAMENTOUS TECHNIQUE

Shoulder Complex

Supine Child

The goal of this technique is to rebalance the muscles and tissue stabilizing the shoulder complex. Treatment should include the glenohumeral joint and clavicle, as previously described. Depending on the size of the child, the physician may to choose to modify this technique by using only one thumb or finger. The contact should be between the serratus anterior and subscapularis muscles.

1. The child is supine. The physician sits on the side to be treated slightly inferior to the shoulder. The physician's hand that is closest to the child's head is placed beneath the child's torso, grasping the scapula with the thumb placed posteriorly in the axilla contacting the lateral margin of the second or third rib.

2. The physician places her other hand over the anterior chest wall, contacting the clavicle with her fingers, while the thumb is placed in the axilla adjacent to her other thumb (see Fig. 4.61 for hand placement).

3. The child's arm is resting at his side (Fig. 4.62).

4. The physician uses her thumbs as a fulcrum, and her hands to elevate, protract, depress, retract and flare the scapula and clavicle, taking the shoulder complex through its planes of motion to achieve balanced tension in the tissues of the scapula and the anterior chest wall (Fig. 4.62).

5. The physician maintains this position until a correction in the mechanical strain or improvement in tissue function is noted.

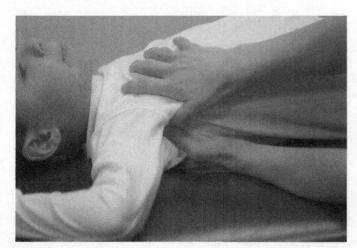

Fig. 4.61

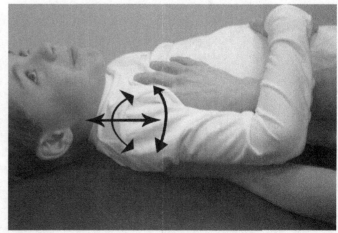

Fig. 4.62

References

Cofield R. Rotator cuff disease of the shoulder: current concepts. J Bone Joint Surg [Am] 1985; 67A: 974–979.

Curtis R. Shoulder injuries. In: Stanitski CL, DeLee J, Drez D, eds. Pediatric and adolescent sports medicine, 3rd edn. Philadelphia: WB Saunders, 1994; 191–215.

Eng GD, Binder H, Getson P, O'Donnell R. Obstetrical brachial plexus palsy (OBPP) outcome with conservative management. Muscle Nerve 1996; 19: 884–891.

Eng GD, Koch B, Smokvina M. Brachial plexus palsy in neonates and children. Arch Phys Med Rehab 1978; 59: 458.

Hill JA. An epidemiological perspective on shoulder injuries. Clin Sports Med 1983; 2: 241–246.

Jobe FW, Jobe CM. Painful athletic injuries of the shoulder. Clin Orthop 1983; 173: 117–124.

Micheli LJ. Overuse injuries in children's sports, the growth factor. Orthop Clin North Am 1983; 14: 337–360.

Rupp S, Berninger K, Hopf T. Shoulder problems in high level swimmers – impingement, anterior instability, muscular imbalance? Int J Sports Med 1995; 16: 557–562.

Tibone J. Shoulder problems in adolescence. Clin Sports Med 1983; 2: 423–426.

Yanai T, Hay JG, Miller GF. Shoulder impingement in front-crawl swimming: I. A method to identify impingement. Med Sci Sports Exerc 2000; 32: 21–29.

Chapter Five

5

Femur, hip and pelvis

CHAPTER CONTENTS

OVERVIEW

The hip undergoes tremendous changes in position, orientation and vascular supply from birth to adulthood. This occurs due to the composite nature of the femur and acetabulum. The femoral head and neck develop as three parts from three separate ossification centers. Likewise, the acetabulum is formed by the convergence of three bones: the ilium, the ischium and the pubes. The composite parts of the acetabulum join at a Y-shaped epiphysis located at the base of the acetabular cup (Fig. 5.1). The acetabulum enlarges by triradiate cartilaginous growth at the junctional Y-shaped intersection and at the circumferential rim. This triradiate growth center is vulnerable to distortion from excessive forces of compression and torsion. The composite parts of the femur – the greater and lesser trochanters and the femoral head – are joined to the femoral shaft by epiphyses, which are vulnerable to compressive and shearing forces. During normal growth the shape and orientation of the femoral head, neck and acetabulum alter in response to external and internal factors. In response to this bony remodeling, the vascular anatomy of the hip joint undergoes a process of division and absorption; it develops collateral circulation, and new areas of anastomosis. As a consequence, at different stages of growth the vascular supply to any of these areas may be vulnerable to damage, with the femoral head supply being the most vulnerable.

At birth, the femur and acetabulum lie in a more anterior position than they do during childhood. This position changes in response to growth, muscle development, weightbearing and gait. In the newborn, the transverse axes of the femoral head and neck are positioned more anteriorly in relation to the femoral condyles than they are in older children. In newborns the femur is said to be in an anteverted position, with the angle between the condyles of the femur and the head and neck at 30°. This anteverted position encourages intoeing. When the child starts to ambulate, the hip is placed in an extended position and loaded. This stresses the anterior aspect of the articular capsule where it inserts on the femoral neck. This mechanical stress results in non-perpendicular and torsional loads that produce rotational growth of the femoral neck. It is the rotational growth that remolds the femoral head and neck into a retroverted position. If standing or walking is delayed or connective tissue laxity is present, then remolding may be incomplete.

In addition to the anteverted position, the femurs are also externally rotated at birth. The resting length of the hip flexor muscles and the external rotator muscles is reduced but the resting tone is increased. As flexor muscle tone in the hip decreases, there is a concomitant reduction in the external rotation. With stance, gait and femoral retroversion,

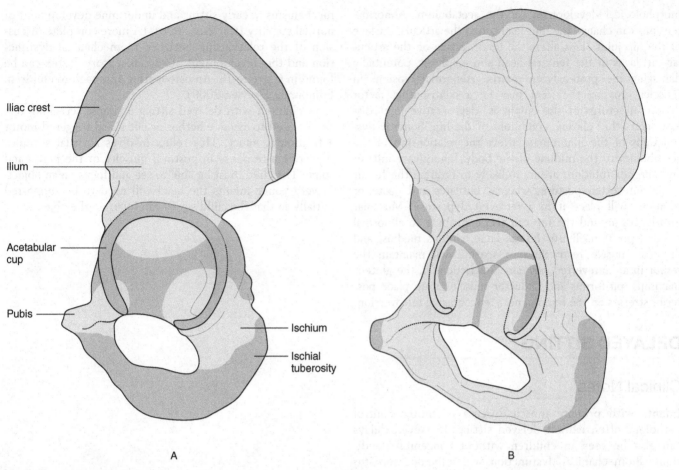

Iliac crest

Ilium

Acetabular
cup

Pubis

Ischium

Ischial
tuberosity

A

B

Fig. 5.1 • Schematic diagram of the innominate (A) at birth and (B) in adolescence. (Adapted from Williams P. Gray's anatomy. London: Churchill Livingstone, 1995, with permission.)

tone in the adductors increases, bringing the femur into a more neutral position so that by the age of 7 the patella lies in the frontal plane. Attendant upon this mature positioning of the limb is the development of the medial longitudinal arch of the foot, which develops as a result of strengthening and maturation of firing patterns in the anterior and posterior tibialis muscles.

In some cases persistent hip anteversion is extreme and quite obvious, but more often it is subtle and does not interfere with the attainment of normal developmental milestones. Children with spasticity affecting the adductor column may develop internal rotation of the femur and persistent anteversion. In milder cases of anteversion, compensations develop in the long bones and feet. Consequently, anteversion should be considered in the differential diagnosis of lower leg problems. Later in life the abnormal positioning of the hip predisposes the patient to degenerative hip conditions.

Abnormal hip positioning may also occur due to a misshapen or malpositioned acetabulum. Normally, growth along the rim of the acetabulum deepens the socket, as growth in the center enlarges it. The shape of the acetabulum is determined by the concerted growth at the Y-shaped epiphysis between the ilium, ischium and pubes. Concurrent growth at the other epiphyses of these bones expands and remodels the innominate, shifting the position of the acetabulum posteriorly and laterally, which accommodates changes in the femur. If the developmental repositioning of the acetabulum is inhibited, the femur will persist in an anteverted position. Although the mechanical forces at play on the femoral neck persist, the bone is unable to respond to them appropriately.

The three composite bones of the innominate act as anchors for the long restrictor and stabilizing muscles of the pelvis, hip and knee. Abnormal tensions and biomechanical dysfunctions in these muscles may interfere with normal morphological development of the acetabulum. Abnormal tensions can change the unit load across the articular surface of the hip joint. This alters the forces acting on the articular cartilages of the femoral head and epiphysis, potentially damaging the proteoglycan matrix. Abnormal tensions in muscles crossing the joint may be a contributing factor in microfractures of the epiphysis, degenerative joint disease, and other chronic conditions of the hip. Somatic dysfunctions of the innominate affect the relationship of the acetabulum to the midline of the body. Innominate inflares and anterior rotations are more likely to position the femur in an anteverted posture, whereas outflares and posterior rotations will place it in a retroverted posture. Muscular imbalances around the hip can also contribute to abnormal femoral position. Tensor fasciae latae, gluteus medius, and iliopsoas muscle restrictions or spasms will maintain the femur in an anteverted position. Restrictions in the gluteus maximus, piriformis and adductor muscle group place posterior stresses on the femoral neck, encouraging retroversion.

DELAYED SITTING

Clinical Notes

Infants with primary muscle disease or motor control pathology often exhibit delayed sitting. However, delays can also be seen in children without congenital conditions. Biomechanical dysfunction will influence somatosensory input as well as muscle response to motor signals. Dysfunction affecting the pelvis, knee extensors, sacrum or lumbar spine can be associated with delayed sitting in otherwise normal infants. Early sitting is dependent on visual input, which activates muscle synergies. It is suspected that visual input maps onto areas of motor cortex before somatosensory input. As the proprioceptive system matures, its influence on motor cortex increases. The shift to non-visual balance in infants requires accurate proprioceptive mapping and motor patterning. Postural and balance strategies in the adult are driven by vestibular, visual and somatosensory input. The somatosensory input has the strongest control. Seated balance and postural mechanisms mature along with the connections between the proprioceptive and motor systems. This requires several things: appropriate muscle resting length and strength, an intact motor system and an intact sensory system. In most children with delayed sitting one or more of these factors is not functioning appropriately. Imbalances in muscle tone or joint biomechanics may disrupt somatosensory mapping and the development of normal motor firing patterns. Abnormal proprioceptive input from the hip may adversely influence balance

mechanisms in early sitting and undermine development of normal stability (Carreiro 2009). (A more complete discussion of the relationship between biomechanical dysfunction and the development of somatosensory cortex can be found in Carreiro JE. An osteopathic approach to children. Edinburgh: Elsevier, 2009).

In children with delayed sitting a simple screening test can be used to assess whether or not visual triggered motor activation is intact. This reflex involves a visual stimulus triggering a response in postural muscles of the pelvis and spine. The child must be able to see and focus on an object. In very young infants the head will need to be supported initially so that the child's eyes can focus on the object.

Assessment of Visual–Motor Integration in Infants

1. The child is placed in a seated position with the clinician supporting the pelvis. The child should face a parent or caregiver who has a toy.

2. If the head is not supported, the infant will not be able to maintain balance and will fall to one side or the other. Typically, the head will stay in line with the shoulders and the lumbar spine will flex as the child loses his balance (Fig. 5.2).

3. If the head is supported so that the child can focus on the toy, the lumbar and pelvic muscles will contract and stabilize the pelvis and lumbar spine. The thorax and cervical muscles will also engage, thereby stabilizing the head (Fig. 5.3).

4. This response is present in infants as young as 6 weeks if the visual–motor system is intact. The clinician can use this response to evaluate visual–motor–proprioceptive integration in older infants who have delayed sitting. If the response is present but the child still shows instability with unsupported sitting, one must consider biomechanical dysfunction affecting normal proprioceptive mapping. If the response cannot be elicited but vision is present, one must consider motor or structural abnormality.

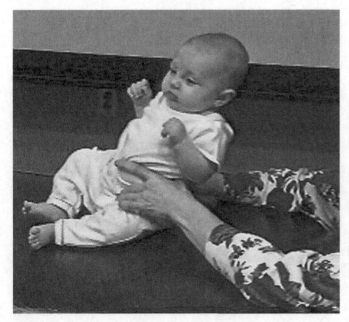

Fig. 5.2

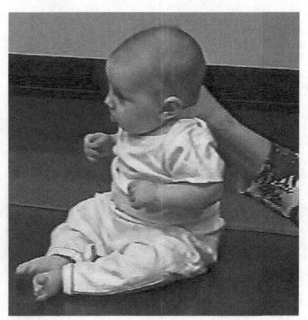

Fig. 5.3

BALANCED LIGAMENTOUS TECHNIQUE

General Approach Lumbosacral Junction, Pelvis and Hip

Toddler or Infant

A general approach to the lumbopelvic and hip mechanism such as the one described below can be used to localize specific areas of biomechanical dysfunction, as well as provide a general regional treatment.

1. The child is seated or supine on the treatment table. The physician sits beside him on the side to be treated. One hand is placed over the innominate. The index finger contacts the lumbosacral junction. The middle finger contacts the sacrum. The ring finger is placed under the ischial tuberosity and the thumb contacts the anterior superior iliac spine (Fig. 5.4).

2. The other hand is used to grasp the femur. The index finger contacts the pubic ramus and the thumb is placed on the femur approximately at the axis of the femoral neck. If the child is supine, the femur should be flexed between 45° and 90°. If the child is seated, the femur is in the appropriate position. The femur is then compressed slightly towards the acetabulum until the rotator cuff muscles of the hip are engaged.

3. The mechanics of the hip, pelvis and lumbosacral areas can be evaluated using this contact. The innominate and sacrum are monitored while dynamic testing of femoral movement is assessed in all planes to evaluate the rotator cuff muscles and position of the femur. Forces should be applied in a slow, steady manner to load the tissues.

4. Innominate movement can then be assessed by monitoring the sacroiliac joint and using the femur as a lever.

5. A stacking technique is employed to establish balanced tension. The femur is then taken through its various positions: internal and external rotation, adduction and abduction, and compression and decompression, while the innominate, sacrum and lumbosacral junction are monitored. Once the femur is positioned in balanced tension, the innominate is moved through anterior and posterior rotation, inflare and outflare as the responses at the sacrum and lumbosacral junction are monitored to establish balanced tension. Finally, the balanced tension is fine-tuned by addressing the sacrum and lumbosacral junction.

6. Once balanced tension is achieved, the position is maintained until a correction in the mechanical strain or an improvement in tissue function is noted.

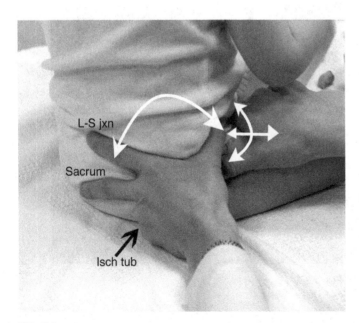

Fig. 5.4

CONDITIONS OF THE FEMORAL HEAD AND EPIPHYSIS

DEVELOPMENTAL DYSPLASIA OF THE HIP (DDH)

Clinical Notes

Developmental dysplasia of the hip is a condition of newborns and infants involving a posterior dislocation of the hip. In most cases the condition is not related to a neuromuscular disorder or syndrome and is called typical DDH. When the dislocation is associated with an underlying congenital condition it is called teratologic DDH. Teratologic DDH usually occurs in utero and is truly a congenital condition. Typical DDH usually occurs after birth or during delivery in a hip that is unstable. DDH appears to be more common in first-born children, presumably because the cervix and vaginal tissues are less compliant and increase the stress on the immature hip.

The structures of the hip in typical DDH are normal in the newborn period except for increased laxity in the ligamentum teres and articular capsule, and a change in the shape of the acetabulum. This is especially true if the fetus was in a breech position or the baby presented in breech. Fetuses in frank breech or breech positions during the last trimester are at greater risk of developing hip instability owing to the excessive adduction and flexion of the hip.

The flexed position stretches the lax posterior capsule and exposes the posterior aspect of the femoral head. In addition, movement of the hips is limited in the breech position, and this interferes with the normal development of the acetabulum. DDH can be associated with metatarsus adductus, congenital torticollis, and general ligamentous laxity. There is also a familial association.

During the neonatal period DDH is usually diagnosed on physical examination. Hip instability can be detected by using the Barlow test, which stresses the posterior components of the hip. If the hip is dislocatable, the femoral head moves posteriorly and returns to its original position when the clinician's force is released. The Ortolani maneuver can be used to correct or diagnose a dislocated hip. If the hip is dislocated, the clinician will feel a 'clunk' as it relocates as opposed to a 'click'. A 'click' may indicate muscular imbalances around the hip joint, or in some cases mild ligamentous laxity due to mechanical strain. In infants, DDH may present as delayed sitting, crawling, or even walking. In ambulating children DDH may present as limping, a waddling gait or toe walking. On physical examination there may be restricted hip abduction, asymmetrical skin folds around the buttocks or hips, or a leg length discrepancy. The Ortolani maneuver is not effective in older infants and toddlers and the Barlow test may be equivocal. Diagnosis is confirmed by ultrasonography in young infants and newborns. Frog-leg views on plain X-ray can be used in older infants and toddlers.

ASSESSMENT OF DEVELOPMENTAL HIP DYSPLASIA

Barlow Test (Fig. 5.5)

1. The newborn is supine. The physician stabilizes the pelvis by contacting the ilium and pubes on the side to be tested, and then grasps the leg to be tested by flexing the knee and contacting the lower leg and femoral shaft.

2. The hip is flexed and abducted. A posterior force is placed through the femur. The physician notes whether the femoral head translates posteriorly. Then the force is removed and the physician notes whether the femoral head returns to its initial position.

3. A positive test occurs when the femoral head is displaced posterior and returns to position.

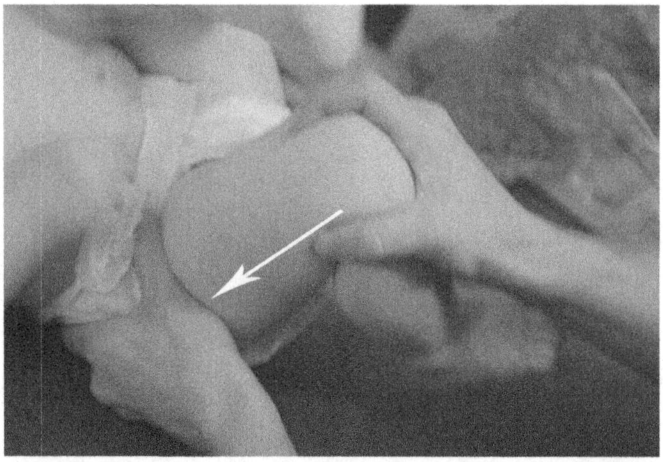

Ortolani Maneuver

1. The infant is supine. The physician contacts the leg by flexing the knee and grasping the lower leg and femoral shaft. The fingers wrap around the hip to contact the femoral head posteriorly (Fig. 5.6).

2. The hips are flexed and abducted as the femoral head is lifted anteriorly (Fig. 5.7).

3. A dislocated hip will make an audible and palpable 'clunk' as it is reduced. A softer 'click' may be felt in hips with somatic dysfunction.

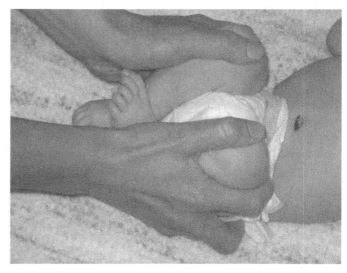

Fig. 5.6

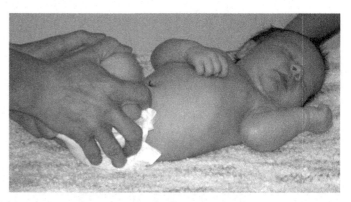

Fig. 5.7

Fig. 5.5

Treatment Notes

Children with DDH should be treated according to stand-ard medical care. In infants less than 6 months of age this involves reducing the femur in the acetabulum. This is done by stabilizing the femur in a flexed and abducted position to promote tightening of the articular capsule and ligaments. Various methods of accomplishing this include use of a Pavlik harness, a Frejka splint or other abduction device. In very young neonates these devices are often too large, so double or triple diapering is used in the first few weeks. After 6 months many infants with DHH require surgical closed reduction. Older infants and toddlers with DDH are at severe risk for developing deformities of the femoral head and acetabulum. They often require open reduction and osteotomy. The most common complication of DDH is avascular necrosis of the capital femoral epiphysis. This usually occurs as a result of compromise of the epiphyseal vessels due to reduction of the femoral head. Children between 4 and 6 months are more at risk for developing areas of necrosis and abnormal growth owing to the vulner-ability of the femoral head.

Osteopathy may be beneficial as an adjunct treatment to address mechanical and somatic strains that are influencing the condition. As mentioned in the chapter overview, intra-osseous strains of the composite innominate will influence the shape of the acetabulum and the relationship of the lig-aments and articular capsule. The long and short restrictor muscles are involved in joint stabilization and movement. Mechanical strains of the composite sacrum or between the sacrum and the innominate will influence their function. Malformations or malpositions of the lower leg and foot have the potential to affect resting tone and function of the quadriceps and hamstring groups, which also play a role in hip function.

In the presence of an equivocal Ortolani or Barlow test and normal joint ultrasound, somatic dysfunction of the short restrictor muscles and fasciae of the hip is the most likely diagnosis. Balancing techniques may be used to address the mechanical dysfunction. All indirect techniques to the hip, sacrum, pelvis and leg are contraindicated in these children.

BALANCED LIGAMENTOUS TECHNIQUE

Rotator Muscles of the Hip

Long Lever Technique

Supine Infant

In this technique the forces are applied into the soft tissue structures, not the articulation.

1. The infant is supine. The physician sits beside the hip to be treated. One hand is placed under the pelvis to stabilize the innominate and sacrum (Fig. 5.8). The fingers contact the PSIS, sacrum (S) and ischial tuberosity (IT). The thumb of this finger contacts the greater tuberosity of the femur (white arrow).

2. The other hand grasps the shaft of the femur as superiorly as possible (Fig. 5.9).

3. The physician will use a stacking method to achieve balanced tension. The physician applies a slow steady compression through the femur into the surrounding

tissues of the hip until there is a slight change in tissue texture.

4. Gentle forces are then introduced into the tissues of the femur and innominate to encourage them into their respective mechanical positions, taking care to stay well within the midpoint of permitted motion. Internal and external rotation, flexion and extension are introduced into the femur. At the same time, anterior and posterior rotation and inflare and outflare are introduced into the innominate.

5. The innominate is positioned to establish balanced tensions in the surrounding myofascial structures. A direct approach is used to establish the balanced tension. An indirect approach is contraindicated in infants and toddlers with hip dysplasia.

6. Once balanced tension is established, the position is maintained until there is a change in tissue texture, a correction of the strain pattern or an improvement in function.

7. Intraosseous strains in the composite innominate, if present, need to be addressed at this time.

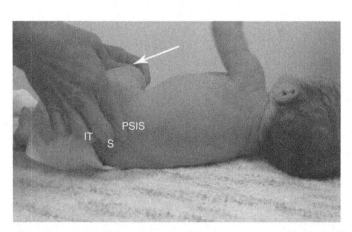

Fig. 5.8

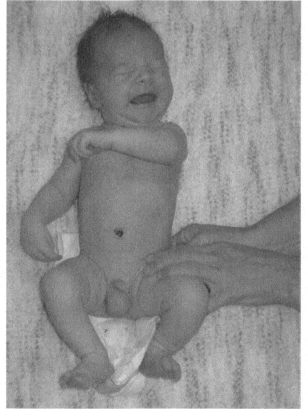

Fig. 5.9

BALANCED LIGAMENTOUS TENSION TECHNIQUE

The Composite Hip Joint

Supine Infant

1. The infant is supine. The physician uses one hand to contact the superior aspect of the innominate. The index finger contacts the anterior superior iliac spine and the middle finger contacts the pubic ramus. The remainder of the hand contacts the femur. The superior aspect of the femur is palpated with the thumbs. (In the infant, the greater trochanter may not be distinctly palpable.) The thumbs are positioned at the approximate level of the long axis of the femoral neck (Figs 5.10 and 5.11).

2. The other hand contacts the posterior aspect of the innominate with a finger placed on each part of the composite bone: the anterior and posterior superior iliac spines and the ischial tuberosity, similar to that in the description for composite hip joint seated toddler.

The thumb contacts the femur. Contact is also made with the sacrum.

3. The forces within the three parts of the composite bone should resolve at the center of the acetabulum in the Y-shaped epiphysis. The axis through the femoral neck and head should align with the center of the Y-shaped epiphysis.

4. Gentle balancing and molding techniques are applied to address any stresses or strains palpated within this system. Once balanced tension is established, the physician maintains that position until a correction in the mechanical strain or improvement in tissue function is noted.

5. The goal of the technique is to resolve somatic stresses that may be contributing to or exacerbating hip instability, femoral head epiphyseal ischemia, degenerative changes in articular cartilage or epiphyseal microtrauma. This approach may be employed in children with internal or external fixation devices. However, greater emphasis is placed on the molding component of the technique.

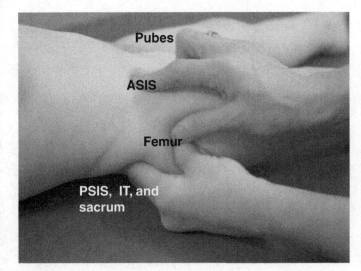

Pubes

ASIS

Femur

PSIS, IT, and sacrum

Fig. 5.10

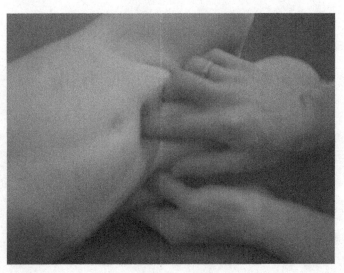

Fig. 5.11

PERSISTENT FEMORAL ANTEVERSION

Clinical Notes

Under normal conditions, once the child begins walking, the tensile forces in the anterior aspect of the articular capsule of the hip and the hip rotator muscles increase. These forces mold the femoral neck so that the femur moves into a more lateral position. This, coupled with the triradiate growth of the acetabulum and pelvis, moves the hip into a retroverted position with the femur facing slightly laterally. In some children, femoral anteversion may persist due to malposition or malformation of the acetabulum, abnormalities of muscle tone or abnormal mechanical forces on the acetabulum or femur. Normal molding of the femoral neck is a mechanical event that can be inhibited by ligamentous contractures, spasticity or mechanical imbalances in the surrounding muscles. Restrictions in the iliopsoas, pectineus and adductor longus muscles can interfere with molding of the femoral neck. Certain positions, such 'W' sitting and sleeping prone with the legs and feet tucked underneath, place the femur in internal rotation and encourage anteversion.

The older child with persistent anteversion will compensate by intoeing and generating a valgus position at the knee. Some children will develop a condition called miserable malalignment syndrome, a series of compensatory adaptations that result in femoral anteversion, an externally rotated tibia with an internal torsion, genu valgus with medially placed patella, and pronation of the subtalar joint. In the standing position, children with miserable malalignment syndrome present with an abnormal appearance of the limb, such as 'kissing patellae', patellae that face each other when the child is standing, and the 'bayonet sign', an acute angulation at the medial aspect of the knee. This abnormal posturing places significant stress on the patella, hip and foot. The problem may arise as an adaptation to femoral anteversion or severe foot pronation. In either case children with this condition are predisposed to degenerative changes in the knee and hip in later life.

There is a significant difference between mechanical restriction of the hip due to functional muscle imbalance and mechanical restriction due to anteversion, although the two often exacerbate each other. Femoral anteversion can be seen on plain X-ray; functional malposition cannot.

Assessing Femoral Anteversion

Child/Athlete

1. The child is prone, with the hip extended and the knees flexed (Fig. 5.12). The physician stands either beside the table or at the foot of the table.

2. The physician compares internal rotation of the hip by moving the child's feet laterally, and external rotation by moving the feet so they cross the body's midline.

3. The range of motion should be bilaterally symmetrical. The anteverted hip will usually assume a more lateral position of the foot (Fig. 5.13) and resist movement of the foot across the midline (external or lateral movement of the femur).

4. Restriction of hip rotator muscles may produce a false positive. Hip rotator muscles should be evaluated and treated as described below, after which femoral position is reassessed.

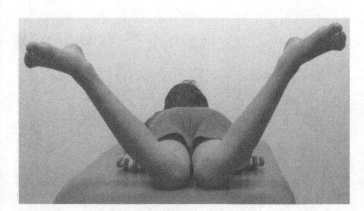

Fig. 5.12

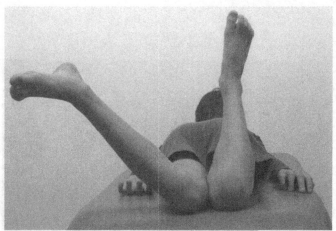

Fig. 5.13

Assessing Femoral Rotation

Child/Adolescent

This is done with the patient supine and the hip and knee extended. Hip flexion (sitting) creates laxity in the anterior hip capsule.

1. The child is supine. The physician stands at the feet. Each ankle is grasped inferiorly and the legs are lifted to approximately 15°. This places the hips in a neutral position. (The hips are in an extended position when the patient is supine.)

2. The physician internally rotates the legs, noting when motion occurs at the innominate (Fig. 5.14).

3. The position of the feet may also be compared. However, dysfunction below the knee, such as tibial rotations and foot malpositions, will distort the findings as they relate to the hip.

4. Internal (Fig. 5.14) and external rotation (Fig. 5.15) of the legs are compared for symmetry. The total degrees of internal and external rotation will change as the femurs move into a retroverted position. In spite of this, the range and quality of motion should be bilaterally symmetrical for each position.

5. A femur that demonstrates greater internal rotation and less external rotation is said to be 'in internal rotation' or 'internally rotated'. A femur that demonstrates greater external rotation and less internal rotation is said to be 'in external rotation' or 'externally rotated'.

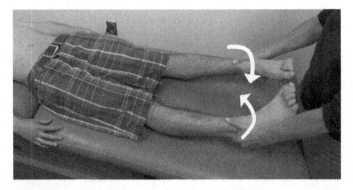

Fig. 5.14

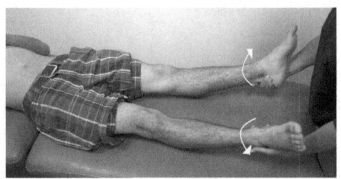

Fig. 5.15

Treatment Notes

Femoral anteversion may be due to congenital malformation or functional mechanical influences. Surgery may be necessary in severe cases of malformation, but in most children conservative treatment is used. Imbalances in the associated musculature need to be addressed. Isometric and isotonic muscle energy techniques can be used in older children to address resting muscle length, strength and firing patterns. Balanced ligamentous techniques can be used to correct fascial and ligamentous dysfunction. Isolytic muscle energy techniques, articular techniques and joint mobilization may be needed in young athletes to correct restricted joint motion. Children should be encouraged to avoid postures such as 'W' sitting that reinforce the anteversion. In most cases, however, the child is choosing these postures because they are most comfortable. Correction of the mechanical dysfunction will often facilitate normal sitting and sleeping postures. Exercises and activities that reinforce core stabilization and postural mechanics need to be added to the treatment regimen in addition to normal play and sports. The activity should be chosen with the child and parents and be appropriate to the child's interests and capabilities. Activities that can achieve the desired end and also be enjoyable include martial arts, horseback riding, yoga, Pilates and some forms of dance. I find that many children, especially boys, brighten up considerably at the suggestion of martial arts. The key component to using martial arts as rehabilitation in children is to find an instructor who is more concerned with form than force. Many of my patients, including those with spasticity and hypotonia, have benefited immensely from karate training with a knowledgeable and kind instructor.

Persistent anteversion and other hip problems that involve the femur–hip–pelvis complex may arise as a secondary compensation to dysfunction in sacropelvic mechanics. Malalignment of the sacroiliac joint can occur due to mechanical dysfunction of the sacrum, the innominate or the associated muscles. Positional strains of the sacrum and innominate will alter sacroiliac mechanics by limiting motion in one or the other bone. Intraosseous sacral strains alter sacroiliac mechanics by changing the articular relationship on the sacral side of the joint. This affects the axis of motion and creates asymmetry of the sacroiliac joints, a not uncommon finding in cadaveric specimens. Intraosseous strains of the composite innominate affect the sacroiliac joint through the sacroiliac ligaments. The joint is located completely in the ilium, but the suspensory and stabilizing ligaments span the posterior aspect of the composite, inserting on the ischial tuberosity. Ligamentous influences may also affect the sacroiliac joint through the interdigitation of the iliolumbar ligaments with the superior bands of the sacroiliac ligament (Fig. 5.16).

When evaluating and treating any problem of the hip in a non-ambulating child, the sacroiliac joint, the rotational and mediolateral mechanics of the innominate, and the long and short restrictors of the hip can all play a role in maintaining or exacerbating the condition. These areas all have the potential to affect the hip joint itself. In addition, the influences of the knee and foot as well as the center of gravity will play an important role in an ambulating child.

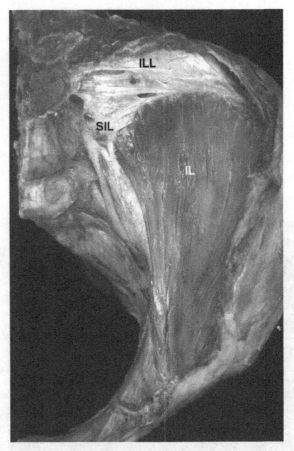

Fig. 5.16 • Anterior view of the right side of a bisected pelvis. The iliopsoas muscle (IL), iliolumbar ligament (ILL) and anterior sacroiliac ligament (SIL) are labeled.

ISOMETRIC MUSCLE ENERGY TECHNIQUE

Functional Malposition of the Femur

Internal Rotation

Child

This technique is performed in the supine position with the hip and knee extended to protect the ligaments of the knee. It should not be performed using the prone posture described to assess femoral position.

1. The patient is supine with the hips and knees extended. The physician may stand ipsilateral or contralateral to the leg to be treated (Fig. 5.17). In this example the left leg is being treated.

2. The leg is contacted on the femur and rotated externally (black arrow) to the restrictive barrier.

3. The child is instructed to turn his leg (or knee, not the foot) towards his other leg (medially, white arrow). The physician resists the child's motion with an equal and opposite force.

4. This isometric contraction is maintained for 4–5 seconds. Then the child is told to stop turning the leg as the physician reduces her force.

5. The physician maintains the position for 4–5 seconds until a change in tissue tension at the hip is perceived. Then the physician externally rotates the leg to the new restrictive barrier.

6. The sequence is repeated twice.

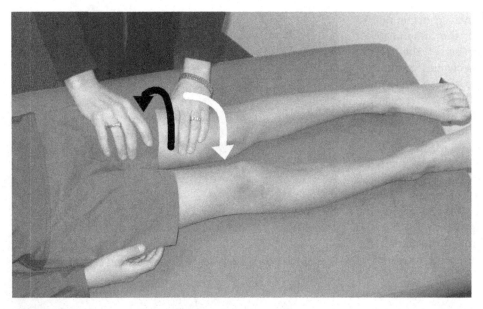

Fig. 5.17

ISOMETRIC MUSCLE ENERGY TECHNIQUE

Functional Malposition of Femur

External Rotation of the Femur (Fig. 5.18)

Child

This isometric muscle energy technique is performed in the supine position with the hip and knee extended to protect the child's ligaments. It should not be performed using the prone posture described to assess femoral position. The technique may be used to address piriformis restriction as well as restriction in the gluteal complex and the quadratus femoris muscle.

1. The patient is supine with the hips and knees extended. The physician stands ipsilateral to the leg to be treated.

2. The leg is contacted just proximal and distal to the knee and gently rotated internally to engage the restrictive barrier (Fig. 5.18).

3. The child is instructed to turn his leg towards the physician (white arrow). The physician resists the child's motion with an equal and opposite force (black arrow).

4. This isometric contraction is maintained for 4–5 seconds. The child is then told to stop turning the leg as the physician reduces her force.

5. The physician maintains the position for 4–5 seconds until a change in tissue tension at the hip is perceived. Then the physician internally rotates the leg to the new restrictive barrier.

6. The sequence is repeated twice.

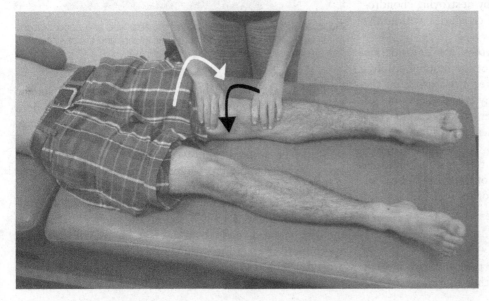

Fig. 5.18

LEGG–CALVÉ–PERTHES' DISEASE

Clinical Notes

Legg–Calvé–Perthes' disease is an idiopathic condition of children involving delayed maturation of and disturbed circulation to the capital femoral epiphysis. It often presents as a limp in boys between the ages of 5 and 8 years. The child may complain of pain and stiffness in the hip, knee or ankle. Symptoms are usually intermittent, and the child may have periods when they are completely symptom free. The classic findings on physical examination are limited internal rotation, extension and abduction of the femur. Tenderness may or may not be present. Leg lengths may be uneven in the supine position.

Legg–Calvé–Perthes' mainly involves the epiphysis, which becomes ischemic. The resulting inflammation causes a synovitis. In severe cases the epiphysis becomes necrotic, which can affect the femoral head, resulting in deformation. Deformation of the femoral head predisposes the child to osteoarthritis as an adult. The primary disease process does not appear to be neoplastic or inflammatory, and in the majority of cases there is no historical or temporal relationship with trauma. Although a disturbance in epiphyseal circulation is present, it is unclear whether this is an associated finding or a contributing factor. The vascular system of the femoral epiphysis is fairly unique. The vessels arise from the somatic tissues of the metaphysis and then enter the articular capsule to penetrate into the epiphysis. Consequently, they are vulnerable to compression along that journey. Furthermore, from an osteopathic perspective one must consider the role of increased or abnormal compressive forces acting on the epiphysis. Wolff's law states that bone will remodel according to the forces to which it is exposed. However, repetitive compressive forces may impede normal growth mechanisms by destroying chondrocytes or causing tamponade of the capillaries within the growth plate.

The hallmarks of Legg–Calvé–Perthes' are deformation of the femoral head and destruction of the femoral epiphysis. The severity of the disease is categorized based on the quantity of involvement of the epiphysis and the extent of deformity of the femoral head, as seen on radiographs (Figs 5.19 and 5.20). In early or mild cases, plain films may be negative and diagnosis requires MRI or bone scans. There are several classifications in use, but in general, children with deformation of more than 50% of the femoral head or 75% of the epiphysis have a worse prognosis.

Treatment Notes

The goals of treatment are to reduce pain, improve motion and, most importantly, prevent further deformity of the

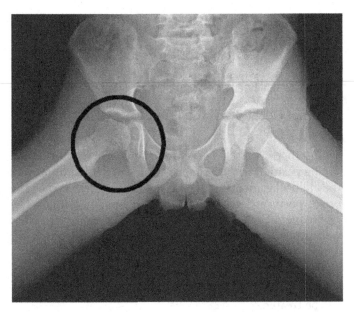

Fig. 5.19 • X-ray. Sclerosis of the epiphysis is present. The femoral head is relatively intact.

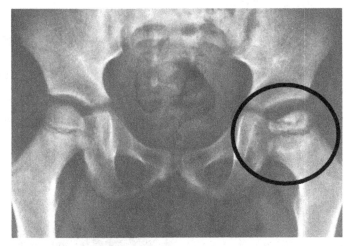

Fig. 5.20 • X-ray. Severe sclerosis of the epiphysis and degeneration of the femoral head. The femoral head is inferior and the child may well present with a long right leg when supine.

femoral head. In children without severe disease and no femoral head involvement, standard medical treatment involves complete rest and no weightbearing until symptoms improve and the synovitis resolves. Occasionally, traction may be applied. Non-weightbearing range of motion exercises in an aquatic program may be beneficial for these children. Children with significant femoral head involvement require containment of the femoral head to control development. This is based on the theory that seating the femoral head correctly in the acetabulum will create the appropriate contact forces to stimulate normal growth. The procedures used to establish this positioning include abduction casts and various osteotomy surgeries. The recovery period in children with significant disease can be quite long; older children with more than 50% femoral head involvement may require repeated casting for 2 or more years after surgery.

Osteopathic manipulative treatment of children with mild to moderate Legg–Calvé–Perthes' disease should be directed at improving motion in the hip, normalizing biomechanical dysfunction that may be contributing to the disease process, and improving circulation. The concept of chronic low-grade biomechanical dysfunction adversely influencing normal bony development is important for the overall treatment plan. At the time of initial presentation the pain of the synovitis may produce reflex contractions, tender points and trigger points of the short restrictor hip stabilizers, whereas the long restrictors are being influenced by compensatory weightbearing adaptations. However, in the context of the disease process these strains represent chronic biomechanical dysfunctions that contribute to the degenerative process. The somatic dysfunction may play a role in maintaining and perhaps exacerbating the underlying problem. Somatic dysfunction of the short restrictor muscles and the articular dysfunctions of the sacroiliac, innominate and knee may respond to indirect or balancing techniques. Direct techniques should be avoided in the hips, pelvis, and lower extremities in children with Legg–Calvé–Perthes' disease.

SLIPPED CAPITAL FEMORAL EPIPHYSIS (Fig. 5.21)

Clinical Notes

Slipped capital femoral epiphysis (SCFE) is a condition of adolescence that usually presents with insidious onset of groin pain or, more typically, knee pain that may radiate into the thigh. The pain is dull and achey and exacerbated by physical activity. Rarely is there a history of an inciting event. More often the symptoms are slow to progress and include a reduced range of motion and the development of a limp. In conditions with slow chronic development the child may present with a short leg in a markedly externally rotated and abducted position that is accentuated with walking. On physical examination there is restricted internal rotation. With passive flexion of the hip the femur may position itself into external rotation. The restriction is articular without muscle contractures. Range of motion testing may be uncomfortable but tolerable. Although in many children both hips are involved, the presentation is typically unilateral. The diagnosis of SCFE is often missed in chronic presentation until the joint integrity is significantly disrupted. In rare cases SCFE presents with acute onset. The child is unable to bear weight on the affected limb and is in

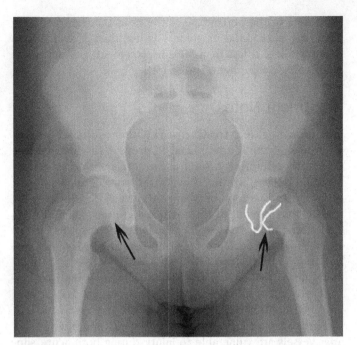

Fig. 5.21

significant pain. The pain is exacerbated by passive motion, which significantly impedes examination. There is spasm of the hip restrictors and the limb is typically positioned in external rotation and slight extension.

Slipped capital femoral epiphysis arises when the integrity of the femoral epiphysis is disrupted and the femoral head is displaced medially and posteriorly. The femoral epiphysis is vulnerable to shearing forces in adolescence because with growth of the femoral neck and pelvis it moves from a horizontal to an oblique orientation. Mechanical imbalances in the long and short hip restrictor muscles may alter the vectors of forces crossing the hip joint. Increasing body mass during times of rapid growth can place a shearing force through the obliquely oriented epiphysis. Microfractures in the epiphysis develop, disrupting the integrity of the femoral head and neck. The femoral head slips posteriorly and medially, while the femoral neck externally rotates and moves cephalad. If the vascular supply to the femoral head is compromised by the slipped position, the femoral head will become ischemic. This sequence of events places the child at risk for avascular necrosis of the femoral head and osteoarthritis of the hip.

SCFE typically presents in adolescent boys during periods of rapid growth, although females are affected as well. There is a familial predisposition, but it does not appear to be inherited. Interestingly, SCFE is more likely to occur in obese children, or in those who are tall and thin. Slipped capital femoral epiphysis is usually diagnosed by plain X-rays in a frog-leg position. CT scans may be needed in early or mild cases. SCFE is graded on a 4-point scale according to the percentage of the head that has displaced from the neck. Mild or grade 1 is less than 25% displacement, grade 2 is less than 50% displacement, grade 3 is less than 75% displacement, and so forth.

Treatment Notes

The primary goal of treatment in children with SCFE is stabilization of the femoral head to prevent vascular damage and further deformity. Surgical correction with open reduction and internal fixation is needed to prevent ossification of the head and femoral neck in an abnormal position. Owing to the vulnerability of the vasculature direct manipulation and closed reduction are contraindicated, except in a surgical setting with an acute displacement. The retinacular vessels supplying the femoral head are vulnerable to damage both during an acute slippage and during the correction.

There are two risks for the postoperative patient that must be considered: avascular necrosis and destruction of the articular cartilage. As previously mentioned, the retinacular vessels are vulnerable to injury during both acute slippage and correction. Gentle osteopathic treatment directed towards improving vascular and lymphatic circulation may

be beneficial in supporting low-pressure circulatory function in the postoperative period. Mechanical dysfunctions in the supporting tissues of the hip and pelvis may be treated using inhibition, balancing or indirect techniques to address extra-articular pain generators. In some children chondrolyis may develop as a result of an intra-articular inflammatory reaction or due to direct damage from the fixation pins. In the latter case, surgical removal of the pins is necessary. In chondrolysis due to an intra-articulatory inflammatory reaction osteopathic treatment may be a beneficial adjunct to pharmaceutical therapy. Balanced ligamentous techniques are the safest and most appropriate to use until the fixation has stabilized.

Long-term management includes rehabilitation of muscle strength, flexibility and functional relationships. Reciprocal inhibition, isotonic concentric and isotonic eccentric muscle energy techniques may be implemented to improve strength and recondition agonist/antagonist muscle relationships in the limb. Muscle energy techniques, motion against resistance and other strengthening exercises may be employed in most children once the hip is stable. If the internal fixator is still in place, the treatment is modified appropriately.

BALANCED LIGAMENTOUS TECHNIQUE

Rotator Muscles of the Hip

Long Lever Technique

Supine Athlete

1. The patient is supine with the knee on the affected side flexed. The physician sits alongside and below the affected hip, facing the patient.

2. The physician's hand furthest from the patient is placed under the innominate, contacting the femur with the thumb and the ilium and ischium with the palm and fingers. The other hand stabilizes the patient's knee as the physician uses her shoulder against the knee to flex the hip slightly (Fig. 5.22).

3. The femur is used as a long lever to assess somatic dysfunction in the myofascial tissues of the hip. The femur is distracted and compressed towards the acetabulum to evaluate flexibility at the joint. Tension in the myofascial structures is then assessed by using a stacking mechanism by which restriction and ease are noted as the femur is moved into internal and external rotation, abduction and adduction, and hyperflexion.

4. The femur is used as a long lever to achieve balance in the long and short restrictor muscles of the hip joint. This is done through a stacking mechanism. Compression is introduced through the femur until a slight slackening is felt in the tissues surrounding the hip. Excessive compression will move the innominate posterior and lock the sacroiliac joint.

5. Balanced tension in the restrictor muscles is achieved by gently introducing different vectors of motion into the hip. The femur is taken into internal and external rotation, abduction and adduction, and hyperflexion. In each position tension in the surrounding tissues is assessed for a progression towards equal tension (not least tension) throughout the myofascial system of the hip.

6. Once balanced tension is established, the position is maintained until there is a change in tissue texture, an improvement in function or a correction of the strain pattern.

Fig. 5.22

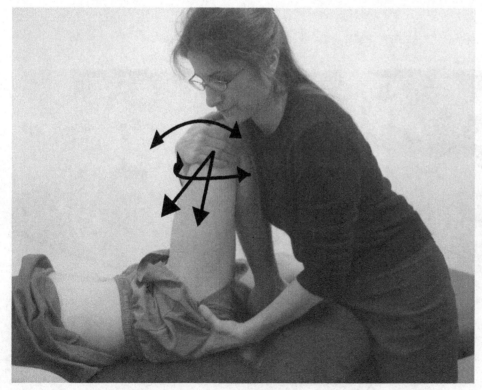

BALANCED LIGAMENTOUS TECHNIQUE

Rotator Muscles of the Hip

Long Lever Technique

Seated Toddler

1. The toddler is seated or supine with the knee on the affected side relaxed or slightly flexed. The physician sits beside the affected hip, facing the child.

2. The superior aspect of the femur is palpated. (In the young toddler, the greater trochanter may not be distinctly palpable.) The thumb is positioned at the approximate level of the long axis of the femoral neck, with the remainder of the hand holding the shaft of the femur (Fig. 5.23). The index finger of the same hand contacts the ipsilateral pubic ramus.

3. The other hand contacts the innominate with a finger placed on each part of the composite bone: the anterior and posterior superior iliac spines, and the ischial tuberosity. Contact is also made with the sacrum (Fig. 5.24).

4. The femur is used as a long lever to assess somatic dysfunction in the myofascial tissues. The femur is distracted and compressed towards the acetabulum to evaluate flexibility at the joint.

5. Tension in the myofascial structures is then assessed by using a stacking mechanism. Restriction and ease are noted as the femur is moved into internal and external rotation, abduction and adduction, and hyperflexion.

6. The femur is used as a long lever to achieve balance in the myofascial tissues of the hip joint. Compression is introduced through the femur until a slight slackening is felt in the tissues surrounding the hip. Excessive compression will move the innominate posterior and lock the sacroiliac joint.

7. Balanced tension in the restrictor muscles is achieved by gently introducing different vectors of motion into the hip. In this age group it is best to use a direct approach to find the position of balanced tension. The femur is taken into internal and external rotation, abduction and adduction, and hyperflexion. In each position, tension in the surrounding tissues is assessed for a progression towards equal tension (not least tension) throughout the myofascial system of the hip.

8. Once balanced tension is achieved, the position is maintained until there is a change in tissue texture.

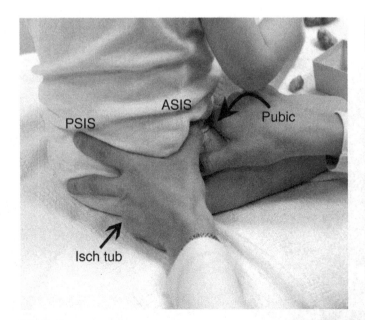

Fig. 5.23

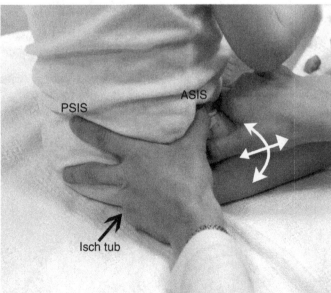

Fig. 5.24

BALANCED LIGAMENTOUS TECHNIQUE

Lumbosacral Junction, Pelvis and Hip

The Differential Technique

Seated Athlete/Older Child

This technique is useful in addressing complicated compensatory adaptation after the primary strain has been treated. It can also be used to identify the location of the primary strain when it is masked by chronic compensatory changes. When treating toddlers and infants, the balanced ligamentous technique for lumbosacral junction, pelvis and hip described at the beginning of this chapter can be used.

1. The athlete is seated upright on his ischial tuberosities, maintaining a slight lordotic curve (no slouching). The physician is seated slightly below the patient so that her feet are at the level of his knees. The physician braces the patient's feet against the lateral aspect of her knees (Fig. 5.25).

2. The physician extends the knees slightly to the point that the patient's center of gravity falls on a plane between the ischial tuberosities and his weight stabilizes the ischial tuberosities. With the ischial tuberosities stabilized, a force applied through the femur will cause the innominate to rock either anteriorly or posteriorly on the ischial tuberosity.

If the knees are extended too far, the patient's center of gravity will fall backwards behind the center of the pelvis, causing the patient to roll off the ischial tuberosities and the sacrum to counternutate.

3. The physician then motion tests the innominates and sacroiliac joint by simultaneously introducing an oppositional force through the legs into the innominate. In Figures 5.26 and 5.27 the right leg is being compressed towards the pelvis to induce a slight

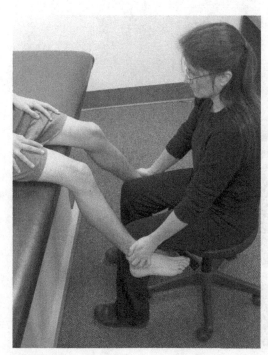

Fig. 5.25

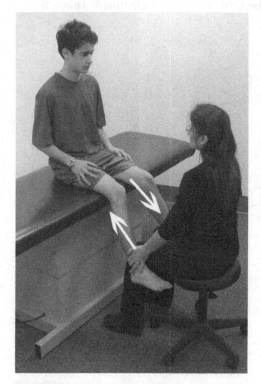

Fig. 5.26

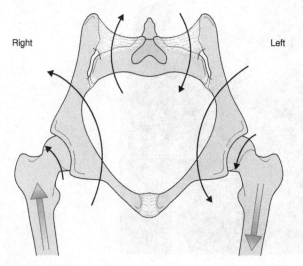

Right   Left

Fig. 5.27

posterior rotation of the innominate (R), while the left leg is being tractioned away from the pelvis to induce a slight anterior rotation of that innominate (L). When these movements are performed simultaneously the sacrum will pivot on its oblique axis. In the example, the sacrum would move anteriorly on the left and posteriorly on the right (Fig. 5.28).

4. The maneuver is repeated using opposite force vectors in each leg (Fig. 5.29). The permitted motion during the two maneuvers is compared. The maneuver that met with the least resistance is identified. This is the

position of ease. The maneuver that met with the greater resistance is the restrictive barrier.

5. The position of ease (least resistance) is reproduced and the legs are held in that position. The leg that is tractioned away from the pelvis is said to be long, whereas the leg that is compressed towards the pelvis is said to be short. In Figure 5.26 the left leg is tractioned away, so it is the long leg.

6. While the physician maintains the position of the legs, the patient is asked to turn his head and torso slowly towards the side of the long leg. In the example this is the left side. The patient must turn the torso so that the lumbar spine rotates. This will engage the sacrum. As the sacrum begins to move, the physician will sense a change in the tensions in the legs. At that moment, the patient stops turning and remains in the position (Fig. 5.30).

7. The physician then fine-tunes the placement of the legs until there is balanced tension between the hips, sacroiliac joints and lumbosacral junction.

8. Once balanced tension is achieved, the physician maintains the placement of the legs and asks the patient to slowly turn back to the neutral position. The physician lets go of the legs. On retesting, the movement of the innominates and sacroiliac joints should be symmetrical.

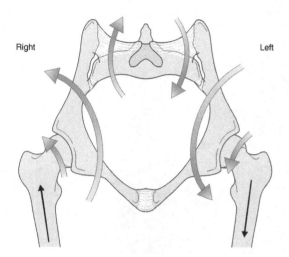

Fig. 5.28

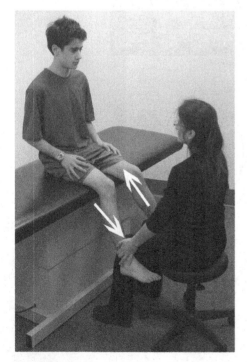

Fig. 5.29

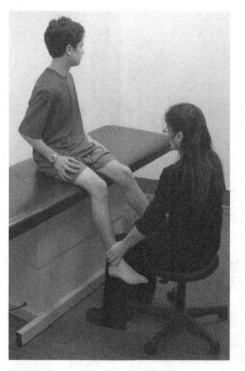

Fig. 5.30

BALANCED LIGAMENTOUS TENSION TECHNIQUE

The Composite Hip Joint

Seated Toddler

1. The toddler is seated. The superior aspect of the femur is palpated. (In the young toddler, the greater trochanter may not be distinctly palpable.) The thumb is positioned at the approximate level of the long axis of the femoral neck, with the remainder of the hand holding the shaft of the femur (Fig. 5.31). The index finger of the same hand contacts the ipsilateral pubic ramus.

2. The other hand contacts the innominate with a finger placed on each part of the composite bone, the anterior and posterior superior iliac spines, and the ischial tuberosity. Contact is also made with the sacrum (Fig. 5.32).

3. The forces within the three parts of the composite bone should resolve at the center of the acetabulum in the Y-shaped epiphysis. The axis through the femoral

neck and head should align with the center of the Y-shaped epiphysis.

4. Gentle balancing and molding techniques are applied to address any stresses or strains palpated within this system. Rotation and flaring are introduced into the innominate as rotation, compression, distraction, adduction and abduction are introduced into the femur. As the force vectors of these motions are introduced into the tissues, the bone is not necessarily moved.

5. Once balanced tension is achieved, the physician maintains that position until a correction in the mechanical strain or improvement in tissue function is noted.

6. The effectiveness of this technique decreases in older children. The goal of the technique is to resolve somatic stresses that may be contributing to or exacerbating hip instability, femoral head epiphyseal ischemia, degenerative changes in articular cartilage or epiphyseal microtrauma. This approach may be employed in children with internal or external fixation devices. However, greater emphasis is placed on the molding component of the technique.

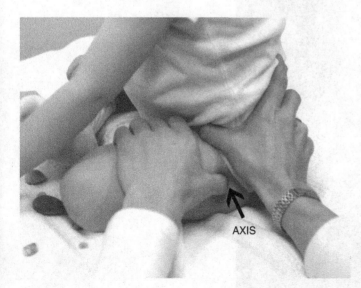

Fig. 5.31

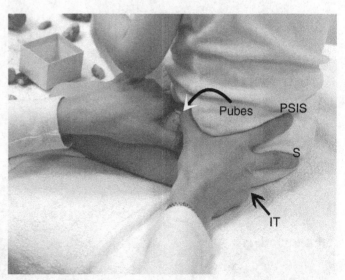

Fig. 5.32

BALANCED LIGAMENTOUS TENSION TECHNIQUE

The Composite Hip Joint

Side-lying Athlete

1. The athlete is lying on the unaffected side with the hips and knees flexed to stabilize the pelvis. The clinician sits beside and behind the patient's legs so that she can contact the anterior and posterior landmarks of the innominate (Fig. 5.33).

2. The greater trochanter (GT) is located and the thumbs are placed just inferior to it, at the approximate level of the long axis of the femoral neck (asterisk). The hands are positioned so that all three parts of the innominate composite bone are contacted. The ileum is contacted through the anterior and posterior superior iliac spines, the ischium through the ischial tuberosity and the pubic bone via the pubic ramus.

3. The forces within the three parts of the composite bone should resolve at the center of the acetabulum in the Y-shaped epiphysis. The axis through the femoral neck and head should align with the center of the Y-shaped epiphysis.

4. Gentle balancing and molding techniques are applied to address any stresses or strains palpated within this system.

5. The effectiveness of this technique decreases in older children. The goal of the technique is to resolve somatic stresses, which may be contributing to or exacerbating femoral head epiphyseal ischemia, degenerative changes in articular cartilage or epiphyseal microtrauma. This approach may be employed in children with internal or external fixation devices. However, greater emphasis is placed on the molding component of the technique.

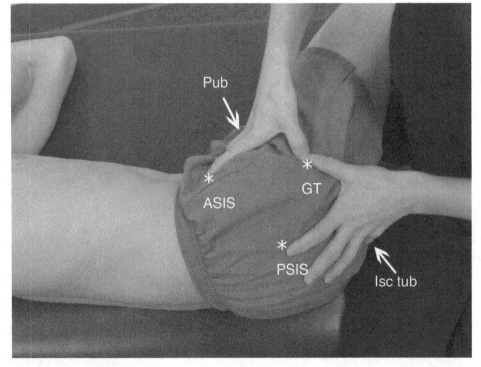

Fig. 5.33

FLUID TECHNIQUE

Hip

Side-lying Athlete/Supine Infant

This technique is used to encourage intravascular and extravascular fluid movement in the structures of the hip. Osteopathic treatment should be used as an adjunct to standard medical care in children with conditions of the femoral head or epiphysis. This approach may be useful when there is edema or effusion in the hip. For the best results this technique should be employed after musculoskeletal strains and imbalances in the lumbosacral, pelvic and hip mechanism have been addressed.

1. The child is supine or laterally recumbent. The physician places her thumbs over the greater trochanter and then uses the fingers of both hands to contact the composite parts of the innominate on the involved side. A gentle fluid fluctuation is initiated using one of two methods.

2. The first method requires the physician to create a lateral fluctuation across the epiphysis using alternating pressures from either side (Fig. 5.34). The second method (Fig. 5.35) is accomplished by alternating the pressures between the thumbs, which are over the greater trochanter (white arrow), and the two hands (black arrows). The method is chosen according to the child's response.

3. The same hand contact and methods can be used in an infant (Fig. 5.36, black and white arrows, or Fig. 5.37).

4. Once the fluctuation begins, the physician observes it through several cycles until the amplitude begins

to weaken. Then the physician gently discourages the fluctuation by introducing a resisting force in the direction of the fluctuation.

5. This continues until the fluctuation subsides and there is a still point. The tissues are allowed to resume normal function without any input from the clinician.

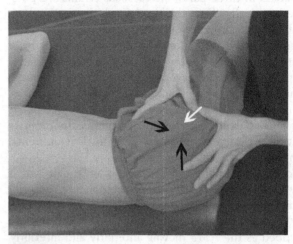

Fig. 5.35

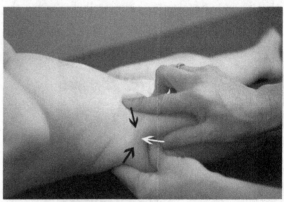

Fig. 5.36

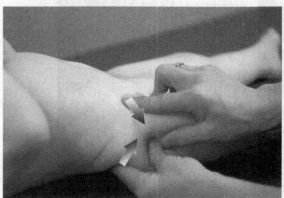

Fig. 5.37

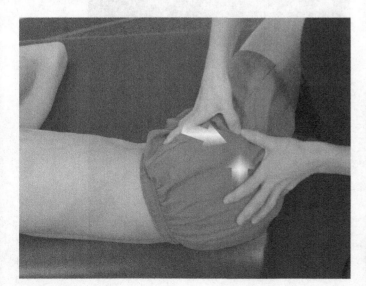

Fig. 5.34

INNOMINATE DYSFUNCTIONS

Clinical Notes

Innominate dysfunctions play an important role in the development of conditions of the hip and leg. Because the innominate is in three parts, intraosseous strains are possible. These typically affect the hip through the acetabulum, rather than the sacroiliac joint. Intraosseous and interosseous innominate dysfunctions can develop as primary or secondary conditions. Innominate dysfunction can alter muscle resting length and agonist–antagonist coordination, affect the gait cycle, create functional leg length differences, contribute to foot and knee abnormalities, influence pelvic stability and contribute to spinal conditions. Innominate dysfunctions in infants may interfere with developmental milestones, especially sitting and standing.

Physiologic innominate motion occurs with gait and is typically described as having two components: anterior and posterior rotation around a transverse axis that passes through the sacroiliac joint (Fig. 5.38). Anterior rotations are described as the ASIS moving anteriorly and inferiorly, as though the innominate were rotating clockwise on the transverse axis (Fig. 5.39). Posterior innominate rotations describe the innominate rotating counterclockwise on the

transverse axis (Fig. 5.40). Medial and lateral flaring occur around a vertical axis that passes through the iliac blade (Fig. 5.41). The medial and lateral flaring are defined by convention as medial flare or inflare when the ASIS moves

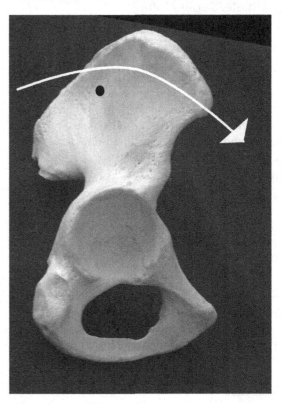

Fig. 5.39

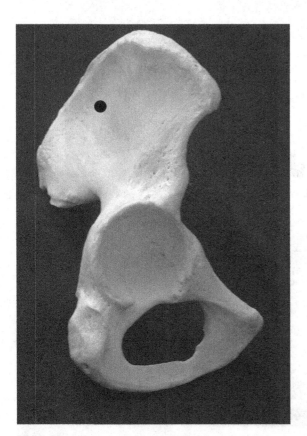

Fig. 5.38

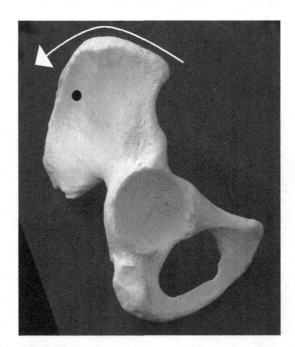

Fig. 5.40

medially and the PSIS moves laterally (Fig. 5.42), versus lateral flare or outflare when the ASIS moves laterally and the PSIS moves medially (Fig. 5.43). These four motions are physiological because they are components of normal gait. Posterior rotation is accompanied by lateral movement or outflare during the swing phase of gait. Anterior rotation is accompanied by medial or inflare during stance and toe-off.

Innominate dysfunctions can also be unphysiological. In this case, they usually involve translation in a caudad or cephalad direction. Caudad translation of the innominate is called downslipped and cephalad translation is called upslipped. These strains are usually traumatic and quite symptomatic, producing pain in the hip, sacroiliac region or back. Leg length difference may be due to strains of the innominate, especially vertical and rotation dysfunctions.

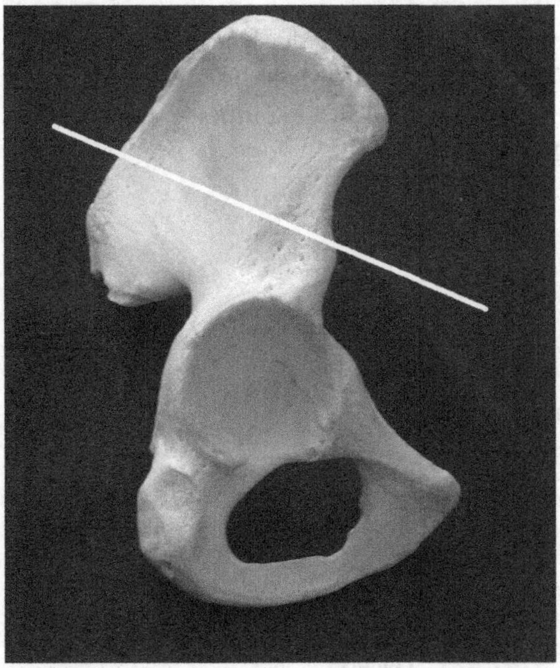

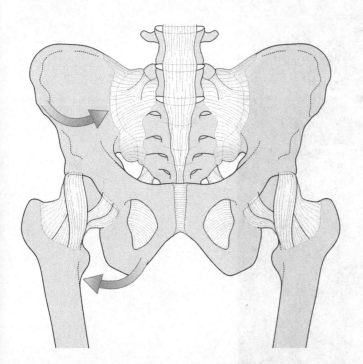

Fig. 5.41

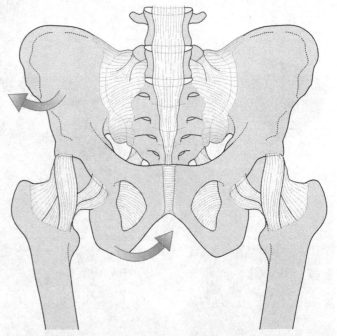

Fig. 5.42 • Schematic diagram of an inflare dysfunction of the left innominate. The anterior iliac spine moves medially as the ischial tuberosity moves laterally.

Fig. 5.43 • Schematic diagram of an outflare dysfunction of the left innominate. The anterior iliac spine moves laterally as the ischial tuberosity moves medially.

Assessment of the Innominate Position

Young Athlete

Static

Innominate dysfunctions can be diagnosed using static or dynamic criteria. Static analysis is based on three pieces of information: the laterality of the standing flexion test, and the positions of the ASIS and PSIS on the ipsilateral side to the positive standing flexion test. Diagnosis may also be made based on the innominate's response to passive motion testing.

Standing Flexion Test (Fig. 5.44)

This test is used to detect the presence and laterality of an innominate dysfunction. The positions of the ASIS and PSIS are then assessed to determine the axis and direction of movement of the innominate.

1. The patient stands facing away from the physician. The physician contacts the posterior superior iliac spines (PSIS) and positions herself so that they are at eye level.

2. The patient is instructed to slowly bend forward, as though he was going to touch his toes.

3. The PSIS which moves first or farthest is the side of the dysfunction.

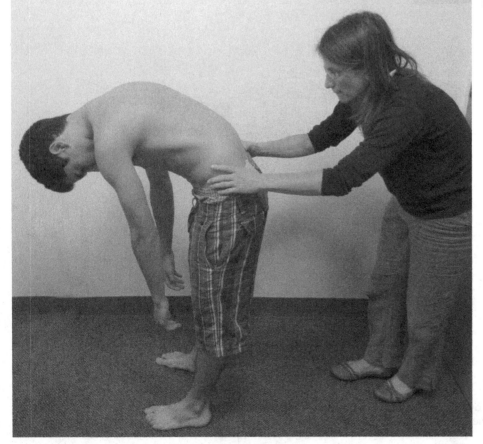

Fig. 5.44

Static Assessment Anterior Superior Iliac Spines (Fig. 5.45)

Young Athlete

1. The patient is supine. The physician stands beside the patient with her dominant eye over the midline of the patient's body. The physician locates the anterior superior iliac spines (ASIS) with the thumbs.

2. The thumbs slide over the ASIS to rest just below the inferior aspect of the prominences. The two sides are compared (Fig. 5.45).

3. In the figure, the left ASIS appears to be more superior and lateral than the right. The actual side of dysfunction is determined by the standing flexion test. In this patient, the standing flexion was positive on the right, so the right ASIS is actually inferior and medial. This is a static test of the position of the innominate.

4. The physician then assesses the position of the PSIS to determine the dysfunction of the innominate.

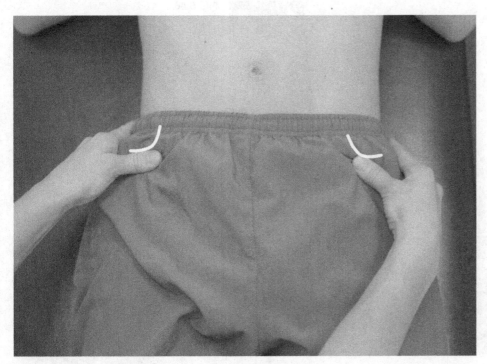

Fig. 5.45

Static Assessment Posterior Superior Iliac Spines (PSIS)

Young Athlete

1. The patient is prone and the physician is standing beside the patient with her dominant eye over the midline of the patient's body. The physician locates the posterior superior iliac spines (PSIS) with the thumbs.

2. The thumbs slide over the PSIS to rest just below the inferior aspect of the prominences. The two sides are compared (Fig. 5.46).

3. In the figure, the right PSIS appears to be more superior and lateral than the right. The actual side of dysfunction is determined by the standing flexion test. In this patient, the standing flexion test was on the right, so the right side is superior and lateral.

4. This information is combined with the information from assessment of the ASIS gathered previously.

5. In this example, the static diagnosis is anterior rotated innominate with slight inflare.

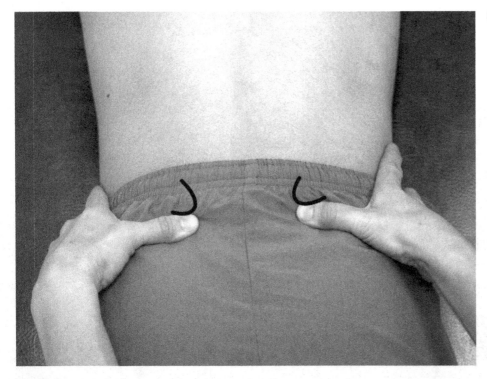

Fig. 5.46

Assessment of the Innominate

Supine Athlete

The physician can perform dynamic testing by evaluating passive motion mechanics and tissue response.

1. The patient is supine. The physician is standing beside the patient with her dominant eye over the midline of the child's body. The physician contacts the innominates bilaterally by placing the palm of her hand over the ASIS and her fingers along the iliac crest, curling around the superior aspect of each innominate (Fig. 5.47).

2. The innominates are motion tested by introducing a posterior lateral force into the left innominate and an anterior medial force into the right innominate. This creates a posterior rotation and lateral flare of the left innominate and an anterior rotation and medial flare of the right innominate (Fig. 5.48).

3. The quality of the response of the tissues and the restrictive barrier is noted.

4. The physician repeats the maneuver alternating the sides so that the left innominate is rotated anteriorly and flared medially and the right innominate is rotated posterior and flared laterally. Again the quality of the tissue response and the restrictive barriers is noted.

5. In this patient the greatest freedom of motion and least tissue resistance are found in posterior rotation of the left innominate (Figs 5.47 and 5.48).

6. An anterior innominate will move more freely in anterior rotation and resist posterior rotation, and vice versa. An inflared innominate will have greater freedom of motion in anterior rotation and inflare. Inflare and outflare dysfunction can be assessed more precisely by increasing the degree of flare and decreasing the degree of rotation when the force is introduced.

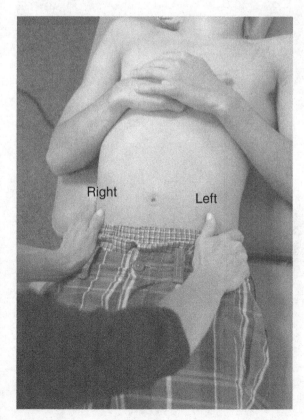

Fig. 5.47

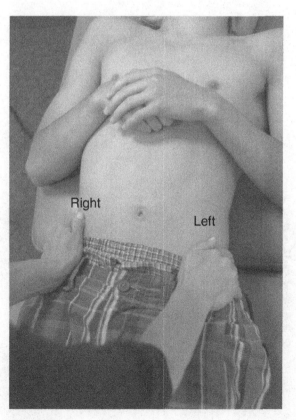

Fig. 5.48

Assessment of the Innominate

Seated Toddler

1. The child is seated on the treatment table facing away from the physician. The physician sits behind the child. The anterior superior iliac spine (ASIS) and the posterior superior iliac spine (PSIS) are contacted with the thumb and fingers of each hand (Fig. 5.49).

2. The child is allowed to play. The degree of accommodation of each innominate bone to the child's active movement is noted. This is active motion testing.

3. Passive motion testing requires that one innominate be stabilized while the other side is assessed. During normal gait each innominate moves into anterior rotation with some degree of inflare, and posterior rotation with some degree of outflare. All four planes of motion should be assessed.

4. In the figure the left innominate bone is stabilized to assess passive motion in the right. The right innominate is gently rotated anteriorly and posteriorly to assess rotational movement (Fig. 5.50). The right innominate is then taken into the positions of inflare and outflare to assess medial and lateral movement (Fig. 5.51). Passive movement on the right is compared to passive movement on the left. It should be symmetrical.

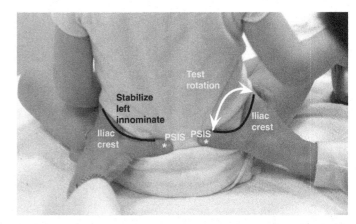

Fig. 5.50

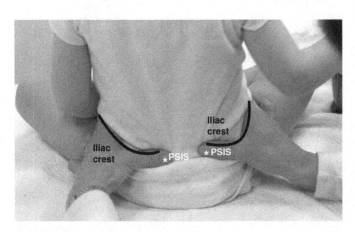

Fig. 5.49

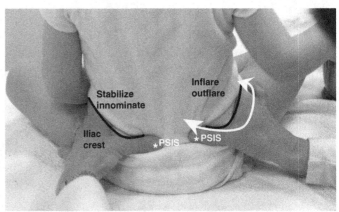

Fig. 5.51

Assessing Femoral–Hip–Pelvic Relationship

Seated Toddler

1. The child is seated. The physician sits beside the patient. The innominate and sacrum are held with one hand. The thumb contacts the anterior superior iliac spine with the remainder of the hand grasping the posterior innominate and sacrum. The index finger monitors the thoracolumbar junction. The other hand holds the femur (Fig. 5.52).

2. The mechanical relations between the innominate and femur are assessed. The innominate is rotated posteriorly with lateral flare as the femur is internally rotated. The quality and quantity of movement between the two bones at the hip joint is noted. Concurrently, the response at the sacrum and thoracolumbar junction is monitored to determine whether compensatory adaptations are occurring.

3. The findings are compared with the opposite side. There should be symmetry of quality and quantity of motion, and the compensatory response at the sacrum and thoracolumbar junction. Asymmetries may be due to dysfunction of the femur, the intraosseous composite innominate, the innominate or sacrum at the sacroiliac joint or the intraosseous sacrum.

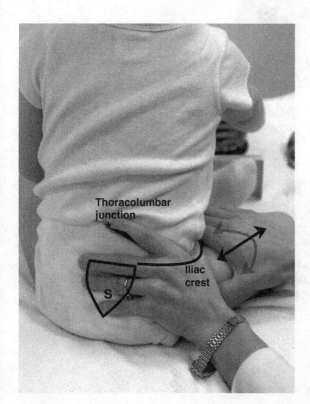

Fig. 5.52

Assessment of the Innominate

Supine Infant

1. The infant is supine. The physician grasps each innominate, contacting the anterior superior iliac spine, the posterior iliac blade and the ischial tuberosity. One finger of each hand is placed on the sacrum (Fig. 5.53).

2. Movement of the innominate at the sacroiliac joint is observed with normal respiration and the voluntary movements of the child.

3. Passive motion is induced by simultaneously rotating one innominate anteriorly and the other posteriorly (Fig. 5.54, white arrows). The procedure is repeated in the opposite direction. Range and quality of motion at the sacroiliac articulation are noted.

4. The hands are then repositioned slightly inferiorly so that the thumb contacts the pubic ramus, and the ilia and ischia are contacted with the other fingers.

5. Involuntary movement of the composite parts is monitored for intraosseous strains.

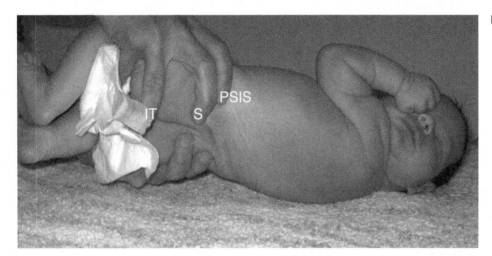

Fig. 5.53

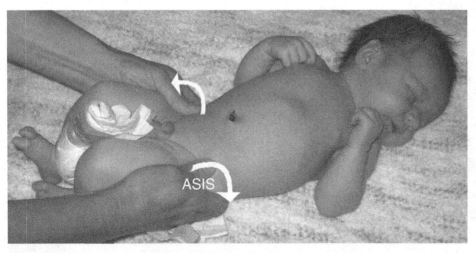

Fig. 5.54

Treatment Notes

Innominate dysfunctions play a role in conditions of the hip, pelvis, sacrum, back and leg. They can be primary or secondary. In newborns with breech presentation or abnormal lie innominate dysfunctions tend to be primary. In an ambulating child with an innominate dysfunction that appears to respond to treatment only temporarily, leg length difference should be ruled out. Children may have a functional or structural leg length difference. Occasionally in children with functional leg length differences, lift therapy can be employed temporarily to address the innominate dysfunction.

ISOTONIC MUSCLE ENERGY TECHNIQUE

Anterior Rotated Innominate

Supine Athlete/Child

This approach is used if the anterior rotation is primarily a result of quadriceps tension. The knee flexor muscles are engaged to rotate the innominate posteriorly.

1. The patient is supine. The physician sits beside the patient ipsilaterally and below the innominate to be treated (Fig. 5.55).

2. The physician flexes the hip and places the patient's foreleg on her shoulder. The hip is then flexed even more to rotate the innominate posteriorly to the restrictive barrier at the sacroiliac joint.

3. The child is instructed to push his leg (bend his knee) into the physician's shoulder (black arrow). The physician resists the motion and monitors for engagement of the innominate (Fig. 5.55, straight white arrow).

4. The knee is prevented from flexing but the innominate is not restricted from moving.

5. This isotonic contraction is maintained for 4–5 seconds. Then the patient is asked to cease contraction while the physician simultaneously rotates the innominate to reposition it to the new barrier (curved white arrow).

6. The sequence is repeated twice.

Fig. 5.55

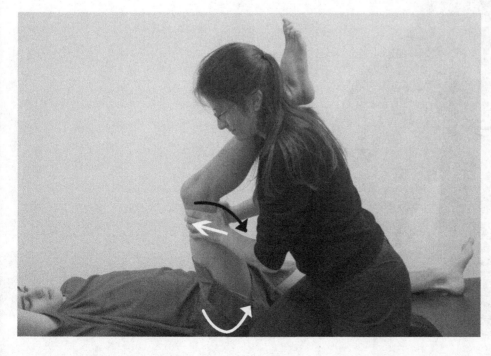

RECIPROCAL INHIBITION/ ISOMETRIC MUSCLE ENERGY TECHNIQUE

Anterior Rotated Innominate

Supine Athlete/Child

Anterior innominate rotations typically occur due to quadriceps or psoas tightness. This isometric approach is used to address the articular strain at the sacroiliac joint and the myofascial component.

1. The patient is supine. The physician sits beside the patient ipsilaterally and below the innominate to be treated.

2. The physician flexes the hip and places the patient's leg against her shoulder (Fig. 5.56). The hip is then flexed to rotate the innominate posteriorly to the restrictive barrier at the sacroiliac joint. The other hand monitors the sacroiliac joint.

3. The child is instructed to push his leg into the physician's shoulder (black arrow). The physician resists the motion and monitors for engagement of the innominate (white arrow).

4. This isometric contraction is maintained for 4–5 seconds, then the patient is asked to cease contraction while the physician simultaneously reduces her counterforce.

5. The physician maintains contact and waits for tissue relaxation (approximately 4–5 seconds).

6. The physician posteriorly rotates the innominate to reposition it to the new barrier (curved white arrow). The sequence is repeated twice.

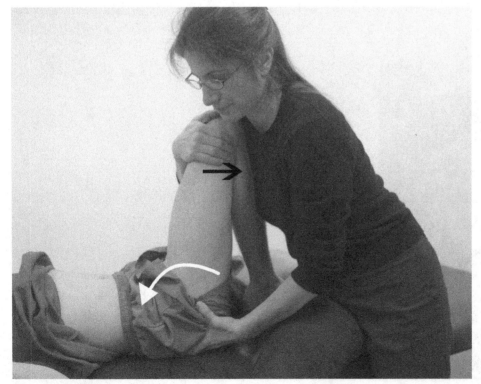

Fig. 5.56

ISOTONIC/RECIPROCAL INHIBITION

Anterior Rotated Innominate

Supine Athlete/Child

This isotonic approach is used to address the articular strain at the sacroiliac joint and the myofascial component of the iliopsoas and hip flexors. The gluteal muscles and hip extensors are used in this approach.

1. The child is supine. The physician sits beside the patient ipsilaterally and below the innominate to be treated.

2. The physician contacts and monitors the innominate with the hand closest to the child's head. The other hand contacts the upper leg just above the knee and flexes the child's hip to posteriorly rotate the innominate to the restrictive barrier (Fig. 5.57).

3. The child is instructed to push his leg towards the table or into the physician's hand (white arrow). The physician resists the motion (straight black arrow) and monitors for engagement of the innominate.

4. The hip is prevented from extending, but the innominate is free to move.

5. This isotonic contraction is maintained for 4–5 seconds, then the patient is asked to cease contraction while the physician relaxes her counterforce.

6. The physician maintains contact and waits for tissue relaxation (approximately 4–5 seconds). Then the physician uses the femur as a long lever to rotate the innominate posteriorly to reposition it to the new barrier (curved black arrow).

7. The sequence is repeated twice.

Fig. 5.57

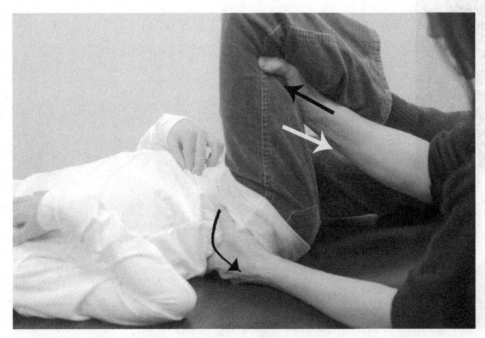

ISOMETRIC MUSCLE ENERGY TECHNIQUE

Posterior Rotated Innominate

Prone Athlete

1. The patient is prone with the knee flexed. The physician stands on the ipsilateral side and grasps the knee from the medial side of the leg. The patient's foot rests against her shoulder. This stretches the quadriceps group. The other hand is placed on the posterior aspect of the affected innominate at the upper pole of the sacroiliac joint and the iliac crest (Fig. 5.58).

2. The patient is instructed to push his leg towards the table (straight white arrow). The physician resists movement at the knee and hip (straight black arrow).

3. This isometric contraction is maintained for 4–5 seconds, then the patient is asked to cease contraction while the physician simultaneously reduces her counterforce.

4. The physician maintains contact and waits for tissue relaxation (approximately 4–5 seconds).

5. The physician anteriorly rotates the innominate using the femur to reposition it to the new barrier (large curved white arrow). The sequence is repeated twice. The innominate motion is then re-evaluated.

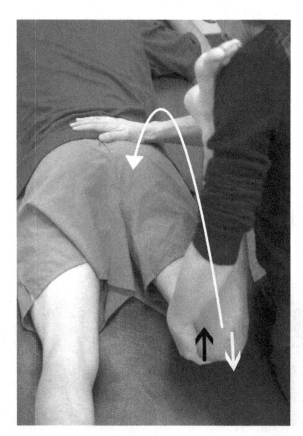

Fig. 5.58

ISOTONIC MUSCLE ENERGY TECHNIQUE

Posterior rotated innominate

Supine Older Child

1. The child is supine. The physician sits beside the child on the affected side. The physician uses the hand closest to the child's head to contact the innominate. The fingers contact the posterior surfaces (PSIS and blade) and the thumb contacts the ASIS. The physician uses the other hand to contact the child's anterior thigh (Fig. 5.59).

2. The physician monitors the innominate and drops the leg on the affected side off the table to engage the restrictive barrier to anterior rotation of the innominate.

3. The physician asks the child to lift his leg towards the ceiling. The physician resists the child's motion with an equal and opposite force until the restrictive barrier is engaged.

4. The physician asks the child to relax, and as he is relaxing she gently increases the extension of the hip and anterior rotation of the innominate to the restrictive barrier.

5. The sequence is repeated twice, and the innominate motion is then re-evaluated.

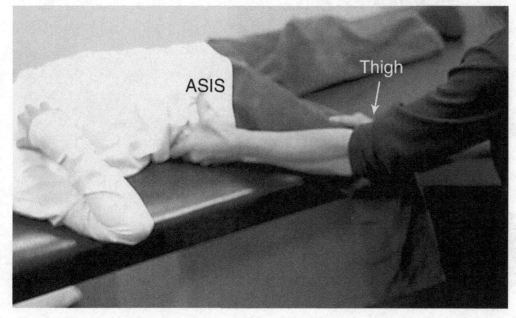

Fig. 5.59

ISOTONIC CONCENTRIC MUSCLE ENERGY TECHNIQUE

Inflare Innominate

Supine Young Athlete/Child

1. The patient is supine. The physician stands beside the patient ipsilaterally and below the innominate to be treated (Fig. 5.60).

2. The physician flexes the patient's knee and places the ankle on the contralateral leg. This externally rotates and abducts the hip and places the innominate in a position of outflare.

3. The child is instructed to lift his knee into the physician's hand (white arrow). The physician resists the motion and gently increases her pressure, which causes the child to increase the strength of his contraction (black arrow). The contraction of the adductors and internal rotators carries the innominate laterally. The physician stabilizes the contralateral innominate.

4. This isotonic contraction is maintained for 4–5 seconds. Then the patient is asked to cease contraction while the physician simultaneously reduces her counterforce.

5. The physician maintains contact and waits for tissue relaxation (approximately 4–5 seconds).

6. The physician then outflares the innominate to reposition it to the new barrier by pushing down on the knee (curved white arrow). The sequence is repeated twice.

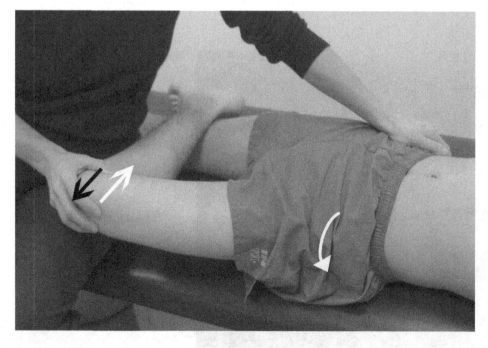

Fig. 5.60

ISOMETRIC MUSCLE ENERGY TECHNIQUE

Outflare Innominate

Supine Young Athlete/Child

1. The patient is supine. The physician stands beside the patient ipsilaterally and below the innominate to be treated (Fig. 5.61).

2. The physician flexes the patient's hip and knee and places the knee against her shoulder. The other hand uses a posterior contact to monitor the innominate (Fig. 5.62). The femur is then adducted to inflare the innominate to the restrictive barrier.

3. The child is instructed to push the knee laterally against the physician (white arrow). The physician resists the motion.

4. This isotonic contraction is maintained for 4–5 seconds. The patient is then asked to cease contraction while the physician simultaneously reduces her counterforce.

5. The physician maintains contact and waits for tissue relaxation (approximately 4–5 seconds).

6. The physician then adducts the femur while using the hand contacting the innominate to carry it to the new restrictive barrier (white arrow on innominate).

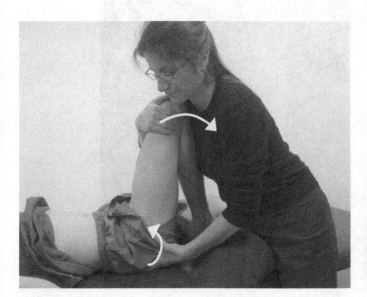

Fig. 5.61

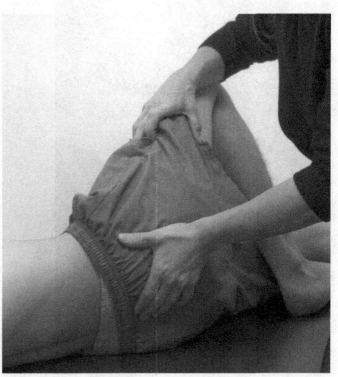

Fig. 5.62

BALANCED LIGAMENTOUS TECHNIQUE

Innominate

Standing Young Athlete

In addition to chronic primary dysfunction, this technique is especially useful in treating traumatic injuries to the pelvis, such as those that produce upslipped or downslipped innominate dysfunctions.

1. The athlete is standing sideways with his hand on a supporting table or countertop. The physician is seated facing the side of the patient. One hand is placed under the ischial tuberosity and the other grasps the anterior superior iliac spine (ASIS). The thumbs contact the femur. A firm contact is made (Fig. 5.63). Care is taken that the patient's back remains straight with no rotation.

2. The athlete is asked to unload the sacroiliac joint by crossing the ipsilateral leg across the opposite leg and rest the foot on the ground. The physician resists any movement of the innominate through the contacts on the tuberosity and ASIS (Fig. 5.64). It may be necessary for the physician to stabilize the hand contacting the tuberosity by leaning her elbow on her knee.

3. The patient is then asked to slowly bend the leg he is standing on until the physician feels the sacroiliac joint disengage (Fig. 5.65). The patient is told to hold this position.

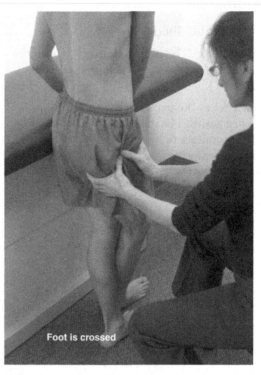

Foot is crossed

Fig. 5.64

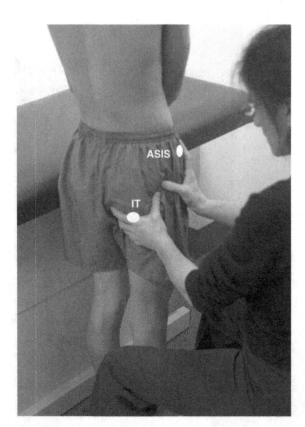

Fig. 5.63

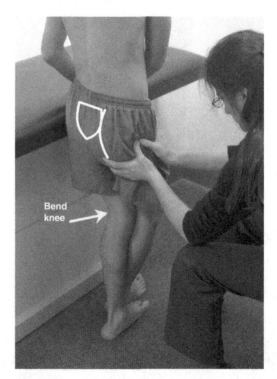

ASIS

IT

Bend knee →

Fig. 5.65

4. The physician then finds balanced tension in the pelvis and sacroiliac joint by using a combination of innominate movements: anterior and posterior rotation, medial and lateral flare, and cephalad and caudad positioning (Fig. 5.66). Balanced tension is maintained until there is an improvement in tissue function or a correction of the mechanical strain.

5. The physician holds the position of the innominate as the patient slowly straightens his leg. Then he is asked to uncross the legs so that equal weight is on both.

6. The technique should be performed on both innominates.

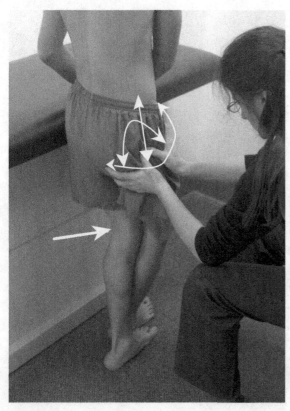

Fig. 5.66

BALANCED LIGAMENTOUS TECHNIQUE

Innominate and Pelvic Bowl Dysfunction

Seated Toddler

1. The child is seated on the treatment table facing away from the physician. The physician is seated behind the child (Fig. 5.67). Both innominates and the sacrum are contacted with both hands. The fingers contact the anterior superior iliac spines (ASIS), and the thumbs are placed across the posterior superior iliac spines (PSIS) and onto the sacrum. The remainder of the hand contacts the iliac crest.

2. The innominates are taken in opposite directions using the hands and fingers (Fig. 5.68). For example, the right innominate is anteriorly rotated as the left is externally rotated, or the right is inflared as the left is outflared. The thumbs control movement of the sacrum to accommodate the innominate position.

3. Balanced tension is established between the sacrum and innominates and within the tissues of the pelvic bowl.

4. Once balanced tension is achieved, the physician maintains that position until a correction in the mechanical strain or improvement in tissue function is noted.

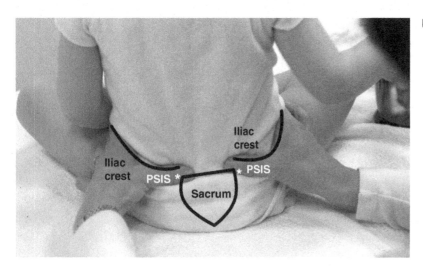

Fig. 5.67

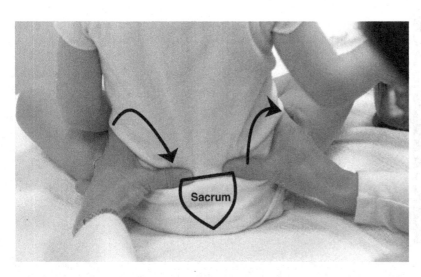

Fig. 5.68

BALANCED LIGAMENTOUS TECHNIQUE

Innominate/Pelvic Bowl

Supine Infant

1. The infant is supine. The physician contacts the ASIS bilaterally with the thumbs. Posteriorly, contact is made with the PSIS, the ischial tuberosity and the sacral base, similar to the hold used to assess innominate motion (Fig. 5.69). Alternatively, one hand can be used to contact both innominates and the sacrum posteriorly as the other hand bridges the ASIS across the lower pelvis anteriorly.

2. The physician uses a stacking method to introduce slow, steady forces into the two innominates and the sacrum to produce rotation and flaring of the innominates and rotation on the oblique axis of the sacrum to achieve balanced tension.

3. Often balanced tension will be found with the innominates rotated and flared in opposite directions and the sacrum nutated slightly on the side of the anterior innominate (Fig. 5.70).

4. Once balanced tension is achieved, the position is maintained until a change in tissue texture, a correction of the somatic dysfunction or improvement in motion mechanics is perceived.

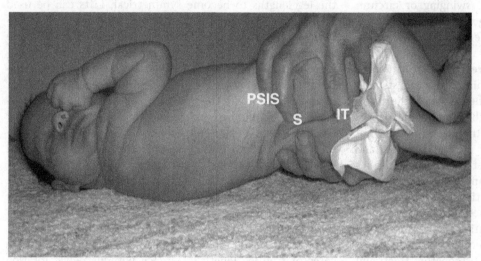

Fig. 5.69

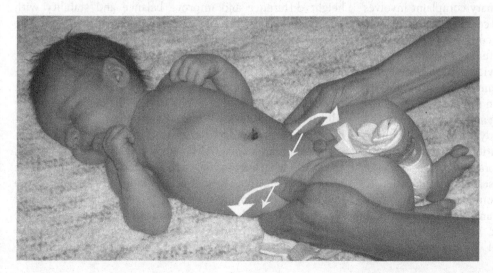

Fig. 5.70

LEG LENGTH DISCREPANCY AND LIFT THERAPY

Clinical Notes

Leg length differences are not uncommon in children. They may be structural and due to discrepancies in tibial or femoral growth or persistent femoral anteversion, or functional and due to muscle imbalances and increased resting tone. Functional leg length discrepancies appear to arise during periods of rapid growth. Although many resolve spontaneously, many trigger compensatory adaptations in the limb and lumbar spine which in themselves may contribute to or exacerbate musculoskeletal conditions. This is especially true in young athletes. Children will compensate for a leg length discrepancy by shifting the center of gravity, toe-walking, flexing the opposite knee, swinging or circumducting the opposite leg, or vaulting over the opposite leg (Song 1997). There is increased mechanical work at the knee and hip.

Leg length discrepancies may correct with treatment of muscle imbalances and articular strains; this suggests that the asymmetry is compensatory and functional. If the asymmetry returns, it may be because the muscle imbalances are of a more chronic nature and retraining is required, or because rotation in the pelvis is the primary problem and is maintaining the leg length asymmetry, or because the leg length difference has a structural component and the child is overcompensating. Whether functional or structural, if leg length equality cannot be sustained, lift therapy should be implemented to avoid the creation of compensatory adaptations. In some children, especially young athletes, a lift may be used as an adjunct to osteopathic treatment of functional leg length discrepancy until muscle and gait retraining are completed. If the primary complaint involves the spine, lift therapy is used to correct the unleveling of the sacral base. If the primary complaint involves the limb, the lift is used to correct the femoral heights. Unless the child has a hemipelvis, the pelvic rotation is typically compensatory and exaggerates or sometimes distorts the leg length difference. The pelvic rotation needs to be corrected with manipulation, muscle retraining and lift support.

A plain film standing postural study X-ray with a plumbline reference will reveal pelvic rotation and the heights of the iliac crest, sacral base and femoral head. These are all useful pieces of information, but a scanogram is needed to determine the true leg lengths. In some cases the legs may be of equal length but the femurs and tibiae are unequal. This creates a much distorted gait, with significant rotation and torque in the pelvis and lumbar spine. Pelvic rotation may produce the appearance of an inferior iliac crest and sacral base on the side ipsilateral to the short leg and low femoral head. If significant pelvic rotation is present, a scanogram is needed to assess the legs.

In most children with leg length discrepancies the somatic dysfunction should be treated first and then the level of response should be assessed. If the asymmetry and pelvic dysfunction resolves their length discrepancy is most likely functional. The child should resume normal activities and be followed up in 1 week. Depending on the degree of pelvic dysfunction and leg length difference that has returned on follow-up, a standing postural study should be done to ascertain pelvic rotation, sacral base, iliac crest and femoral head unleveling. There are several parameters to consider when using a lift in growing children, especially those who have entered puberty. In children who have not finished growing, there is still an opportunity for the leg lengths to become symmetrical. Lifts can be used as an adjunct to osteopathic treatment to correct mechanical adaptations and strains that can influence growth. Some authors believe that lift therapy should be reserved for children with differences greater than 1.5 cm. I think that postural stability and balance mechanisms are a better indicator of the need for lift therapy than the actual height difference. Lifts should be employed as an adjunct to osteopathic treatment and muscle retraining whenever postural instability is related to the leg length difference, regardless of whether it is functional or structural.

The use of the lift is based upon several parameters, the most important of which is postural stress testing. If lift therapy corrects the leg length difference but creates postural instability, it is not therapeutic. The degree of pelvic compensation will alter the child's response to the lift. In cases of true leg length difference without pelvic rotation and diagnosed by scanogram, the lift should correct for the height difference and improve balance and stability with postural stress testing. When pelvic rotation is present, the lift height is determined by a combination of the sacral base unleveling and postural stress testing. In many children, with continued osteopathic treatment and muscle retraining, the pelvic compensation resolves. This will change the postural study and the height of the lift will need to be adjusted. In children with tibial and femoral height disparity, lift therapy should be employed to address gait mechanics rather than stance. Although the leg lengths are equal, the stride length from heel strike to toe-off and the degree of pelvic tilt differ. Toe-off occurs later on the side of the long femur, prolonging the swing phase of the contralateral leg. As the leg with the short femur moves into swing phase the ipsilateral pelvis needs to elevate to avoid dragging the foot. The leg with the short femur begins toe-off earlier.

POSTURAL STRESS TESTING

Functional Balance

1. The child stands with feet hip width apart and the arms abducted to shoulder level. The physician stands either directly behind or in front of the child. Balance and stability are tested using each arm independently.

2. The physician places a hand over one of the child's arms just above the elbow (Fig. 5.71). The child is instructed to resist the physician's downward force (black arrow). The physician says, 'Don't let me push your arm down.'

3. As the physician pushes down on the arm, the placement of the feet, pelvis and torso is noted. The physician then repeats the procedure on the other arm, noting any differences in posturing or balance mechanisms.

4. In Figure 5.71 the child has good stability while stressing the left arm, but stressing the right arm (Fig. 5.72) results in adaptations in foot and pelvic placement (white circle).

5. A child with instability due to a leg length disparity, sacral unleveling or pelvic compensation will demonstrate significant asymmetry in the balance strategies used to stabilize the arm. Depending upon the associated problem, the child may supinate the foot, translate the pelvis and/or rotate and side-bend the torso on the ipsilateral side. In some children the arm will collapse owing to their inability to stabilize the body.

6. The child is asked to drop the arms to his sides and a lift is placed under the foot of the short leg or side of instability with stress. In this example there is instability when the right arm is tested, so the lift is placed under the right foot. Usually two or three lifts within a range of 4–8 mm are compared.

7. The procedure is repeated. With the proper lift in place, the child should show symmetrical balance strategies and improved ability to resist the physician's pressure (Fig. 5.73).

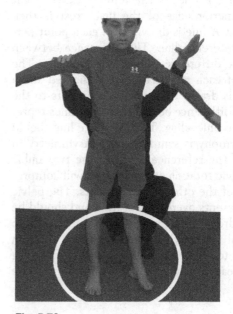

Fig. 5.72

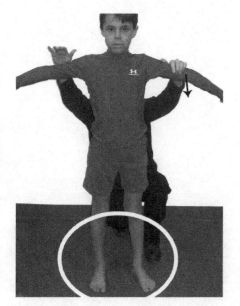

Fig. 5.71

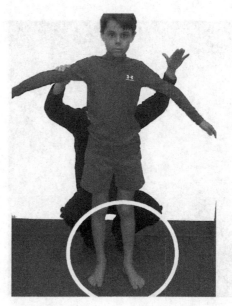

Fig. 5.73

POSTURAL STUDY

A postural study is a radiographic study used to assess sacral base leveling, pelvic rotation, iliac crest heights and femoral head heights. The study is performed by asking the child to stand in front of a plumb-line aligned with the vertical midline of the body. The X-ray is taken with an anterior posterior projection (Fig. 5.74). The plumb-line acts as a reference line. The most superior aspect of the femoral heads is identified bilaterally and marked. A line is drawn from each point perpendicular to the reference line. The difference between the lines is the femoral head height difference. The superior edge of the iliac crest is then identified bilaterally. A line is drawn from each point perpendicular to the reference line. The difference between the two lines is the difference in iliac crest heights. The superior junction of each sacroiliac joint is marked and a perpendicular line is drawn from these two points to the reference line. The difference between the two lines represents the sacral base unleveling. The reference line should bisect the pubic symphysis symmetrically. Asymmetry in the relationship of the reference line and the two pubic rami represents pelvic rotation or torsion and will compromise the accuracy of the other measurements. The pelvic rotation often represents overcompensation and should be addressed. In children, scanograms may be necessary to ascertain the actual leg length difference. Pelvic rotation can be so severe as to create the appearance of a short leg (inferior femoral head, iliac crest and sacrum) on the side of the long leg.

STRESS FRACTURES

Clinical Notes

In young athletes, repetitive activities may lead to microstresses at the transitional area between the epiphysis and the diaphysis of a bone. Transitional areas also exist at the insertion of ligaments, tendons and muscles on the bone. With repeated stress, macrofailures develop. In bone these are called stress fractures, and in connective tissue they result in sprains, strains and ruptures. In either case, the tissue is responding to the abnormal load placed on it. In most cases this abnormal load is a result of a combination of altered mechanics and repetitive stress. Typically, this is a biomechanical issue involving either joint mechanics, muscle tone or firing patterns. Treatment should be focused on correcting joint mechanics, removing fascial restrictions, balancing resting length of muscles and retraining movement patterns.

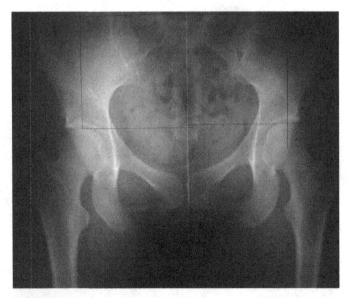

Fig. 5.74

APOPHYSEAL AVULSION FRACTURES AND ENTHESOPATHIES

Clinical Notes

The apophyses are ossification centers responsible for circumferential growth in bones. They develop after birth, and in some cases do not emerge until early puberty. As cartilaginous growth centers they are vulnerable to trauma and excessive muscular forces.

Apophyseal avulsion fractures are more common in adolescent boys between 14 and 17 years of age. They are also more common in the hip and pelvis, because of the significant number of apophyses that serve as the insertion sites for the large, long restrictor muscles of the hip and knee, such as the iliopsoas, quadriceps and adductor groups. In many young athletes these long restrictor muscles are stronger than their bony anchors, which are still growing. The ossification centers are subjected to excessive tensile forces of muscles contracting and stretching during activities that require rapid stops, starts and turns. This is especially true if the athlete is wearing cleated footwear.

Athletes with avulsion fractures typically present acutely with localized pain and swelling. There is point tenderness to palpation and a restricted range of motion. Active motion is painful, as is passive stretch and contraction against resistance. Avulsion fractures are usually visible on plain X-ray, although in some cases a bone scan needs to be performed.

In contrast to avulsion fractures, enthesopathies occur when there is derangement of the ligament or periosteum at the site of attachment. This affects the presenting pain pattern. Whereas an avulsion fracture will tend to present with pain localized to the site of injury, because enthesopathies involve the ligament and periosteum the pain pattern is often diffuse and may refer to the associated muscle. For example enthesopathy of the straight head of the rectus femoris on the anterior inferior iliac spine refers into the deep belly of the muscle and the knee. Enthesopathies are typically not visible on plain film radiographs and require a bone scan or MRI for diagnosis.

The most common sites for avulsion fractures and enthesopathies in the pelvis are the anterior superior and inferior iliac spines, the ischial tuberosity and the iliac crest. In many cases the same mechanical stress that might result in a muscle strain in a mature athlete may produce an avulsion fracture or enthesopathy in a teenager.

Treatment Notes

Treatment of acute avulsion fractures and enthesopathies initially involves rest and ice. The limb should be positioned to maximally reduce stretch in the involved muscle. Indirect techniques may help to alleviate pain generators in surrounding tissues and to improve vascular and lymphatic circulation. Gentle passive range of motion exercises may be introduced to tolerance. Once the pain improves the patient should move to active range of motion. Once full range of motion is re-established, strengthening and firing rehabilitation needs to be initiated. These exercises can initially be enhanced by the application of isometric and then isotonic muscle energy techniques. Additionally, activities that reinforce the functional relationships of the limb, such as stationary cycling and aquatic therapy, should be part of the rehabilitation program. Return to full competition needs to be delayed until normal strength and functional capabilities are achieved.

Occasionally, enthesopathies and avulsion fractures will go undiagnosed resulting in chronic muscle adaptations, persistent pain generators and, in extreme cases, instability. In these cases, trigger point injection may need to be employed to address chronic pain generators. In the most severe cases, prolotherapy at the site of the enthesopathy may need to be considered.

ILIAC APOPHYSITIS

Clinical Notes

Iliac apophysitis is an inflammation of the apophysis of the iliac crest caused by repetitive microtrauma. It typically develops as a result of increased tensile forces at the insertion of the tensor fascia latae or external oblique muscles. Iliac apophysitis is an overuse condition more commonly seen in young athletes who are engaged in running sports, although it can also be seen in downhill skiers, dancers and gymnasts. The pain usually develops gradually as a deep ache with intermittent sharp or stabbing sensations, and intensifies over time. Symptoms are exacerbated in certain positions and aggravated with activity. In the early phases rest may alleviate the symptoms completely. On examination, there is tenderness over the iliac crest. Mild swelling may also be present. In chronic cases the involved muscles may have areas of fibrosis and edema near the site, as well as tender points and/or trigger points. If left untreated, continued trauma may result in an enthesopathy. Acute iliac apophysitis may also develop from direct trauma to the anterior pelvis; in these cases avulsion fracture may need to be ruled out.

In most cases, apophysitis arises as a result of the oppositional forces acting on the pelvis during gait. As the pelvis and torso rotate and tilt away from each other, repetitive stress is placed on the apophysis superiorly by the abdominal muscles and inferiorly by the tensor fascia latae muscle. In an adult, this same mechanism may result in muscular or periosteal microtrauma because the apophysis is fused. However, in the immature athlete the growth plate of the iliac crest is vulnerable to microfractures from shearing and distraction stresses.

Treatment Notes

The goals of treatment in the young athlete with iliac apophysitis are resolution of the inflammation, correction of associated biomechanical dysfunctions, reconditioning of muscle groups and gradual return to the activity. The inflammation can be addressed by eliminating the recurrent stress, and by the use of ice and anti-inflammatory medications when necessary. In the initial presentation, osteopathic treatment should address the vascular and lymphatic circulation in the area to facilitate wound healing. Indirect or balancing techniques can also be used in the early phase of recovery to correct biomechanical dysfunction. Once the inflammation and pain have improved, muscle reconditioning can be performed using muscle energy techniques and a stretching protocol. The athlete's return to the activity should be monitored closely for recurrence of symptoms. In rare cases, changes in footwear or orthotics may be necessary.

PAIN PATTERNS WITH COMMON PELVIC ENTHESOPATHIES

The pain pattern of an enthesopathy may be similar to that of a trigger point. However, the primary site of tenderness will be at the apophysis, not in the belly of the muscle.

Anterior Superior Iliac Spine/Tensor Fascia Latae (Fig. 5.75)

Enthesopathy of the anterior superior iliac spine is usually a result of injury or overuse of the tensor fascia latae. There is pain along the anterolateral aspect of the thigh and it may radiate to the knee. Pain and tenderness can be elicited by adducting the leg across the body midline and asking the child to abduct it against resistance.

Anterior Inferior Iliac Spine/Rectus Femoris (Fig. 5.76)

Enthesopathy of the anterior inferior iliac spine often presents as a deep ache in the anterior thigh which may radiate to just above the knee (speckled pattern). The pain is exacerbated with eccentric contraction of the rectus femoris muscle or concentric contraction against resistance. There is point tenderness over the AIIS which can be elicited with knee extension against resistance.

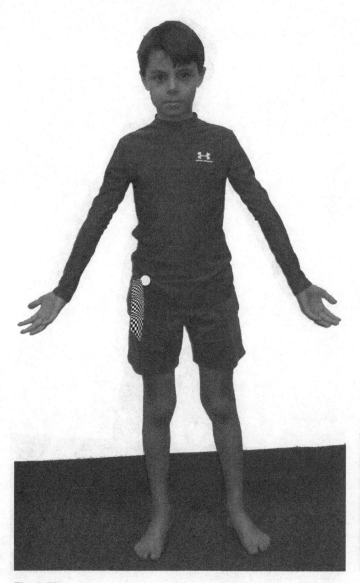

Fig. 5.75

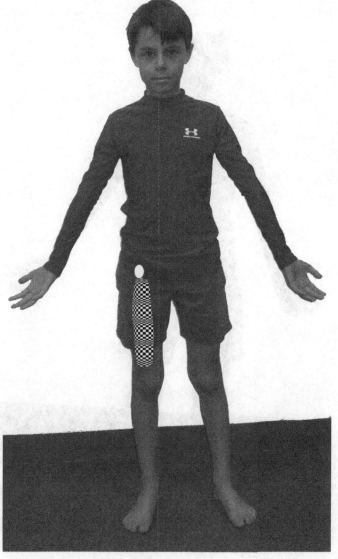

Fig. 5.76

Ischial Tuberosity/Biceps Femoris (Fig. 5.77)

Enthesopathy of the ischial tuberosity is typically a result of damage to the biceps femoris muscle. The pain presents as a deep ache in the posterior thigh, which is exacerbated with eccentric contraction such as climbing the stairs. On examination, the pain pattern can be reproduced with the patient supine with hip flexed and knee extended. Knee flexion against resistance will exacerbate the pain.

Iliac Crest/Abdominal Oblique (Fig. 5.78)

Enthesopathy of the iliac crest results from overuse or strain of the oblique abdominal muscle. There is tenderness over the anterior and lateral aspect of the crest. Pain is exacerbated with side-bending of the torso away from the injury, or reaching overhead with the ipsilateral arm.

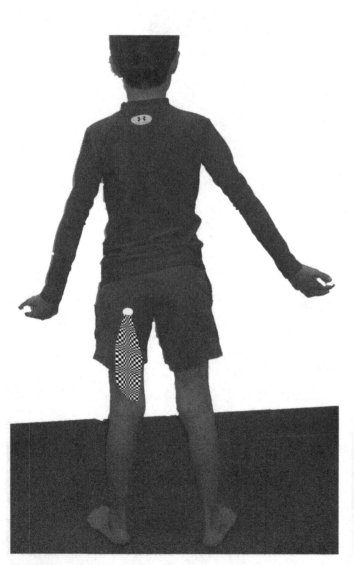

Fig. 5.77

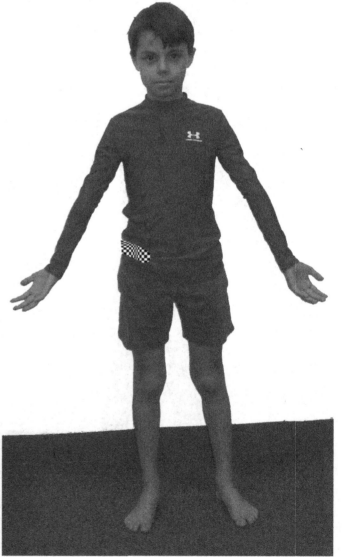

Fig. 5.78

ILIOTIBIAL BAND CONDITIONS

Snapping Hip Syndrome/Runner's Knee

Clinical Notes

Iliotibial band (ITB) conditions usually present in adolescents or young athletes. There are three named conditions. Athletes who complain of a snapping or popping of the proximal hip that is not associated with pain have a condition called snapping hip syndrome. When the condition presents as pain along most of the length of the iliotibial band, it is called iliotibial band syndrome. Finally, when the pain is localized to the distal attachment of the ITB, it is called runner's knee. Regardless of the name, in each case the problem is a syndrome of overuse of the iliotibial band. The ITB becomes inflamed from repeated microtrauma, usually due to overstretching or direct contusion. There are four degrees or grades of ITB syndrome: symptoms occur following activity; symptoms occur with activity but do not interfere with play; symptoms occur with activity and interfere with play; symptoms prevent participation in play. Rest, ice and anti-inflammatory medication may provide short-term relief of acute exacerbations, especially in milder cases. Soft tissue manipulation can be performed to improve circulation in the area. Osteopathic treatment of the contributing biomechanical dysfunctions needs to be augmented by rehabilitation of the associated muscular relationships.

In snapping hip syndrome the sensation typically occurs during running, especially if there is a sudden turn. There is no swelling or tenderness over the joint. The snapping may be reproduced when the hip moves rapidly through the sequence of flexion, internal rotation and extension. Snapping hip syndrome usually arises when tautness of the iliotibial band causes it to compress against the trochanteric bursa. The condition may progress to a trochanteric bursitis with continued irritation. Iliotibial band syndrome represents an overuse problem of the ITB. Initially, the pain, which is low grade and localized to the lateral aspect of the thigh, will resolve when the activity stops. Many athletes will attempt to 'play through the pain.' Unfortunately, sustained activity results in recurrent microtrauma. Ice and rest may help, but symptoms typically resume with activity. Runner's knee occurs when the ITB is irritated at its distal attachment on the lateral femoral condyle. Fibers of the ITB interdigitate with the lateral aspect of the articular capsule of the knee to form part of the arcuate ligamentous complex. As a result, distal ITB irritation (runner's knee) can extend into the lateral aspect of the knee.

Iliotibial band irritation develops due to shortening or overstretching of the tensor fascia latae muscle, prolonged contraction or spasm of the gluteus maximus and medius, or stretch on the iliotibial fascial complex. Iliotibial band conditions may develop in athletes due to biomechanical dysfunction in the pelvis, hip, leg, knee or foot. The localization of the pain – proximal, shaft or distal – reflects where the primary strains are resolving. The iliotibial band complex acts as a lateral stabilizer for the hip and knee. The tensor fascia latae (TFL) muscle inserts on the anterior margin of the ITB and the gluteus maximus and medius insert on its posterior margin. These muscles provide a counterforce across the proximal portion of the band (Fig. 5.79) that helps to stabilize the pelvis during single leg stance. During gait, contraction of the TFL and gluteal muscles flexes and extends the hip. Their counterforce maintains the position of the ITB. These opposing forces increase the tensile forces in the ITB that stabilize the knee laterally and support it in extension. This myofascial column supports

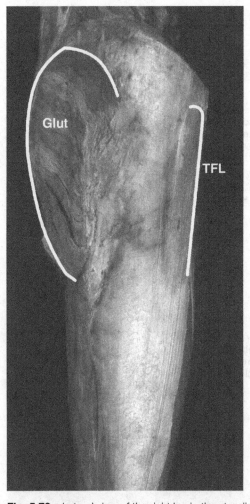

Fig. 5.79 • *Lateral view of the right leg in the standing position. The gluteus maximus (Glut) and tensor fascia latae (TFL) muscles are identified. Fibers from the gluteus and TFL interdigitate with the iliotibial band.*

the lateral weight displacement that occurs with heel strike and acts as a compressive counterforce over the trochanter to balance the compressive load on the femoral head and neck. In very young athletes, this is especially important to protect the capital femoral epiphysis and femoral neck.

The proximal portion of the ITB will glide anteriorly and posteriorly in response to alternating contraction of the TFL and the gluteal muscles. During the swing phase, the TFL contracts to flex the hip and the proximal ITB moves anteriorly. The concomitant knee flexion causes maximum stretch on the ITB. As the athlete moves from heel strike to midstance, the gluteal muscles increase their contractile force to stabilize the sacroiliac joint and pelvis as the leg is loaded. The ITB is pulled posterior by the gluteal muscles. If the TFL and gluteal muscles are working together, the

forces across the hip will be balanced and the hip stabilized (Fig. 5.80). If, however, biomechanical dysfunction is present, then one or the other muscle may be at a mechanical advantage and the proximal ITB will suddenly 'slip' in one direction or the other, resulting in a snapping sensation at the hip. This is called snapping hip syndrome. If the biomechanical dysfunction causes excessive stretch or loading of the ITB, the tight band will rub against the greater trochanter and, with repetition, the trochanteric bursa can become inflamed, resulting in trochanteric bursitis. Snapping hip syndrome is associated with ipsilateral short leg, anterior or posterior innominate rotation (depending on which muscle is involved), outflared innominate, increased Q angle, femoral anteversion, externally rotated femur, piriformis spasm, imbalances in agonist–antagonist coordination

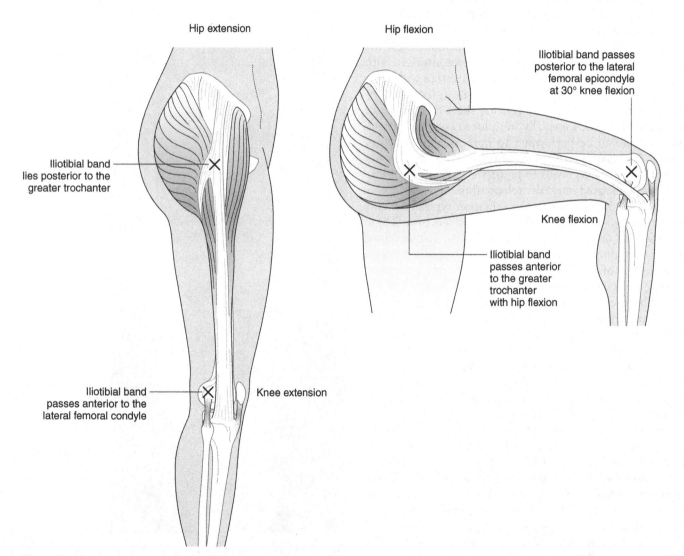

Hip extension

Hip flexion

Iliotibial band passes posterior to the lateral femoral epicondyle at 30° knee flexion

Iliotibial band lies posterior to the greater trochanter

Knee flexion

Iliotibial band passes anterior to the greater trochanter with hip flexion

Iliotibial band passes anterior to the lateral femoral condyle

Knee extension

Fig. 5.80 • Schematic diagram comparing normal position of iliotibial band during knee and hip extension and flexion. Note that the iliotibial band moves posteriorly to the femoral condyle during knee and hip flexion and anterior during knee and hip extension. (Adapted from Saidoff DC, Mcdonough AL. Critical pathways in therapeutic intervention: extremities and spine. St Louis: Mosby, 2001, with permission.)

of hip stabilizer muscles, abnormal foot mechanics and weakness of the tensor fascia latae muscle (Fig. 5.81). In some cases a snapping sensation may be felt more medially and anteriorly. If the sensation occurs with rotation of the femur, both with and without weightbearing, it may be due to displacement of the iliopsoas tendon over the femoral head. This condition is more common in dancers and gymnasts. It may be due to spasm of the psoas or iliacus, contraction of the contralateral erector spinae muscles, external rotation of the femur or an outflared innominate. If left untreated, a greater trochanteric bursitis may develop.

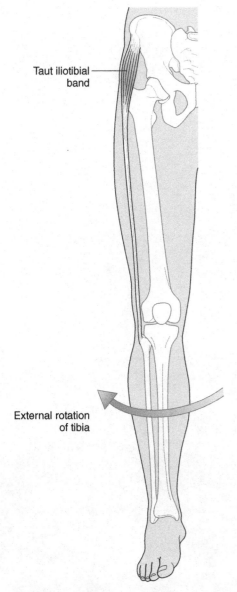

Taut iliotibial band

External rotation of tibia

Fig. 5.81 • Excessive foot supination promotes lateral (external) rotation of the tibia, which may increase the tension on the iliotibial band. Adapted from Saidoff DC, Mcdonough AL. Critical pathways in therapeutic intervention: extremities and spine. St Louis: Mosby, 2001, with permission.)

Runner's knee develops when the forces of stress summate at the distal portion of the iliotibial band. The distal aspect of the ITB freely crosses the lateral femoral epicondyle before merging fibers with the articular capsule of the knee and inserting on the anterolateral tibial condyle. The ITB is free to translate anteriorly and posteriorly over the lateral femoral epicondyle as the knee flexes and extends. Throughout the gait cycle the translation of the distal ITB is in the opposite direction to the proximal component. The distal ITB is initially posterior to the lateral femoral condyle at toe-off when the knee is flexed more than 30°. As the leg moves into swing phase and the knee extends, the ITB passes over the condyle into an anterior position. It returns to the posterior position during much of heel strike and remains there for midstance and terminal gait. During running and most running sports, however, more of the gait cycle is spent with the knee flexed, even during stance. As a result, even when the hip is extended the distal ITB is positioned posterior to the condyle. The contraction of the TFL muscle during hip flexion places an anterior stress on the posterior positioned distal ITB. This loads the ligament. When the knee finally moves into extension the ligament snaps forward. With repetition the tendon becomes irritated and inflamed. The strain may extend into the lateral joint space owing to the interconnection of the distal ITB with the articular capsule. Runner's knee may develop secondary to inappropriate training practices, such as inadequate stretching, increasing distance too quickly and poor footwear. It is also associated with running on irregular surfaces, such as the curvature of a road or beach, and increased stride length. Athletes who overextend their stride exacerbate the strain on the TFL by forceful knee extension and exaggerated hip flexion. Running down inclined surfaces results in over-pronation, internal tibial rotation and an increased load on the anterior articular capsule and ligaments. Running on a sloping surface causes the foot positioned on the upslope to assume a supinated posture, placing a varus stress across the knee. The varus stress loads the distal ITB. Athletes with pes cavus and over-supination compensate by externally rotating the tibia, which widens the lateral aspect of the knee joint during flexion, creating a varus stress.

Iliotibial band friction syndrome occurs when the iliotibial band complex is stressed throughout its entire length, resulting in microtrauma to the myofascial tissue along the shaft of the femur. The pain is usually generalized along the lateral thigh. Iliotibial band syndrome is slightly more common in females due to the increased Q angle and the tendency towards genu valgus, the combination of which lengthens the distance between the iliac crest and the tibia. ITB friction syndrome is also associated with over-pronation of the foot and vertical innominate dysfunctions, particularly upslips. Patients with untreated snapping hip or runner's knee syndromes may develop ITB friction syndrome as the area of inflammation extends through the length of the ITB. ITB friction syndrome occurs in runners, skiers and cyclists. Cyclists are more likely to develop ITB friction syndrome due to the excessive and persistent stretch placed on the ITB during the pedaling cycle. This is exacerbated if the pedals have toe clamps or cleats, or if the knees are positioned medially. Direct trauma to the lateral thigh predisposes the ITB to friction syndrome due to the associated swelling and inflammation. Trigger points in the tensor fascia latae and gluteus minimus muscles can present as iliotibial band friction syndrome.

In most cases of iliotibial band overuse syndrome the history, clinical presentation and associated findings are sufficient to make the diagnosis. Nevertheless, there are several maneuvers that can be performed to confirm the diagnosis. In athletes with milder symptoms, the tests may produce false negative results.

Ober Test for ITB Restriction

1. The patient is lying on the unaffected side facing away from the physician. The physician stands behind him. One hand is placed on the innominate on the affected side and the other contacts the same leg below the tibial tuberosity (Fig. 5.82).

2. The pelvis is supported so that there is no rotation at the lumbosacral junction. The physician passively extends the hip while moving the femur into external rotation, extension and adduction so that the leg is suspended off the table behind the patient (Fig. 5.83).

3. The leg should be able to adduct so that the level of the foot is below or at the level of the table. Inability to let the leg adduct or pain in this position confirms ITB restriction and inflammation. (Note: Many patients will feel stretch in this position but they should not feel pain.)

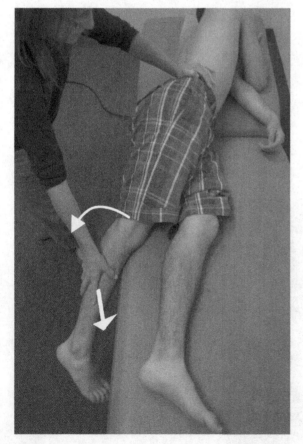

Fig. 5.82

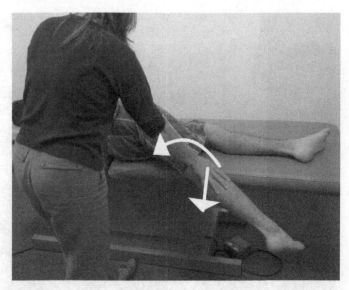

Fig. 5.83

Supine Test for Proximal ITB Restriction

1. The patient is supine. With one hand, the physician stabilizes the pelvis on the affected side. With the other hand, the physician grasps the affected leg at the ankle.

2. With the knee in extension the hip is slightly flexed and adducted over the opposite leg (Fig. 5.84). This position should be painless. The degree of adduction is noted.

3. Deep palpation along the length of the ITB may elicit tenderness at the site of friction and inflammation.

(Proximal tenderness associated with an anterior rotated innominate suggests TFL spasm.) The tissue superior to the greater trochanter should be palpated with the patient in this position to determine whether or not trochanteric bursitis is also present.

4. This maneuver is repeated on the contralateral leg. Both sides should be compared for symmetry.

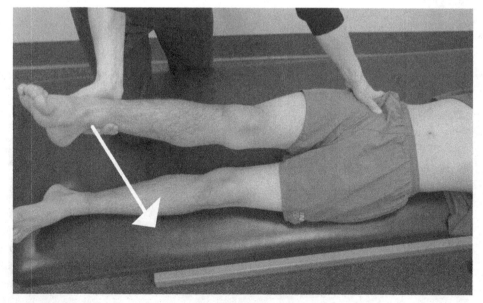

Fig. 5.84

Treatment Notes

Once the diagnosis of one of the iliotibial band conditions has been made, the etiology needs to be uncovered. Tibial rotations, innominate dysfunctions, knee strains, muscle imbalances and foot mechanics all need to be assessed. Stretching and reconditioning exercises targeting the ITB will be completely ineffective if the underlying problem is not corrected. Foot orthotics or running shoes that correct the athlete's foot mechanics need to be employed. Leg length discrepancies should be addressed with lift therapy. In chronic conditions, the presence of trigger points may contribute to a cycle of muscle spasm, altered mechanics, gait imbalances and ITB irritation. In these cases trigger point injections can relieve nociceptive triggers and facilitate correction of the biomechanics and muscle retraining.

ISOMETRIC/MUSCLE ENERGY TECHNIQUE

Abductors/Tensor Fasciae Latae

Supine Athlete

This technique should be performed after innominate dysfunctions have been corrected. This approach is used to lengthen tightened muscles and address fascial strains in acute or chronic conditions. This specific technique can be used to treat the shortened TFL.

1. The patient is supine with the hip and knee extended. The physician stands on the affected side. The physician stabilizes the innominate with one hand and grasps the distal tibia just above the ankle with the other (Fig. 5.85).

2. The hip is slightly flexed and the leg is crossed medially (adducted) to engage the restrictive barrier of the TFL. The physician may internally rotate the leg to further localize the TFL (curved white arrow).

3. The patient is instructed to push his leg laterally (abduct, black arrow) into the physician's hand. The physician resists this motion with an equal and opposite counterforce (white arrow).

4. This isometric contraction is maintained for 4–5 seconds. The patient is then asked to cease contraction while the physician simultaneously reduces her counterforce.

5. The physician maintains contact and waits for tissue relaxation (approximately 4–5 seconds).

6. The physician adducts the leg to reposition it to the new barrier (curved white arrow). Again, internal rotation may be added to localize the TFL. The sequence is repeated twice.

Alternative Position for Isometric Muscle Energy

If the child is unable to tolerate adduction with the knee extended, the technique may be performed with the knee flexed and the foot resting on the table (Fig. 5.86).

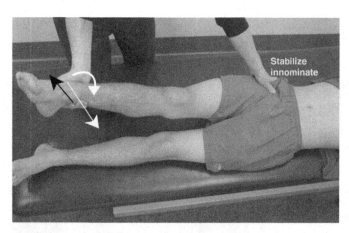

Fig. 5.85

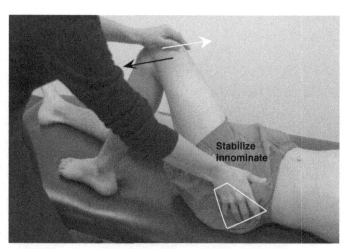

Fig. 5.86

ISOTONIC ECCENTRIC MUSCLE ENERGY

Tensor Fasciae Latae Muscle

Side-lying Athlete

Isotonic eccentric techniques are used to rehabilitate the eccentric contractile function of the muscle, to lengthen the muscle and to address fibrosis. Eccentric contraction techniques may aid in improving muscle coordination. This is a relatively more aggressive technique and should be employed to tolerance after the isometric approach has been used successfully. If the child is unable to tolerate this position the technique can be adopted for use in the supine position until the condition improves enough for the side-lying approach.

1. The athlete is lying on the unaffected side. The physician stands behind the patient or on the side to be treated. The hips are stacked over each other. The physician stabilizes the pelvis with one hand as the affected leg is adducted (dropped off the table) to the restrictive barrier (Fig. 5.87).

2. The patient is instructed to gently abduct his leg against the physician's resistance (lift his leg to the ceiling). The physician initially resists this motion with an equal and opposite counterforce.

3. Then the physician slowly and gently overcomes the patient's abduction and moves the leg towards adduction (towards the floor); this increases the load on the TFL muscle and ITB during contraction.

4. This is an isotonic eccentric contraction. The tone in the child's muscle should not change. The eccentric contraction occurs as the physician increases her force and stretches the contracting muscle. The physician should move the leg 1 or 2 cm.

5. The child is asked to stop his force as the physician reduces her force. The physician waits 5–6 seconds until she feels a change in tissue texture at the hip. Then the leg is adducted to the new restrictive barrier.

6. The procedure is repeated twice. The physician should overcome the child's force and move the leg 1 or 2 cm or to tolerance.

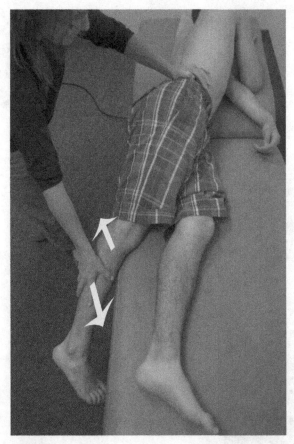

Fig. 5.87

ISOTONIC ECCENTRIC MUSCLE ENERGY

Tensor Fasciae Latae Muscle

Supine Athlete

1. The athlete is supine and the physician stands on the side to be treated. The physician stabilizes the pelvis with one hand as the affected leg is adducted to the restrictive barrier for abductor stretch (Fig. 5.88).

2. The patient is instructed to gently abduct his leg against the physician's resistance. The physician initially resists this motion with an equal and opposite counterforce.

3. Then the physician slowly and gently overcomes the patient's abduction and moves the leg towards adduction (large white arrow); this increases the load on the TFL muscle and iliotibial band during contraction.

4. This is an isotonic eccentric contraction. The tone in the child's muscle should not change. The eccentric contraction occurs as the physician increases her force and stretches the contracting muscle. The physician should move the leg 1 or 2 cm.

5. The child is asked to stop his force as the physician reduces her force. The physician waits 5–6 seconds until she feels a change in tissue texture at the hip. Then the leg is adducted to the new restrictive barrier.

6. The procedure is repeated twice. The physician should overcome the child's force and move the leg 1 or 2 cm or to tolerance.

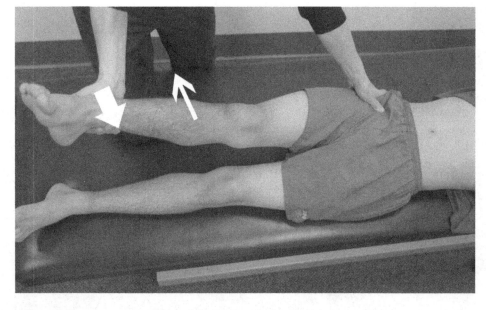

Fig. 5.88

MUSCLE STRAIN/SPASM

Clinical Notes

Muscle strains, sprains and spasms may develop as a result of rapid stretching, over-training or improper training which emphasizes eccentric contraction. Muscle strains occur at the musculotendinous junction due to rapid or forceful contraction. Strains can be categorized into three degrees: first degree results in tenderness to palpation and stretch; second degree results in muscle spasm which alters joint position; and third degree presents with significant pain, spasm and tearing of the tissue. Third-degree muscle strains are more likely to occur in children in late puberty. Younger children are more susceptible to avulsion fractures owing to the weakness of the growth plate. Muscle strains and spasms typically occur in the long restrictor muscles involved in eccentric contraction. The biceps muscle in a tennis player or pitcher, the hamstrings or tibialis muscles in a runner, and the quadriceps in a dancer are common examples.

In the acute phase, rest, ice, compression and elevation (RICE) are the hallmarks of treatment for muscle strains. Pain should resolve between 48 and 72 hours after initiating RICE. If pain persists, an intramuscular hematoma needs to be considered. In severe cases intramuscular hematoma can increase compartment pressures, resulting in compartment syndrome, which typically presents as paresthesias distal to the injury, decreased pulse pressure and changes on neurological examination. Immediate surgical treatment is required. In general, however, surgery is unnecessary for the treatment of muscle strains unless complete rupture of the tendon has occurred, an exceedingly rare event in the pediatric population.

Reciprocal inhibition, balancing and indirect techniques can also be helpful in the acute phase. Once the pain has improved, heat, passive stretching and soft tissue techniques are added. Active stretching, dynamic loading exercises, isometric and concentric isotonic techniques can be introduced to tolerance. Aquatic therapy is very helpful in patients with muscle strains of the lower extremity or back.

Treatment Notes

In general, isometric muscle energy, myofascial and balanced ligamentous techniques work well in acutely injured spastic muscles. Many of the techniques described in Chapter 6, Lower Leg, can be used to address the long restrictors of the hip. Once normal tone has been re-established and the pain has decreased, muscle retraining should begin. Isotonic eccentric and concentric techniques can be employed in the rehabilitation phase.

ISOTONIC ECCENTRIC MUSCLE ENERGY

Knee Flexors

Supine Athlete

1. The patient is supine. The hip is flexed and the knee is extended to engage the restrictive barrier in the hamstrings (Fig. 5.89).

2. The patient is instructed to flex his knee against the physician's resistance (white arrow). The physician initially resists this motion with an equal and opposite force. Then the physician slowly and gently increases her resistance (black arrow) to move the patient's knee 3–5° into extension against the contracting hamstrings.

3. This is an isotonic eccentric contraction, so the tone of the child's knee flexor muscles should not change as the knee is extended. The eccentric contraction occurs as the physician increases her force.

4. The child is asked to stop his force as the physician reduces her force. The physician waits 5–6 seconds until she feels a change in tissue texture at the hip. The knee is then extended to the new restrictive barrier.

5. The procedure is repeated twice.

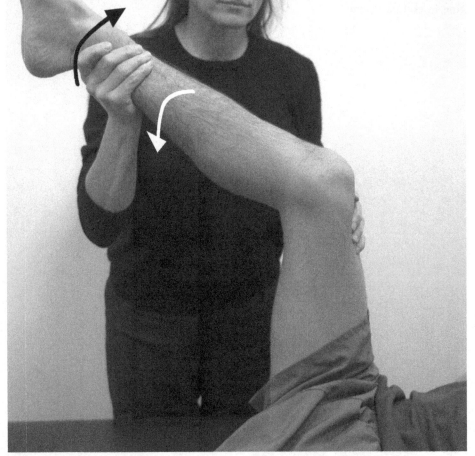

Fig. 5.89

ISOTONIC CONCENTRIC MUSCLE ENERGY

Treatment of Abductors

Supine Athlete

Isotonic concentric techniques allow the muscle to shorten against resistance. This is used to strengthen the muscle, or it can be used to address an articular dysfunction with significant myofascial involvement. This approach may be useful in treating children with abnormalities in muscle tone, overuse strains, and as a general approach to articular dysfunction. This specific technique can be used in the management of children with lower extremity spasticity involving the lateral column.

1. The leg is positioned so that the restrictive barrier to abductor stretching (adduction) is engaged (Fig. 5.90).

2. The patient is instructed to gently abduct his leg against the physician's resistance. The physician initially resists this motion with an equal and opposite counterforce. Then the physician slowly and gently decreases her resistance (small white arrow), which allows the patient to move the leg into abduction as the muscles are contracting (large white arrow). The physician reduces the load on the abductors while they are contracting.

3. This is an isotonic contraction, so the tone of the child's muscle should not change. The concentric contraction occurs as the physician reduces her force. The physician should allow the leg to move through an arch of approximately 20° while stabilizing the pelvis.

4. The child is asked to stop his force as the physician reduces her force. The physician waits 5–6 seconds until she feels a change in tissue texture at the hip. Then the leg is adducted to the restrictive barrier.

5. The procedure is repeated twice.

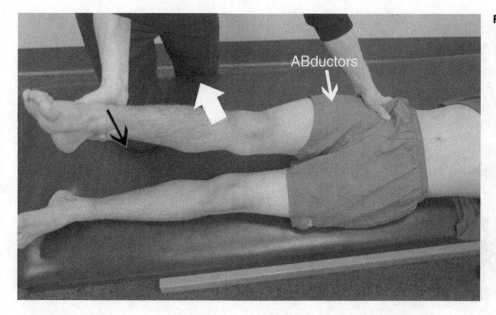

Fig. 5.90

ABductors

ISOTONIC ECCENTRIC MUSCLE ENERGY

Treatment of Abductors

Supine Athlete

Isotonic eccentric techniques are used to rehabilitate the eccentric contractile function of the muscle, to lengthen the muscle and to address fibrosis. Eccentric contraction techniques may aid in improving muscle coordination. This is a relatively more aggressive technique and should only be employed after the child has shown improvement with other approaches. In this example, the abductors are the focus of the treatment.

1. The leg is positioned so that the restrictive barrier to abductor stretching (adduction) is engaged (Fig. 5.91).

2. The patient is instructed to gently abduct his leg against the physician's resistance (small white arrow). The physician initially resists this motion with an equal and opposite counterforce. Then the physician slowly and gently overcomes the patient's abduction and moves the leg towards adduction (large white arrow). This increases the load on the abductors while they are contracting.

3. This is an isotonic contraction so the tone of the child's muscle should not change. The eccentric contraction occurs as the physician increases her force and stretches the contracting muscle. The physician should move the leg 1 or 2 cm.

4. The child is asked to stop his force as the physician reduces her force. The physician waits 5–6 seconds until she feels a change in tissue texture at the hip. Then the leg is adducted to the restrictive barrier.

5. The procedure is repeated twice. Initially, the physician should overcome the child's force and move the leg 1 or 2 cm or to tolerance. However, on subsequent attempts the distance the physician moves the leg should increase.

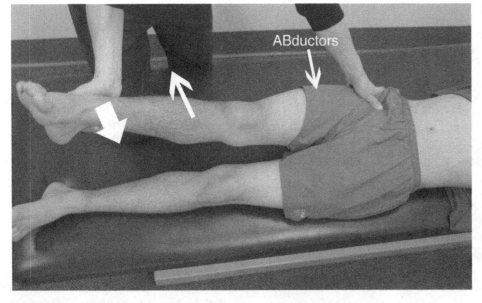

Fig. 5.91

LOWER EXTREMITY SPASTICITY

Clinical Notes

In children with cerebral palsy spasticity interferes with muscle growth, resulting in intraosseous bowing and torsion. Spasticity can influence primary somatosensory mapping, motor firing patterns and movement strategies. In children with spasticity, abnormal biomechanical relations affect postural and balance mechanisms (Woollacott 1998). In addition, there is some evidence to support the role of motor function in cognitive development. Abnormal cognitive function in children with spasticity may be related to altered motor function, which affects somatosensory mapping and ultimately influences components of cognition such as spatial mapping.

Treatment Notes

Lower extremity spasticity is one of the most common presentations in cerebral palsy. Depending on the area of involvement, pelvic stabilizers, adductor muscles, knee flexors and ankle plantar flexors may be affected. Depending on the severity of the spasticity, different techniques can be employed. In children with severe spasticity myofascial and soft tissue techniques can be useful in addressing the long muscles of the limbs. Joint stiffness in these children may respond to balanced ligamentous tension or facilitated positional release techniques. In older children with mild and moderate spasticity, isotonic eccentric contraction and isometric muscle energy techniques can also be used. Counterstrain techniques as described by Jones (Ward 2003) can be used to lengthen and relax tone in long restrictor muscles. Facilitated positional release can be used to address short restrictor muscles, and balanced ligamentous techniques may be useful to attend to articular, ligamentous and membranous components.

Children with spasticity will also benefit from assistance devices and interventions that provide stability without compromising the movement and postural strategies they have developed. A wonderful example of this is an assistance dog that can counterbalance a child's tendency to lean due to an altered center of gravity (Fig. 5.92).

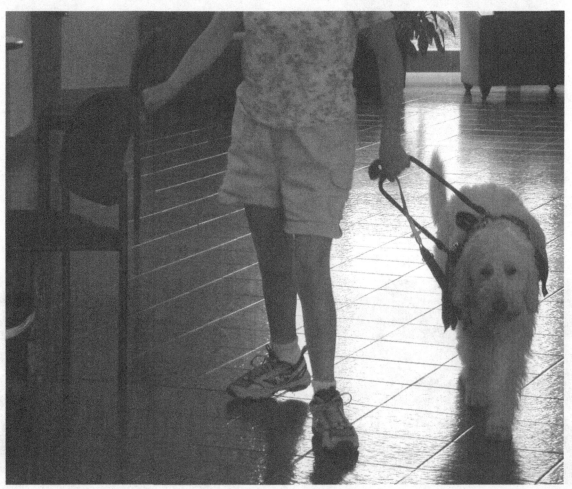

Fig. 5.92

RECIPROCAL INHIBITION MUSCLE ENERGY

Abductors

Athlete

Reciprocal inhibition is used to relax a muscle, lengthen it, and improve agonist–antagonist coordination. In this example the abductors are shortened. This approach may be useful in children with mild to moderate spasticity.

1. The patient is supine. The physician grasps the lower leg with one hand and monitors the ipsilateral hip with the other.

2. The leg is moved medially so that the restrictive barrier to abductor stretching (the adducted position) is engaged (Fig. 5.93).

3. The patient (white arrow) is instructed to gently adduct his leg against the physician's resistance (black arrow). This engages the adductors. The antagonist muscle group, the abductors, should be inhibited (Fig. 5.94).

4. This isometric contraction is maintained for 4–5 seconds, then the patient is told to relax his force as the physician relaxes hers.

5. The physician waits 5–6 seconds until she feels a change in tissue texture at the hip. Then the leg is adducted to the restrictive barrier.

6. The procedure is repeated twice.

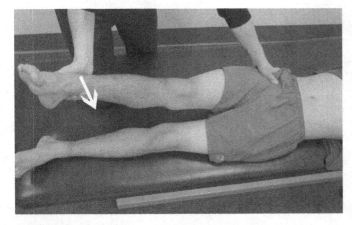

Fig. 5.93

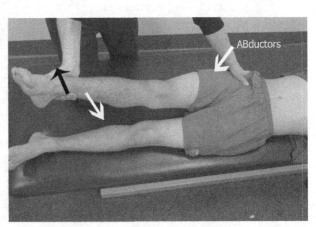

Fig. 5.94

RECIPROCAL INHIBITION MUSCLE ENERGY

Adductors

Athlete

Reciprocal inhibition is used to relax a muscle, lengthen it and improve agonist–antagonist coordination. In this example, the adductors are being treated. This approach may be useful in children with mild to moderate spasticity. Following reciprocal inhibition, the physician may choose to employ isotonic concentric contraction techniques to the adductor muscles to reinforce muscle-firing patterns.

1. The patient is supine. The physician grasps the lower leg with one hand and monitors the ipsilateral hip with the other.

2. The leg is abducted (taken laterally, white arrow) until the restrictive barrier in the adductors is engaged (Fig. 5.95).

3. The patient is instructed to gently abduct his leg (move it laterally) against the physician's resistance (small stippled arrow). This engages the abductors. The antagonist muscle group, the adductors, should be inhibited (Fig. 5.96).

4. This isometric contraction is maintained for 4–5 seconds, then the patient is told to relax his force as the physician relaxes hers.

5. The physician waits 5–6 seconds until she feels a change in tissue texture in the adductors. Then the leg is abducted to the new restrictive barrier in the adductors.

6. The procedure is repeated twice.

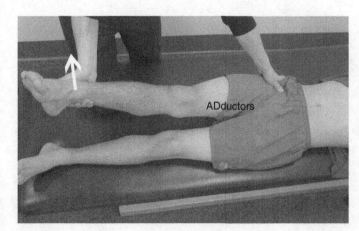

Fig. 5.95

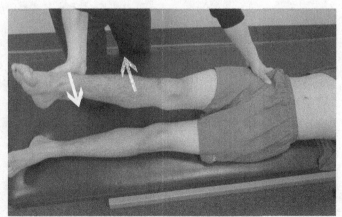

Fig. 5.96

LOWER EXTREMITY HYPOTONIA

Clinical Notes

Hypotonia in children may be due to primary muscle disease, peripheral neuropathy, endocrinopathy or neuromuscular junction anomalies. In cases of acute hypotonia electrolyte imbalance and anemia need to be considered. In many children with low muscle tone the etiology is unknown. These children may also have ligamentous laxity. Boys appear to be affected more than girls. Fortunately, most children with idiopathic hypotonia have moderate to mild disease.

Children with hypotonia create balance and stability mechanisms by locking weightbearing joints and shortening antigravity muscles. Many children with hypotonia often develop stiffness and myofascial restriction in the antigravity muscles. There is shortening of the adductor and quadriceps muscles, which produces an anterior tilt to the pelvis. Tibial rotation and torsion can be present, and depending on the severity of the hypotonia, femoral anteversion may persist. Children with hypotonia often have pes planus and genu valgus functional deformities. Recurrent ankle sprain is a hazard that can be helped by wearing high-top sneakers or ankle foot orthotics if necessary. Knee, hip and back pain are recurrent and frequent complaints owing to the postural mechanisms employed by the child. The cervical lordosis is often reduced, with a compensatory extension of the occiput on the atlas. This gives the child a head-forward posture. This shortening of the suboccipital muscles is typically the basis for the recurrent cervicogenic cephalgia from which many of these children suffer. Suboccipital muscle tightness may trigger cervicomandibular reflexes in the muscles of mastication, leading to bruxisms. (This same mechanism can also be a problem in children with spasticity.)

Isotonic eccentric and concentric techniques are useful in older children with hypotonia. Isotonic eccentric techniques can be used to address shortening of antigravity muscles. Concentric muscle energy techniques may help to strengthen and improve firing patterns in deconditioned flexors and long restrictors. Isometric techniques can be used to address articular dysfunctions that develop secondary to abnormal motor functioning. Facilitated positional release, balanced ligamentous technique and other indirect techniques are appropriate in children of all ages with hypotonia.

The child with hypotonia will benefit from activities or exercises that reinforce appropriate postural and balance strategies while strengthening muscles. Examples of these include horse riding, martial arts and some forms of dance. It goes without saying that the activity needs to be customized to the capabilities of the child and should foster self-confidence. Any activity that employs balance, form and movement can be used to reinforce the core stabilizing mechanisms while strengthening. The author had one 8-year-old patient with primary muscle disease who benefited from a love affair with duckpin bowling. He eventually learned to play ambidextrously, because we insisted that he had to practice rolling the ball with each hand.

ISOTONIC CONCENTRIC MUSCLE ENERGY

Knee Flexors

Isotonic concentric techniques allow the muscle to shorten against resistance. In addition to children with increased tone, isotonic concentric contraction can be valuable to use in children with deconditioning or mild hypotonia. In this example the hamstrings are being treated, but as with the other forms of muscle energy, the same procedure can be applied to any muscle group.

1. The patient is supine. The hip is flexed and the knee is extended to engage the restrictive barrier in the hamstrings (Fig. 5.97).

2. The patient is instructed to gently flex his knee against the physician's resistance (white arrow). The physician initially resists this motion with an equal and opposite force. Then the physician slowly and gently reduces her resistance, which allows the patient to move the knee into flexion as the muscles are contracting (black arrow).

3. This is an isotonic contraction, so the tone of the child's knee flexor muscles should not change. The concentric contraction occurs as the physician reduces her force. The physician should allow the leg to move through an arch of approximately 20°.

4. The child is asked to stop their force as the physician reduces her force. The physician waits 5–6 seconds until she feels a change in tissue texture at the hip. Then the knee is extended to the new restrictive barrier.

5. The procedure is repeated twice.

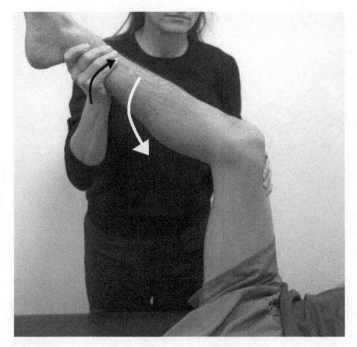

Fig. 5.97

MYOSITIS OSSIFICANS

Clinical Notes

Myositis ossificans is a calcification within the muscle belly that occurs as a result of a severe or repetitive contusion to the same muscle area. Severe or repetitive trauma produces internal hemorrhage and muscle hematoma. Tissue necrosis occurs resulting in the formation of fibrotic scar tissue. The area undergoes ossification. The most common sites for occurrence are the quadriceps and biceps muscles. Differential diagnosis includes fibrodysplasia ossificans progressive and osteosarcoma.

Myositis ossificans is a benign condition, but it can progress if re-injury occurs before the ossification process has completed, which usually takes a year. Athletes should be counseled to avoid activities that may result in re-injury. Exercise, stretching, eccentric isotonic muscle energy techniques may aid in improving and maintaining functional ability of the involved muscle. Surgery is rarely necessary, and if performed too early can exacerbate the condition through postoperative scarring.

PIRIFORMIS SYNDROME

Clinical Notes

Piriformis syndrome is a compressive neuropathy that occurs in athletes due to muscle hypertrophy, muscle spasm, trauma, contracture and mechanical dysfunction. In the early phase it typically presents as buttock pain that may or may not radiate into the posterior thigh and leg. Tingling or paresthesias may also be present. Activity and certain postures usually exacerbate the symptoms. A mild to moderate sensory loss may be present on physical examination. Piriformis syndrome typically involves compression or irritation to the common peroneal nerve or the sciatic nerve. The classic explanation involves an anatomic anomaly whereby the nerve pierces through the piriformis muscle, dividing it in two. Contraction or stress placed on the muscle impinges on the nerve. The piriformis will undergo increased stress with sacroiliac dysfunctions, anteverted femurs, vertical innominate dysfunctions, leg length differences and adaptations to gait abnormalities. The compression neuropathy can be addressed by correction of the underlying mechanical dysfunctions, stretching of the piriformis and muscle reconditioning. Although this may be the case in some patients and is probably the cause in the most recalcitrant cases, it does not explain all cases.

The sciatic trunk and common peroneal nerves lie adjacent to the short restrictors of the hip (Fig. 5.98). These nerves can be compressed between the piriformis and gemelli and obturator muscles. They can also be irritated by contractures or hypertrophy of the quadratus femoris. The muscles of the hip are both short and long restrictors. They can be thought of as a rotator cuff. They contribute to motion, stabilization and proprioception of the hip.

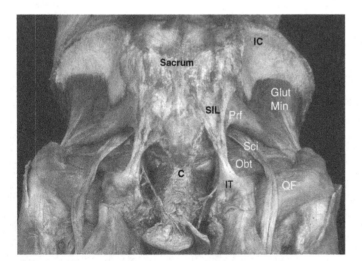

Fig. 5.98 • Posterior dissection of the pelvis. The multifidus, tensor fascia latae, gluteus maximus and gluteus medius have been removed to reveal the complex sacroiliac ligament (SIL) and deep posterior pelvic structures. Iliac crest (IC) ischial tuberosity (IT), coccyx (C), piriformis (Prf), gluteus minimus (GlutMin), sciatic nerve (Sci), obturator externus (Obt), and quadratus femoris (QF) are labeled.

Assessment of Piriformis

Supine Child

When the hip is in neutral or extended, the piriformis muscle is an external rotator of the femur. With the hip flexed 90° the piriformis muscle becomes an internal rotator. It is tested in both positions.

1. The child is supine. The physician stands at the patient's feet. The physician contacts both ankles and lifts the legs to 15°. This is postural neutral for the hip (Fig. 5.99).

2. The physician compares internal rotation of the femurs by turning the feet medially.

3. Then the physician sits ipsilateral to the hip to be tested. The physician contacts the femur proximal to the knee with one hand, while the other holds the foot and ankle (Fig. 5.100).

4. The hip is flexed and the knee is abducted to externally rotate the femur. The degree of external rotation is assessed and compared with that of the other leg.

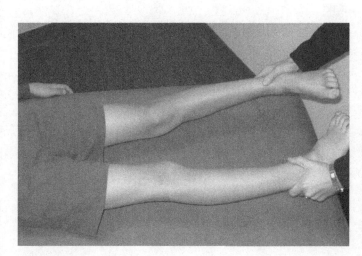

Fig. 5.99

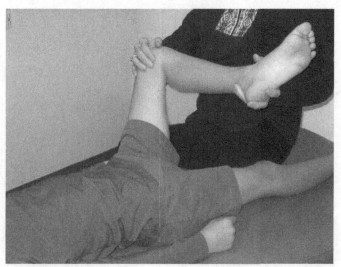

Fig. 5.100

Treatment Notes

Biomechanical dysfunctions between any of the corresponding osseous structures influence the normal function of this rotator cuff. Most of the rotator cuff muscles are short restrictors. The quadratus femoris, the internal and external obturator muscles and the superior and inferior gemelli muscles control the hip joint only. The piriformis is a long restrictor crossing the sacroiliac and hip joint. Consequently, the piriformis is affected by dysfunction of the sacrum, innominate or femur, whereas the other muscles are influenced by dysfunction of the innominate and femur only. In addition to mechanical dysfunction altering the tone or the rotator cuff of the hip, dysfunctions can also affect the tension in the nerves. For example, anterior rotation or upslip dysfunctions of the innominate have the potential to increase the tension on the sciatic and common peroneal nerves.

The rotator cuff can be treated using the balanced ligamentous technique for the hip muscles as previously described. Isometric and isotonic muscle energy techniques may be beneficial for stretching and reconditioning the piriformis muscle.

ISOMETRIC MUSCLE ENERGY TECHNIQUE

Piriformis

Child/Athlete (Fig. 5.101)

This isometric muscle energy technique can be used to lengthen the piriformis muscle. It is usually more easily tolerated than the isotonic eccentric technique that follows.

1. The physician resists this motion with an equal and opposite force (white arrow).

2. This isometric contraction is maintained for 4–5 seconds. Then the patient is asked to cease contraction while the physician simultaneously reduces her counterforce.

3. The physician maintains contact and waits for tissue relaxation (approximately 4–5 seconds).

4. Then the physician externally rotates the femur to reposition it to the new barrier (curved white arrow). The sequence is repeated twice.

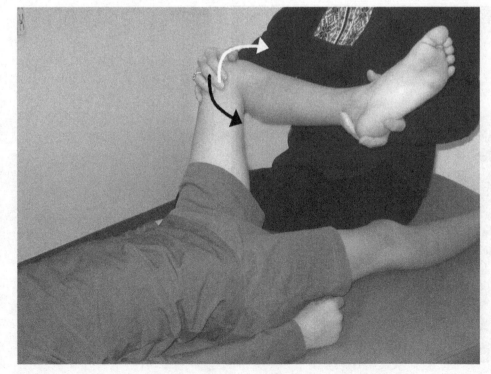

Fig. 5.101

ISOTONIC ECCENTRIC MUSCLE ENERGY TECHNIQUE

Piriformis (Fig. 5.102)

Child

This isotonic eccentric muscle energy technique can be applied to actively stretch the piriformis muscle and retrain it. If the patient cannot tolerate this, begin with the isometric technique previously described. This technique is contraindicated in children with epiphyseal or femoral head damage.

1. The child is supine. The hip and knee are flexed. The femur is externally rotated to the restrictive barrier (Fig. 5.102).

2. The physician contacts the medial aspect of the femur proximal to the knee. The child is instructed to move his knee against the physician's hand (black arrow). This internally rotates the femur.

3. The physician resists this motion with an oppositional force and gently overcomes the child's force (white arrow). The physician's oppositional force should be applied at the distal femur, not the knee joint or tibia.

4. This contraction is maintained for 3–4 seconds. Then the patient is asked to cease contraction while the physician simultaneously decreases her counterforce.

5. The physician maintains contact and waits for tissue relaxation (approximately 4–5 seconds).

6. Then the physician externally rotates the femur to reposition it to the new barrier (curved white arrow). The sequence is repeated twice.

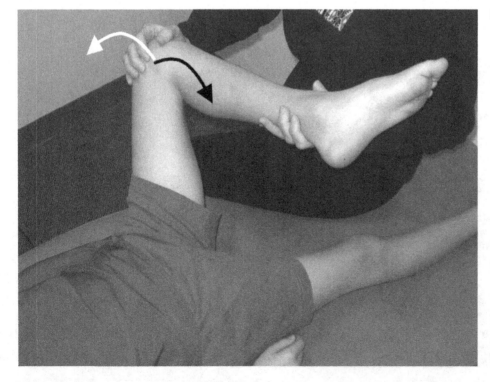

Fig. 5.102

MERALGIA PARESTHETICA

Clinical Notes

Tingling or numbness over the anterior aspect of the thigh just distal to the inguinal ligament without pain or motor loss is known as meralgia paresthetica (MP). Meralgia paresthetica is due to compression of the lateral femoral cutaneous nerve, a sensory branch of the lumbar plexus which passes between the psoas and quadratus lumborum and under the inguinal ligament to innervate the skin of the anterior thigh (Fig. 5.103). Symptoms may present with activity or at rest. Lymphadenopathy of the inguinal area needs to be ruled out. Compression of the lateral femoral cutaneous nerve by enlarged inguinal lymph nodes may be a hallmark of lymphoma or a pelvic neoplasm. More often, the compression is created by muscular or ligamentous structures and does not represent organic disease.

Symptoms may be exacerbated by activities such as running or climbing stairs. There may be a history of trauma with acute onset, but more often the symptoms begin gradually. Hypertrophy of the psoas or sartorius muscles can compress the nerve against the inguinal ligament. Spasm of the psoas may also trigger nerve compression. Meralgia paresthetica may be caused by innominate strains such as outflares, upslips and posterior rotations, which increase stretch on the inguinal ligament. Externally rotated femurs may also be associated with lateral cutaneous nerve compression. Extending the hip and flexing the knee with the patient in the prone or supine position may reproduce symptoms. Compression of the lateral cutaneous femoral nerve may also occur more proximally between the psoas and quadratus lumborum muscles. If this is the case, symptoms may be reproduced by asking the patient to lie prone and lift the chest and arch the back. On physical examination a depressed 12th rib or tenderness in the quadratus lumborum muscle may be present.

Techniques addressing these areas have been described earlier in this chapter and in Chapter 3.

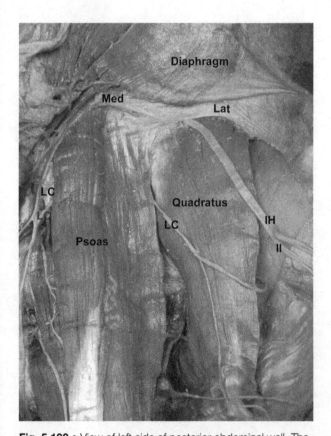

Fig. 5.103 • View of left side of posterior abdominal wall. The diaphragm is lifted to reveal the medial (Med) and lateral (Lat) arcuate ligaments. The lateral cutaneous nerve (LC) can be seen passing between the psoas and quadratus muscles. It will travel inferiorly and pass under the inguinal ligament. The iliohypogastric (IH) and ilioinguinal nerves are also labeled.

References

Carreiro JE. An osteopathic approach to children, 2nd edn. Edinburgh: Churchill Livingstone, 2009.

Song KM, Halliday SE, Little DG. The effect of limb-length discrepancy on gait.

J Bone Joint Surg Am 1997; 79: 1690–1698.

Ward R. Foundations for osteopathic medicine. St Louis: Lippincott, Williams & Willkins, 2003.

Woollacott MH, Burtner P, Jensen J, et al. Development of postural responses during standing in healthy children and children with spastic diplegia. Neurosci Biobehav Rev 1998; 22: 583–589.

Chapter **Six**

Lower leg

6

OVERVIEW

When diagnosing and treating problems in the lower extremity, one must consider the entire leg and hip as a functional unit. Injuries to the knees, ankles and hips do not occur in isolation. If the child is weightbearing at the time of impact, the forces are transmitted throughout the limb. Whereas bony fractures and strained or ruptured ligaments need immediate medical attention, full recovery and return to optimal function depend upon normalization of limb biomechanics. The stability and flexibility of the limb are affected by compensatory changes in the surrounding tissues in response to trauma. For example, when an inversion ankle sprain occurs, the ipsilateral fibula is often displaced posteriorly by the sudden stretch on the peroneus longus muscle. This may be accompanied by an external (lateral) rotation of the ipsilateral tibia. The externally rotated tibia will increase tensile forces on the patellar tendon and tibial tubercle during knee flexion, as well as altering meniscus loading. The posterior fibula increases tensile loading through the iliotibial band, resulting in a lateral flaring of the ipsilateral innominate, which is often associated with a posterior rotation. This in turn influences biomechanics in the sacroiliac and lumbosacral areas. If the inversion occurs with enough force and speed, the fascial strain can be transmitted into the thorax. The ankle may heal nicely, but if the mechanics in the fibula, knee and upper leg are not addressed, the athlete's performance will be hampered, she may be more susceptible to re-injury, and over time may experience patellar or hip pain from irritation to these tissues.

Chronic problems such as Osgood–Schlatter syndrome or patellofemoral syndrome are typically associated with localized biomechanical dysfunction. Over time, however, the child adapts his gait mechanics to compensate for the dysfunction. These compensatory changes in limb and gait biomechanics will maintain or even exacerbate the child's problem. For example, patellofemoral syndrome is often associated with strength imbalance between the vastus lateralis and vastus medialis muscles. During knee extension, the vastus lateralis pulls the patella laterally by overcoming the contractile force of the vastus medialis. Usually these patients will also have somatic dysfunction of the ipsilateral innominate and sacroiliac joint. A posterior innominate causes increased resting tone of the ipsilateral quadriceps muscles, further exacerbating the lateral traction on the patella. Bracing the patella or encouraging the child to strengthen the vastus medialis is of limited benefit if the functional mechanics of the rest of the limb are not corrected.

In very young children, somatic dysfunction in the foot, limb or pelvis may influence the development of optimal gait mechanics, balance and stability. Somatosensory mapping, postural strategies and motor patterning are all influenced by early movements and reflexes in the extremities. According to Wolfe's law, abnormal muscle tensions and resting tone influence bone growth. This all needs to be considered in children with congenital musculoskeletal abnormalities. Some congenital conditions, such as clubfoot, metatarsus adductus and bowlegs, may be associated with abnormal uterine lie. The skeletal tissues have 'grown' in response to altered or restrictive pressures on the limb. The soft tissues of the extremity have adapted to the skeletal changes, and as the child grows the abnormal tensions in fasciae and muscles alter the tensile forces acting on the growing bone. This will contribute to maintaining and frequently exacerbating the deformity. As the child grows, fascial stresses, muscle contractions and mechanical strains will develop to compensate for the deformity. Depending on the severity of the deformation, adaptations may even extend into the pelvis, lumbar spine and thoracolumbar junction. Consequently, limb growth is subjected to the direct effect of the deformity and the tensile effects of the compensatory changes in adjacent tissues. Casting may be used to counterbalance the abnormal tensile forces in the surrounding tissue. In severe cases, surgical correction and casting may be combined. In all cases the compensatory soft tissue restrictions need to be addressed to promote normal growth and alignment.

Q (QUADRICEPS) ANGLE (Fig. 6.1)

The quadriceps or Q angle describes the vector of pull exerted by the quadriceps muscles on the patella. The components of the quadriceps complex attach at the anterior superior and anterior inferior iliac spines (ASIS and AIIS) of the pelvis and converge to form the patellar tendon. The Q angle is measured by dropping a plumb-line through the tibial tubercle and middle of the patella and another from the ASIS to intersect with the first line at the mid-patella. The angle created by the intersecting lines is the Q angle. With growth the pelvis widens, displacing the ASIS and AIIS laterally in relation to the knee. This places a lateral pull on the patellar tendon. During puberty the pelvis widens more in girls than boys owing to hormonal influences. The wider gynecoid structure results in Q angles that are greater in females than in males. The Q angle in males is typically between 8° and 14°, whereas that in females ranges from 11° to 20°. The Q angle typically increases a degree with weightbearing owing to a valgus adaptation of the knee. In general patients with Q angles greater than 14° are vulnerable to patellar conditions, particularly abnormal tracking and instability. The Q angle can be functionally increased in genu varum, genu recurvatum and overpronation of the subtalar joint.

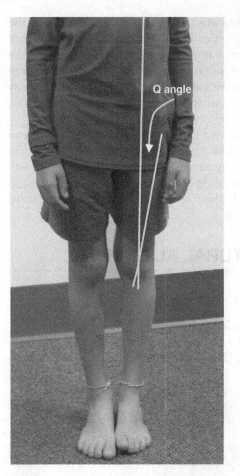

Fig. 6.1

KNEE MECHANICS

The biomechanics of the tibiofemoral joint during gait are very complicated. To put it simply, during the phases of heel strike and stance the knee is extended with the tibia in a relatively lateral position and the femur in a medial position. This occurs partly through the influence of the hip stabilizers, the contours of the articular surfaces of the tibia and femur, and the actions of the quadriceps, hamstring and tibialis muscles. These movements of the tibia and femur combined with the presence of the menisci accommodate the asymmetry of the femoral condyles. During the toe-off and swing phases the tibia moves to a relatively medial position in relation to the femur.

Abnormal motion mechanics in the relative positioning of the tibia and femur may increase loading on the menisci, alter tensions on the collateral, patellar and cruciate ligaments, and affect the resting lengths of the muscles acting on the knee. Altered mechanics of the tibia also influence ankle and foot mechanics, and vice versa. An internally rotated tibia is often associated with pes planus and excessive supination of the foot, especially during running activities. Internal rotation of the tibia may arise from increased tone in the adductor muscles, which limits its external rotation. When the tibia is restricted in an internally rotated position, the medial meniscus is subjected to greater compressive force and loading during the extension phase. Over time this may lead to inflammation of the meniscus, midline joint pain on the medial aspect, and eventual meniscal degeneration.

An externally rotated tibia is typically associated with an over-supinated foot or a pes cavus during stance. However, during gait, especially running, the over-supinated foot will compensate by pronating at the subtalar joint and forefoot. Externally rotated tibias are also found with genu varus posture and bowlegs.

KNEE POSTURAL ALIGNMENT

Clinical Notes

The posture of the leg is determined by comparing the position of the knee to an imaginary plumb-line dropped from the femoral head (Fig. 6.2). This should be done in both

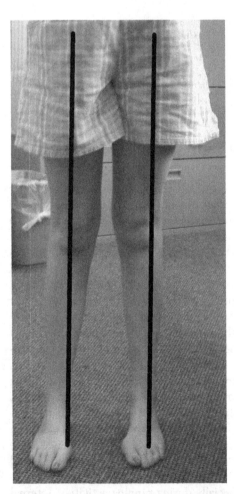

Fig. 6.2

supine and standing positions because in some conditions a valgus posture will only present with weightbearing. Infants and early walkers normally have a varus posturing of the leg. This is partly due to the position of the hip and the increased tone of flexor muscles in the extremities at this age. As the child continues to ambulate, the varus posture becomes more valgus. Between the ages of 2 and 3 years many children will develop a genu valgus. This alignment should straighten by the age of 6 or 7 years. Some girls have a recurrence of the genu valgum as they enter puberty, probably due to the increasing gynecoid shape of their pelvis.

GENU VALGUS (Fig. 6.3)

Clinical Notes

Genu valgus develops as a normal variation in some toddlers and in most resolves by 5 or 6 years of age, although it can persist until 8 years. Genu valgus may also be seen in early adolescence, when it is thought to be a result of rapid growth. Children with significant spasticity involving the adductor column may develop a valgus deformity, and those with weakness of the lateral hip rotator muscles, such as the gluteus maximus and piriformis, are also at risk. Genu valgus posture during standing may be associated with pes planus, everted calcaneus, an internally rotated femur, lower limb compensation for persistent femoral anteversion, internally rotated tibia, or an anteriorly tipped pelvis. Valgus posturing during gait only suggests compensation for an inverted calcaneus (varum calcaneus), abnormal muscle firing patterns, leg length discrepancy, increased adductor tone or spasticity.

GENU VARUS (Fig. 6.3)

Clinical Notes

Genu varus is the normal position of the knee from birth to early walking. It resolves spontaneously in most children before 2 years. In neonates the appearance of genu varum is often magnified by the normally increased flexor tone of the hips and knees, although it may also be exacerbated by true internal torsion of the tibia or femur. The genu varum of the neonate is accompanied by a physiological bowing of the tibia. This is due to the intrauterine lie, where the hips are flexed and the feet and legs are turned medially. This position creates an external rotation of the femur and an internal rotation of the tibia. As the tone in the flexor muscles of the leg decreases, the femur and tibia assume a more neutral position. Both the physiological bowing and the genu varum should resolve spontaneously. However, if the associated muscles and ligaments remain restricted due to concomitant biomechanical dysfunction, the growth pattern of the leg will

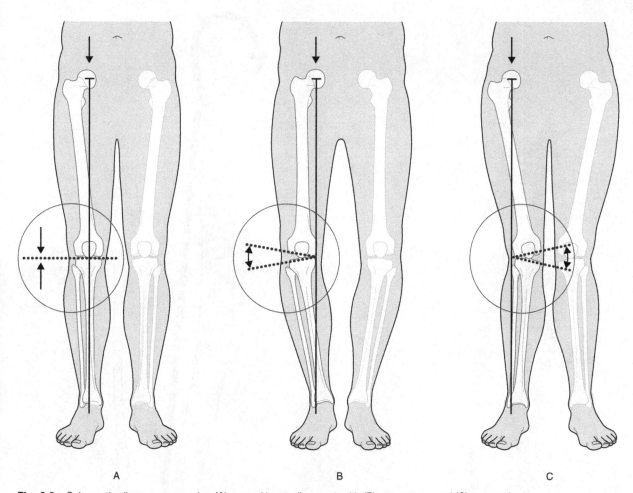

Fig. 6.3 • Schematic diagram comparing (A) normal knee alignment with (B) genu varus and (C) genu valgus.

be affected. Resolution of the bowed leg may be delayed, and in severe cases the varum deformity may worsen as the child grows, rather than improve. Varum deformities are usually categorized as infantile or late onset. Late-onset varum may develop in response to biomechanical strains. However, if it is severe, rickets or Blount's disease must be considered.

Some children will develop a genu varum posture of the legs when running. This causes the lateral aspect of the foot to contact the ground on heel strike rather than the full calcaneus. Then, as the body is carried forward the foot moves into dorsiflexion and over-pronates in compensation for the varum. This places excessive stress on the knee and ankle, and may contribute to the development of shin splints.

OSGOOD–SCHLATTER SYNDROME

Clinical Notes

Osgood–Schlatter syndrome is a condition whereby the epiphyseal plate of the tibial tuberosity becomes inflamed.

Abnormal tensile forces acting on the tibial tuberosity through the patellar ligament result in microfractures in the vulnerable epiphyseal plate. Symptoms usually arise during times of rapid growth, such as adolescence. Once the epiphyseal plate fuses, the symptoms resolve. Although the condition is self-limiting it can be quite painful and may interfere with the child's activities. In milder cases (called type I disease) the child will complain of pain and there may be tenderness, but there are no radiographic changes. In more severe conditions, disruption and inflammation of the epiphyseal plate are evident on plain X-ray and there is tenderness to palpation over the tubercle. This is called type II disease.

The biomechanical influences on the patellar tendon and tibia need to be considered when managing a child with Osgood–Schlatter's disease. During adolescence the immature tibial tuberosity is vulnerable to abnormal biomechanical forces, probably because of its active growth plate. (In the mature knee the meniscus and intra-articular surface of the patella appear to be more susceptible.) Osgood–Schlatter disease seems to be more prevalent in children who play

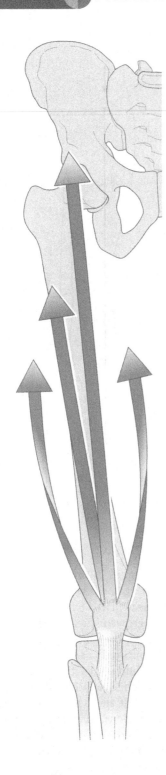

Fig. 6.4

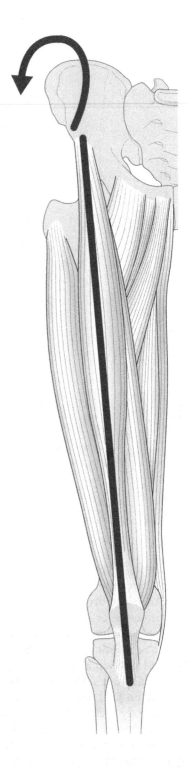

Fig. 6.5

sports that involve rapid stopping and turning, as these movements may exacerbate the forces converging at the tubercle.

The tensile forces of the patellar tendon and the tracking of the patella are governed superiorly by the contraction of the rectus femoris, vastus medialis and vastus lateralis muscles (Fig. 6.4). Anterior and posterior rotations of the innominate will alter the tensile forces through the quadriceps

and hamstrings. For example, a posteriorly rotated innominate coupled with a weak vastus medialis or an externally rotated tibia increases the stretch on the quadriceps during knee flexion, thereby increasing the tensile forces on the patellar tendon (Fig. 6.5). Another condition whereby the tensile load on the patellar tendon and tubercle is increased is pes planus. Pes planus encourages internal rotation of the tibia and limits lateral (external) rotation during the extension phase of gait. This situation is exacerbated during running, because the foot over-pronates to compensate for the restricted motion of the tibia placing more strain on the patellar tendon. The anterior tibialis muscle is often weak and partly responsible for the dropped medial arch. This is correctable through reconditioning of the muscles supporting the plantar arches. In pes planus caused by an articular mechanical dysfunction or bony deformity, the increased tension on the tibialis anterior muscle will create resistance to external rotation of the tibia as the foot is loaded. This may indeed be the etiology for the restricted tibial motion.

In problems of the knee and leg the biomechanics of the pelvis, femur, tibia and foot should be evaluated. The mechanics of the tibia and femur should be addressed initially, followed by the pelvis, the foot, and finally the patella. As a sesamoid bone the patella often becomes the point of convergence for many of the forces acting on the limb. Abnormal foot mechanics need to be managed through manipulation and, when necessary, an appropriate orthotic should be introduced for stability and support (see Foot and Ankle section). The strength and resting tone of the vastus lateralis and medialis muscles can be reconditioned using the retraining exercises described later in this chapter.

ROTATED TIBIA/TIBIAL TORSION

Clinical Notes

True tibial torsion refers to an intraosseous twisting of the tibia on its long axis. A rotated tibia refers to the position of the tibia in relation to the femur. Rotation of the tibia on the femur is a normal component of the gait cycle. Tibial torsion is a normal component of growth and development in humans. As we move from quadripedal to bipedal stance, the tibia molds into external torsion and the femur assumes a less anteverted position. Unfortunately, in discussions regarding clinical conditions involving abnormal torsion or rotation, these terms are often used interchangeably. In reality, most patients have an abnormally rotated tibia rather than an abnormal torsion. A rotated tibia may result from imbalances in muscle strength, altered gait mechanics or trauma. Children may develop true tibial torsion when normal growth is distorted by chronic or severe abnormalities in muscle tone, such as one might see in spasticity. Torsions may also arise as a developmental response to chronic abnormal biomechanics at the foot, knee or hip.

In neonates and infants there is significantly more glide and rotation of the tibia in both the flexed and extended positions than in toddlers and older children. The rotatory and translatory movements at the knee will decrease as the surrounding muscles and ligaments mature. If, however, there are significant asymmetries in resting length, tone or strength between the medial and lateral columns, the knee will develop with a preferential internal or external position of the tibia. The former will give the appearance of an intoed foot, the latter an abducted foot. In toddlers and infants the rotation of the tibia influences the appearance of the foot but not the patella. When the knee is extended, the patella remains on the frontal plane although the foot is in a medial or lateral position. With internal tibial rotation the foot may be adducted during gait, and younger children may have some clumsiness with running or climbing stairs.

A rule of thumb is to evaluate the mechanics of the tibia and femur in all children with problems of the distal leg. This is especially true with complaints related to traumatic injury, repetitive activity, or symptoms associated with generalized midline joint pain, locking of the knee, abnormal foot mechanics, pain in the fibular head or lateral compartment pain. During toe-off the tibia is externally rotated and the femur internally rotated. This represents the 'screw home' mechanism of the knee, which helps to stabilize the joint during weightbearing. The mechanics of the tibia and femur may be assessed with the patient seated or supine. The motion should be relatively smooth and constant until the very end of extension, when there may be a sudden increase in velocity. It is best assessed actively, but in small children or uncooperative patients it can be assessed passively. With the patient in a seated or supine position the tibia appears to rotate externally (move away from the patient's midline) as the knee is extended. (The rotation of the femur is less evident in the non-weightbearing position.) As the knee is flexed, the tibia internally rotates.

Screening of Intraosseous Tibial Torsion

Infant and Toddler

1. The child is seated, supine, or in the parent's lap. The physician sits facing the child. The physician grasps the leg just inferior to the knee and contacts the attachment of the patellar tendon with the thumb. The other hand grasps the distal tibia with the thumb placed at the midpoint of the ankle mortise (Fig. 6.6).

2. The tibial shaft and the two thumbs should lie in the same vertical plane. If there is excessive torsion in the tibia, the thumbs will appear to lie in parallel planes.

Passive Range of Motion Assessment of the Tibia (Fig. 6.7)

Seated Athlete

1. The patient sits with his knees flexed and legs suspended from the table. The thighs should be parallel.

2. The physician grasps the proximal tibia with both hands just inferior to the joint line. The tibia is gently rotated internally and externally.

3. Passive external and internal rotation of the tibia should be bilaterally symmetrical. With the knee in flexion, passive external rotation should be slightly greater than internal rotation.

4. Lateral translation, and anterior and posterior glide are assessed. Lateral translation should be minimal in the young athlete compared to a younger child. Anteroposterior glide should be bilaterally symmetrical.

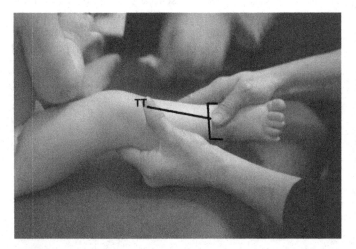

Fig. 6.6

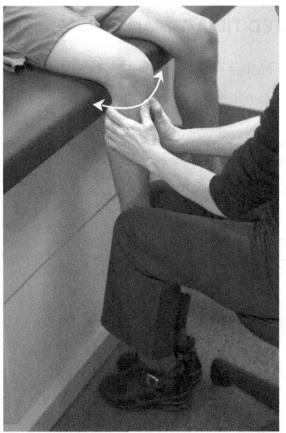

Fig. 6.7

Passive Functional Motion Assessment of the Tibia

Infant/Toddler (Fig. 6.8)

1. The child is seated, supine, or held in the parent's arms. The physician contacts the patella between the thumb and middle finger of one hand (Fig. 6.8), using the index finger to mark the approximate midpoint in the bone (MP). The other hand grasps the tibia with the thumb contacting the insertion of the quadriceps tendon (QT).

2. The physician passively flexes and extends the tibia on the femur, noting the rotatory motion of the tibia and the relationship between the insertion of the quadriceps tendon and the midpoint of the patella.

3. The motion of the tibia should be smooth and symmetrical in both knees. In a non-ambulatory child the rotation will be minimal and equal. The tibia should not internally rotate more medially than the midpoint of the patella.

4. In an ambulatory child external rotation will be slightly greater than internal rotation. With knee flexion the tibia should be aligned with the midpoint of the patella and not positioned medial to that point (Fig. 6.9).

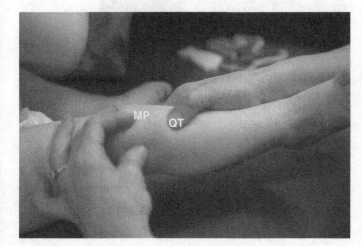

Fig. 6.8

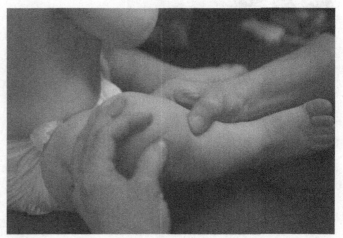

Fig. 6.9

Functional/Active Assessment of the Tibia

Supine and Seated Athlete

1. The patient is supine with the knee flexed. One hand grasps the patella and monitors the center or midline of the bone. The other hand grasps the proximal tibia with the thumb on the tibial tuberosity (Fig. 6.10). The relationship between the positions of the two points is noted. In the flexed position the tibial tuberosity should be in the same plane as the center of the patella. The figure depicts the correct plane of relationship (gray arrow) and the actual plane of relationship (black line).

2. The knee is moved into extension. The tibia should rotate laterally (away from the patient's midline). It is important to stabilize the patella through this motion because abnormal patella tracking will create a false finding. The movement of the tibia is observed through the extension phase. The quality of motion and range of motion are noted. At the end of extension, the tibial tuberosity should be lateral to the midline of the patella (Fig. 6.11).

3. The strain is diagnosed and named according to the position of ease, not the restrictive barrier. If in the flexed position the tubercle is medial to the midline of the patella, this is described as internal rotation of the patella. Likewise, if the tuberosity is in the midline of the patella but does not move laterally during extension, this is also described as internal rotation of the tibia. Conversely, if the tuberosity is positioned lateral to the midline of the patella during flexion, or if it does not move towards the midline of the patella during flexion, this is described as an externally rotated

tibia. Either case can be treated using direct thrust, muscle energy, or the balanced ligamentous technique described under posterior tibia.

4. The test can also be performed in a seated position (Figs 6.12 and 6.13).

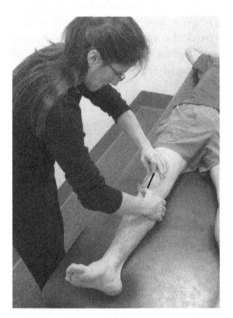

Fig. 6.11

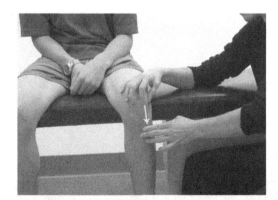

Fig. 6.12

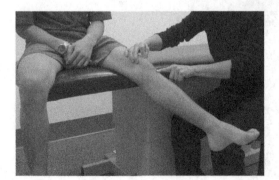

Fig. 6.13

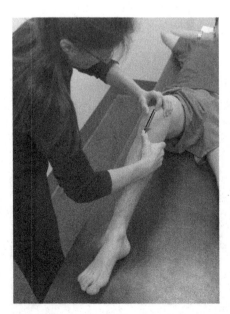

Fig. 6.10

Treatment Notes

Tibial torsion is an intraosseous phenomenon. In infants and very young children the tensile forces acting on the shaft of the tibia can interfere with normal torsional accommodation of femoral development. Treating the soft tissue (muscles and fascia) and biomechanical dysfunctions can eliminate those aberrant forces and may allow the bone to remodel correctly. In older children and young adults the torsional component may have become an inherent component of the bone's structure, and it may not remodel even if the mechanical influences are normalized. In these patients the compensatory strain patterns that arise at the joints and in the stabilizing muscles of the limb and pelvis need to be addressed to prevent secondary problems developing.

DIRECT MYOFASCIAL RELEASE

Long Restrictor Muscles

Infant

1. The infant is supine, seated, or held by the parent. The physician sits beside the child on the affected side.

2. The physician uses one hand to contact the posterior tissues at the proximal end just inferior to the knee, and the other to contact the column at the distal end (Fig. 6.14).

3. The physician slowly introduces compression and distraction and notes the response of the tissue. The physician introduces the appropriate force to engage the restrictive barrier. The physician maintains that tissue tension and slowly introduces torsional forces into the tissue to fine-tune to the restrictive barrier.

4. As the barrier changes, the physician reintroduces the appropriate vector to engage the new restrictive barrier. This is repeated until there is a significant change in tissue tension, or an improvement in the somatic dysfunction.

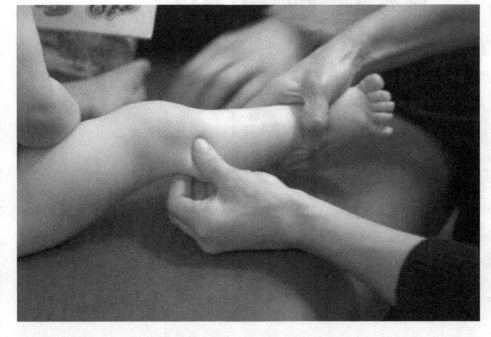

Fig. 6.14

ISOMETRIC MUSCLE ENERGY TECHNIQUE

Externally Rotated Tibia (Fig. 6.15)

Isometric contraction is used to correct the mechanical dysfunction.

1. The patient is seated with the leg passively extended and resting across the physician's knees. The physician should be seated somewhat below the patient, allowing for a slight flexion in the patient's knee.

2. The tibia is rotated internally to the barrier, without causing any rotation in the thigh.

3. The patient is asked to gently turn his leg towards external rotation, thereby externally rotating the tibia. The physician resists this movement to the extent that the long restrictors of the knee are engaged. Care is taken that there is no undue stress placed on the ligamentous structures of the knee.

4. This isometric contraction is maintained for 4–5 seconds, and then the patient is asked to cease contraction while the physician simultaneously reduces her counterforce.

5. The physician maintains contact and waits for tissue relaxation (approximately 4–5 seconds).

6. The physician internally rotates the tibia to reposition it to the new barrier. The sequence is repeated twice.

Fig. 6.15

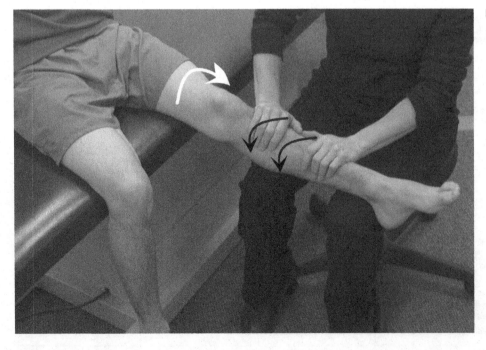

ISOMETRIC MUSCLE ENERGY TECHNIQUE

Internally Rotated Tibia (Fig. 6.16)

1. Isometric contraction is used to correct the mechanical dysfunction.

2. The patient is seated with the leg passively extended and resting across the physician's knees. The physician should be seated somewhat below the patient, allowing for a slight flexion in the patient's knee.

3. The tibia is rotated externally to the barrier, without causing any rotation in the thigh.

4. The patient is asked to gently turn his leg towards internal rotation, thereby internally rotating the tibia.

The physician resists this movement to the extent that the long restrictors of the knee are engaged. Care is taken that there is no undue stress placed on the ligamentous structures of the knee.

5. This isometric contraction is maintained for 4–5 seconds. The patient is then asked to cease contraction while the physician simultaneously reduces her counterforce.

6. The physician maintains contact and waits for tissue relaxation (approximately 4–5 seconds).

7. The physician externally rotates the tibia to reposition it to the new barrier. The sequence is repeated twice.

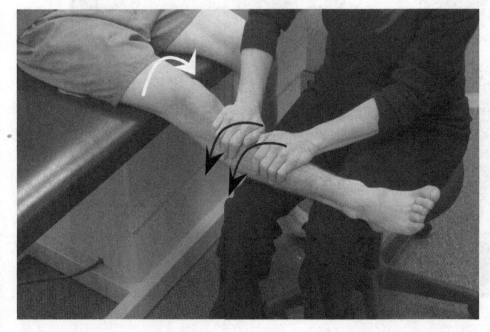

Fig. 6.16

THRUST TECHNIQUE ('J' TECHNIQUE)

Thrust technique may be applied in older children and adolescents to correct abnormal rotation of the tibia during flexion and extension of the knee.

THRUST TECHNIQUE ('J' TECHNIQUE)

Internally Rotated Tibia (Fig. 6.17)

Athlete/Older Child

1. The patient is supine with the knee flexed.
2. The physician places her hand behind the tibia, contacting its posterior surface. The other hand grasps the distal tibia.

3. The tibia is externally rotated to the restrictive barrier.
4. A short, firm thrust in a 'J'-shaped direction is made, moving the tibia laterally to medially towards the ischial tuberosity, exaggerating external rotation.

Externally Rotated Tibia (Fig. 6.18)

Athlete/Older Child

1. The patient is supine with the knee flexed.
2. The physician places her hand behind the tibia, contacting the posterior surface. The other hand grasps the distal tibia.
3. The tibia is internally rotated to the restrictive barrier.
4. A short, firm thrust in a backward 'J'-shaped direction is made, moving the tibia medially to laterally towards the ischial tuberosity, and exaggerating internal rotation.

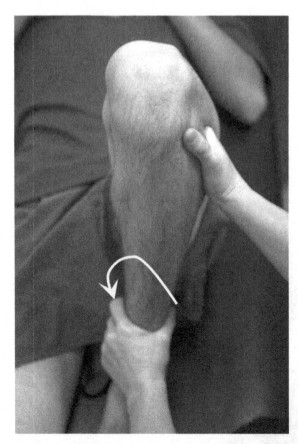

Fig. 6.17

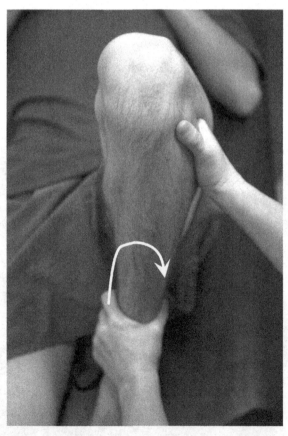

Fig. 6.18

DIRECT TECHNIQUE
ARTICULATORY – SHORT LEVER

Tibia

Toddler

This approach can be used in a toddler or older infant with a true articular dysfunction of the tibia on the femur that does not resolve with correction of the soft tissue dysfunction. Articular tibial strains are less common in infants and toddlers. When they do occur they are more likely to develop as a result of compensatory changes or adaptations to congenital malpositions, bony deformity or abnormal muscle tone. This is a short lever technique and should not be used as a long lever technique.

1. The toddler is supine, seated, or held by a parent. The physician sits beside and facing the child on the affected side. The child's knee is flexed. The physician grasps the proximal tibia in one hand with the thumb contacting the insertion of the patellar tendon (Fig. 6.19). The other hand holds the distal femur between the middle finger and thumb, and marks the midpoint of the patella with the index finger.

2. The physician carries the knee into extension, noting the restrictive barrier to external rotation of the tibia in full extension. The physician flexes the knee, allowing the tibia to rotate medially, and then carries the knee back into extension, engaging the restrictive barrier of the tibia to external (lateral) rotation but not moving through it (Fig. 6.20).

3. During each knee extension the physician meets the restrictive barrier with an equal and opposite force, but not a force that is greater than the restrictive barrier.

4. In Figure 6.20 the black arrow represents the physician's force marrying into, but not through, the restrictive barrier. The tip of the arrow has not stopped at the restrictive barrier: it has entered the resistance of the barrier.

5. The physician flexes the knee again, allowing the tibia to rotate medially, and then extends the knee and laterally rotates the tibia, engaging the restrictive barrier but not moving through it.

6. This sequence is repeated three to four times. With each subsequent extension the restrictive barrier should move a little, increasing the lateral rotation of the tibia.

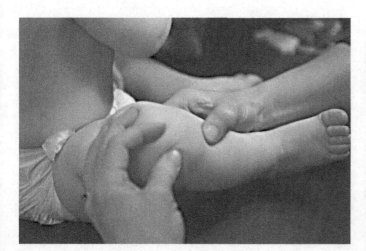

Fig. 6.19

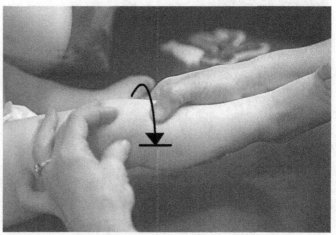

Fig. 6.20

BALANCED LIGAMENTOUS TENSION TECHNIQUE

Knee Joint

Toddler/Infant

This approach can be used in children with lower extremity deformities or dysfunction to address the tensile forces around the knee joint as well as its mechanical function.

1. The child is seated, supine, or held in the parent's arms. The physician sits on the involved side. The physician contacts the proximal tibia with one hand, using the thumb to contact the attachment of the quadriceps tendon (Fig. 6.21). The other hand contacts the distal femur, with a contact on the patella also.

2. The physician monitors the tissue tension at the mid-joint line.

3. The physician attempts to bring the ligamentous articular relations into balanced tension by moving the tissues of the knee through all planes of motion using a stacking method. The structures are moved sequentially through each plane of motion until equal or balanced tissue tension is felt.

4. The physician begins the technique by balancing the tibia and femur in relation to the compressive or distractive forces in the knee. This is done by gently and slowly introducing traction or compression into the joint.

5. The physician can introduce flexion, extension, internal and external rotation at the joint by using her hands to directly move the tibia and femur in opposite directions.

6. Valgus and varus stresses can be introduced by gently exaggerating these stresses into the tissues.

7. A combination of these movements is used to create balanced ligamentous tension throughout the tissues of the knee joint. Once balanced tension is achieved, the physician maintains that position until a correction in the mechanical strain or improvement in tissue function is noted.

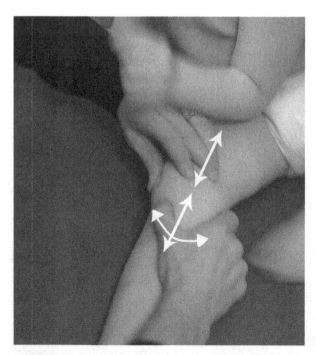

Fig. 6.21

PATELLAR SYNDROMES (Fig. 6.22)

Clinical Notes

At birth the patella is in a relative lateral position and moves into the frontal plane as the femur moves into its mature position. By 6 years, the patella should lie in the frontal plane. Deformities of the tibia, femoral torsion, hip dysplasia and displacement of the acetabulum may all be associated with abnormal patellar position. By and large, most problems concerning the patella are related to patellar misalignment or instability, and are associated with biomechanical dysfunction in the knee, hip or foot rather than a true deformity.

Any strains affecting the mechanics of the tibia and femur will influence the patella. Abnormal patellar tracking leads to increased pressure on the deep cartilaginous surfaces of the patellar facets. The subchondral bone in this area is heavily innervated with primary nociceptors. Continued pressure has the potential to also affect the cartilage of the femoral condyles, disrupting the proteoglycan molecules and leading to a breakdown in the articular cartilage. The resulting inflammation and surface deformity may exacerbate the tracking problems and cause pain. In conditions of the patella such as patellofemoral syndrome, chondromalacia patellae, patellar bursitis and subluxating

patella, the mechanics of the knee, foot and hip need to be considered before treating the patella. Alternatively, when treating dysfunctions of the knee or hip, especially those involving the quadriceps, one should address patellar mechanics as a potential means of preventing problems later in life. Symptoms of patellar dysfunction usually arise after recurrent or prolonged strain. However, there are cases of acute injury resulting in patellar dysfunction.

The patella should glide smoothly between the anterior parts of the two femoral condyles. It is influenced from above by the quadriceps. Innominate rotations will alter the resting length of the quadriceps and may thus influence patellar tracking. One of the most common findings associated with patellar conditions is abnormal function of the vastus medialis and vastus lateralis muscles. Typically, the vastus lateralis is significantly stronger than the medialis muscle. As the quadriceps contracts, the medialis is unable to counterbalance the force of the lateralis and the patella is carried laterally, resulting in lateral tracking. This vastus imbalance is often present in young women and is probably further exacerbated by the increased Q angle in that population. These two factors account for the prevalence of patellar dysfunction in adolescent women.

When the knee is actively extended, the oblique head of the vastus medialis muscle should be visible and firm to palpation (Fig. 6.23). If this is not the case, then the vastus medialis is deconditioned, or in extreme cases dysplastic. In addition to osteopathic treatment, the management plan for

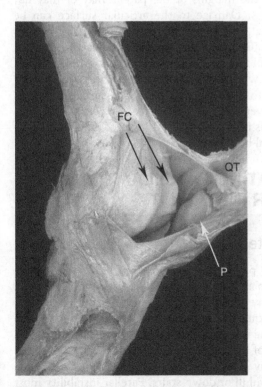

Fig. 6.22 • Medial view into the dissected knee joint. The skin and musculature have been removed. The quadriceps tendon (QT) is pulled away, lifting the patella (P) from its position between the femoral condyles (FC).

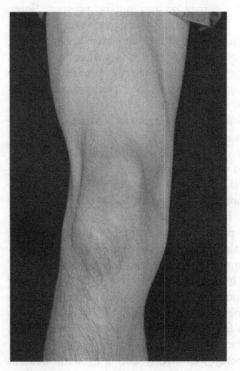

Fig. 6.23

these patients should incorporate muscle rebalancing and strengthening exercises, such as those described below.

Iliotibial band dysfunction may also play a role in patellar conditions. The iliopatellar ligament extends anteriorly from the distal iliotibial band just superior to the lateral femoral condyle. The band crosses from anteriorly and inferiorly to merge with the vastus lateralis muscle and inserts on the lateral border of the patella. In cases of lateral patellar tracking, the components of the iliotibial band need to be assessed for biomechanical dysfunction. This includes the tensor fascia latae, gluteus maximus, and gluteus medius muscles, as well as the ipsilateral innominate and tibia. Strengthening of vastus medialis alone will not be sufficient to overcome the mechanical forces of the iliotibial band if dysfunction persists (see Chapter 5, Femur, Hip and Pelvis). Surgical release of the iliopatellar ligament is sometimes necessary in recalcitrant cases.

CHONDROMALACIA PATELLAE/ PATELLOFEMORAL SYNDROME

Clinical Notes

Chondromalacia and patellofemoral syndrome are non-specific terms used to describe anterior knee pain of unspecified etiology. The patient usually complains of crepitus, grinding, and retropatellar pain, especially after prolonged knee flexion or flexion combined with weight-bearing, such as climbing the stairs or getting out up a chair. Stiffness of the knee may or may not be present. Some patients describe the knee as 'giving out' when loaded. Patellofemoral syndrome can be associated with trauma, but is more commonly insidious in onset. It is common in runners, especially teenage girls, where it tends to be more chronic and is probably influenced by the increased Q angle in that population.

There is considerable controversy surrounding the nomenclature of anterior knee pain. Chondromalacia patellae is a general term that can be used to describe idiopathic anterior knee pain or disruption of the articular surface of the patella. The disruption of the articular surface arises as a result of abnormal compressive forces on the patellar facet, resulting in breakdown of hyaline cartilage. In most cases the primary problem is misalignment of the patella as it travels through the femoral condyles in flexion and extension. The articular surface of the patella has seven distinct facets that allow it to move in different directions during flexion and extension of the knee. The most obvious motion of the patella is the superior and inferior glide in the trochlear groove of the femur as the knee moves through flexion and extension. In addition, the patella glides laterally during mid-flexion and rotates externally during extreme flexion. These movements are carried out as the different patellar

facets come in contact with the articular surface of the condyles. The patella provides leverage to the quadriceps muscle as the knee moves into extension. Hypertonicity of the quadriceps will increase the compressive load on the patella, whereas quadriceps weakness may undermine the stability of the patella.

Patellar tracking is influenced by the patellar ligaments, the rectus femoris, vastus lateralis, and vastus medialis muscles, particularly the oblique head of vastus medialis. These structures stabilize and guide the patella as the tibia is moved on the femur. Weakness of the vastus medialis, especially the oblique head, results in lateral tracking and rotation of the patella. This increases the compressive forces on the facets, particularly the medial facet. Ligamentous laxity or tightness can result in patellar tilt when the knee is in the flexed position. This can also produce excessive compression on the surfaces of the medial facets.

The undersurface of the patella is cartilaginous and vulnerable to trauma. Abnormal tracking places excessive pressure on the soft cartilage, which can eventually break down, resulting in edema, areas of compression, and even dents. This disruption of the smooth cartilaginous surface further exacerbates the tracking problem. When the condition is acutely exacerbated, the patient may present with infrapatellar edema and swelling about the knee. Often there is no clear history of injury or other exacerbating events. Palpation over the margins of the patella may or may not elicit tenderness. Damage to the articular surface can be described using four levels of severity. Stage 1 involves localized softening and inflammation of the cartilage: if not addressed it will lead to breakdown of the hyaline cartilage. Stage 2 occurs when the hyaline cartilage breaks down and fissures begin to appear on the articular surface. The fissures spread over the articular surface and neovascularization occurs; this is stage 3. Stage 4 involves inflammation of the subchondral bone.

SUBLUXATING PATELLA/ PATELLAR INSTABILITY

Clinical Notes

In subluxating patella the knee becomes unstable as the patella moves in and out of the trochlear groove of the femur. The patient may describe popping, instability, crunching or grinding with knee movement, especially when the joint is loaded. Swelling is usually present and may be accompanied by a sensation of locking. The knee often feels unstable, and the patient may avoid activities that stress the knee, such as walking downhill or down stairs. Patellar instability most often involves lateral subluxation. In extreme cases there can be a true dislocation with rupture of the patellar capsule. In recurrent conditions, effusions are common. Joint effusion can worsen the situation by reflexively inhibiting activation of the oblique head of the vastus medialis muscle. In cases of chronic joint effusion with distension of the articular capsule the femoral nerve is inhibited, resulting in atrophy of the oblique head of vastus medialis.

Like other patellar conditions, patellar instability is more common in females than males. This is probably due to the prevalence of genu valgus and increased Q angles in females. Patellar instability is also associated with external tibial rotation, femoral anteversion, weakness of the vastus medialis, tightness of the lateral patellar ligaments, shortening of the rectus femoris or vastus lateralis muscles, tightness of the iliotibial band, and posterior rotation of the innominate. These associated findings may be primary or contributory to the instability.

In addition to manipulative treatment and rehabilitation, bracing during activities is often required to prevent further injury. As one would expect, following an acute exacerbation, wrapping or bracing the knee, rest, ice, and elevation are essential.

PATELLAR BURSITIS

Clinical Notes

Patellar bursitis usually develops from a repetitive strain or microtrauma. Commonly known as 'housemaid's knee' and associated with prolonged kneeling, it is not uncommon in unconditioned but enthusiastic athletes who begin enthusiastic cycling about the time of the seventh stage of the Tour de France. Whereas with patellofemoral syndrome the pain is behind the patella, in patellar bursitis the pain is prepatellar and often accompanied by erythema and focal defined swelling over the anterior surface of the knee. There is tenderness to palpation over the patella. Pain is typically present in full flexion and full extension of the knee, although there is usually no pain with moderate amounts of movement. The inflammation may affect any of the knee bursae, but the prepatellar, infrapatellar and pes anserinus bursae are most frequently involved. The location of the pain, tenderness and swelling is indicative of the kind of bursitis. The infrapatellar and prepatellar bursae act as friction reducers between the tendons of the quadriceps and the skin. With prolonged compression or repetitive motion the bursa swells to produce more fluid for lubrication. As it enlarges, the friction placed on it increases, causing chafing and microtrauma. This leads to inflammation. Quadriceps spasm, posteriorly rotated, outflared and upslipped innominate dysfunctions all predispose the bursa to friction during knee movement. The pes anserinus bursa becomes susceptible to irritation with persistent externally rotated tibia, genu valgus and medial hamstring spasm.

In athletes, especially those with improper training techniques, trigger points, as described by Travell and Simons (1983), need to be included in the differential diagnosis of patellar pain. These authors describe a trigger point at the proximal musculoligamentous junction of the rectus femoris which produces suprapatellar pain. Another trigger point in the distal belly of the vastus medialis muscle will refer to the medial aspect of the patella. Those in the adductor brevis muscle refer to the superior aspect of the patella.

ASSESSMENT OF THE PATELLA

Clinical Notes

Static and dynamic evaluations should be carried out to ascertain the factors contributing to the patellar symptoms. Contraction of the quadriceps should carry the patella superiorly along the trochlear groove of the femur. This should be a smooth and symmetrical movement. Deviation of the patella from the midline of the leg is usually due to an imbalance between the vastus medialis and vastus latera-lis muscles. If the patella moves laterally, then the vastus lateralis is overpowering the vastus medialis.

An internally rotated tibia will produce compressive forces on the medial patellar facet when the knee moves into extension. These forces may converge at the tibial tubercle or on the patella. An externally rotated tibia increases tension on the patellar tendon and the patella during knee flexion. Pes planus of the foot produces a valgus strain in the knee, which may also play a role in patellar dysfunction.

Abnormal movement between the tibia and femur during flexion and extension may also play a role in conditions of the patella. For example, if the tibia is locked in a relatively externally rotated position, then during knee flexion there will be increased tension on the patellar tendon which will compress the patella into the trochlea. Dysfunction of the tibia on the femur should be treated prior to treatment of the patella.

Assessment of the Patella

Static Alignment (Fig. 6.24)

1. The patient stands facing the clinician with the feet facing forward.

2. The center of the patella should fall between the great toe and the second toe. If the patella appears to be medial when the feet are straight, this suggests femoral neck anteversion with internal rotation of the upper leg.

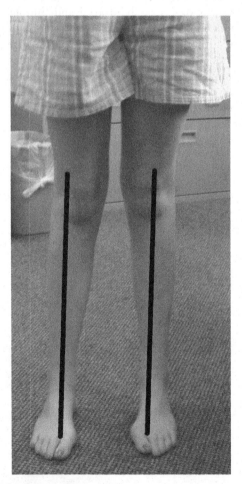

Fig. 6.24

Assessment of Patellar Tracking – Active

Full Range of Motion (Figs 6.25 and 6.26)

1. The patient is seated with the knee flexed. The patella is lightly palpated with one hand (Fig. 6.25).

2. The patient is asked to extend the knee and the patella is monitored through the motion (Fig. 6.26).

3. The quality and plane of movement are noted. The quality of motion is assessed for smoothness, and the presence of crepitus, grinding, clicking or restrictions. The plane of motion should be parallel with the long axis of the trochlear groove of the femur.

Alternate Technique (Fig. 6.27)

1. The knee is placed in passive extension and the patella and posterior tissues are lightly palpated.

2. The patient is asked to forcefully contract the quadriceps muscles.

3. The quality and plane of movement are noted. The quality of motion is assessed for smoothness, and the presence of crepitus, grinding, clicking or restrictions. The plane of motion should be parallel with the long axis of the trochlear groove of the femur.

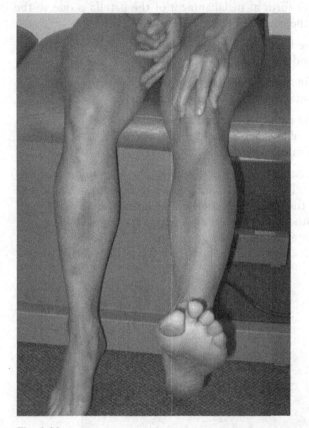

Fig. 6.26

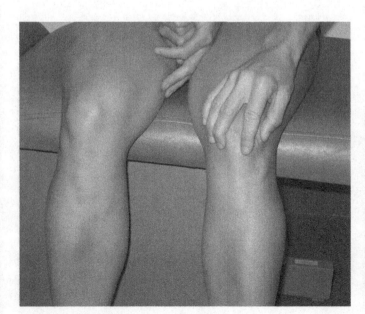

Fig. 6.25

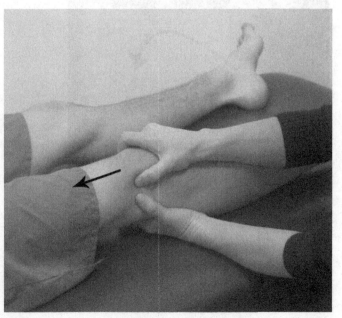

Fig. 6.27

Assessment of Patellar Tilt – Passive

(Fig. 6.28)

Another form of malalignment of the patella is due to the tilt of the patella in the trochlea.

1. The knee is in a passive extension position with the quadriceps relaxed.

2. The medial and lateral borders of the patella are contacted with the thumb and fingers.

3. The patella is assessed for freedom of motion. There should a small amount of give when the patella is lifted from the femur.

4. In patients with malalignment, the lateral aspect of the patella will not lift and passive movement of the patella in the medial direction will be limited. In patients without mechanical dysfunction the patella will be quite mobile.

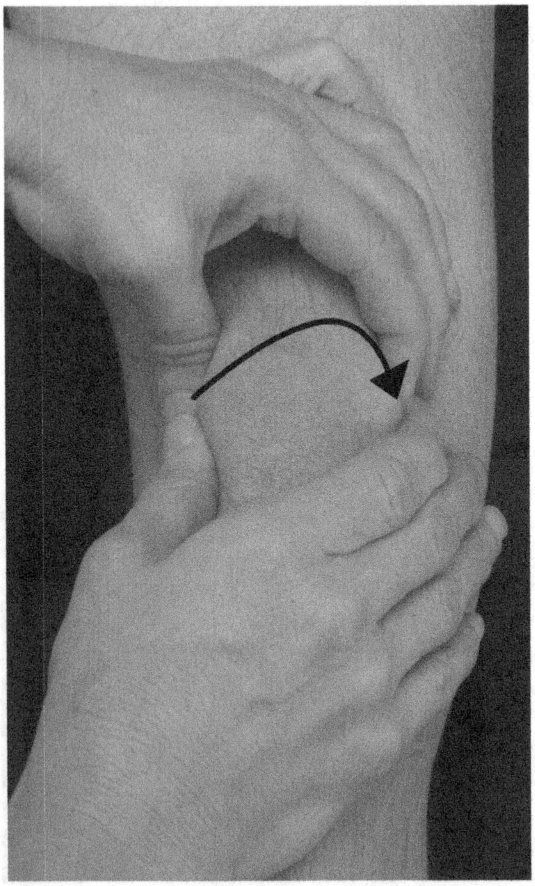

Assessment of Patellar Motion – Passive

Toddler (Fig. 6.29)

1. The child is seated with the legs extended in front of him. The physician contacts the superior margins of the patella while stabilizing the femur, and the inferior margins while stabilizing the tibia (Fig. 6.29).

2. The physician can then apply the appropriate forces to tilt, rotate and translate the patella, assessing range and quality of motion in each plane (Fig. 6.30).

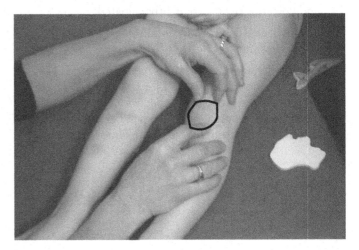

Fig. 6.29

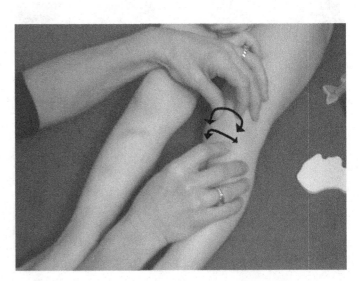

Fig. 6.30

Fig. 6.28

Assessment of Quadriceps Muscle Group
(Fig. 6.31)

The quadriceps group should be assessed for flexibility, tone and strength. Each of these components will influence patellar function.

1. The patient is prone.

2. The physician places one hand on the pelvis to monitor its movement. The other hand grasps the leg just proximal to the ankle.

3. The knee is passively flexed to bring the heel towards the buttocks. In this position, the rectus femoris as well as the vastus group is being stretched.

4. Flexion of the knee continues until a motion barrier is noted. Typically the pelvis will begin to tilt as the barrier in the rectus femoris muscle is reached. If the restriction is in the vastus group, then knee flexion will be limited before there is tilt in the pelvis. The distance between the heel and the buttocks is noted.

5. The same maneuver is repeated on the opposite leg and the findings are compared. The young man in the figure has normal flexibility for this maneuver.

Alternative Testing

Quadriceps Group

1. The patient is supine and the hip is flexed to 90° (Fig. 6.32). In this position the rectus femoris is relaxed and the restricted motion is more likely due to the vastus group. One of the physician's hands is placed over the knee and the other grasps the leg just proximal to the ankle.

2. The knee is passively flexed to bring the heel towards the buttocks until the motion barrier to knee flexion is reached. The distance between the heel and buttocks is noted.

3. The same maneuver is performed on the opposite leg and the findings are compared. The boy in the figure has normal flexibility for this maneuver.

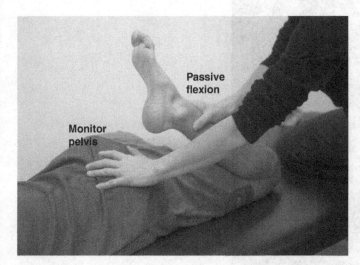

Passive flexion

Monitor pelvis

Fig. 6.31

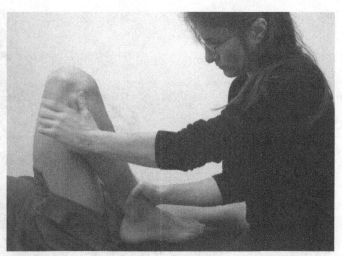

Fig. 6.32

ISOMETRIC MUSCLE ENERGY TECHNIQUE

Quadriceps (Fig. 6.33)

Athlete Prone

1. The patient is prone with the knee flexed. The physician stands on the side to be treated.

2. The physician uses one hand to monitor the pelvis and the other to grasp the distal tibia proximal to the ankle. The knee is flexed to the restrictive barrier.

3. The patient is asked to extend the knee towards the table (gray arrow) as the physician applies an equal but opposite force (black arrow). The patient's contraction should be localized to the quadriceps. The physician monitors the pelvis for motion.

4. This isometric contraction is maintained for 4–5 seconds. Then the patient is asked to cease the contraction while the physician simultaneously reduces her counterforce.

5. The physician maintains contact and waits for tissue relaxation (approximately 4–5 seconds). The physician flexes the knee to the new barrier. The sequence is repeated twice.

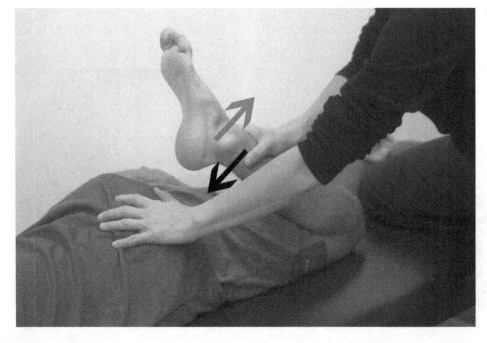

Fig. 6.33

Retraining of the Vastus Medialis Muscle
(Figs 6.34 and 6.35)

The vastus medialis can be retrained using a modified straight leg raising exercise.

1. The patient is seated on a firm surface with her back supported and her legs extended in front. One leg is maintained in a straight, extended position while the other is turned slightly into external rotation.

2. The leg that is externally rotated is then raised for three counts (Fig. 6.34), held for seven more counts and lowered for three counts (a total of 13 counts).

3. There are two points that are necessary for this exercise to be effective: first, when the leg is raised it needs to be sufficiently externally rotated that the vastus medialis is loaded and the vastus lateralis has less input (Fig. 6.34, white arrow). If, however, there is too much external rotation then the adductors will take over. (It is useful if the child can be taught to feel the vastus medialis working.) Second, the leg needs to be raised and lowered slowly to take advantage of both concentric and eccentric activity.

4. In Figure 6.35 the leg raise is performed with the leg in a neutral position (not externally rotated). The white arrow indicates the vastus medialis muscle. Compare this with the vastus medialis in Figure 6.34, when the leg is externally rotated to isolate the vastus medialis.

5. If weight training is employed for quadriceps strengthening it should be done with the knee in a flexed position at no less than 30° to avoid stressing the patella.

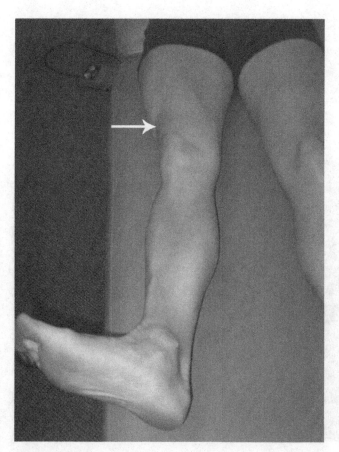

Fig. 6.34

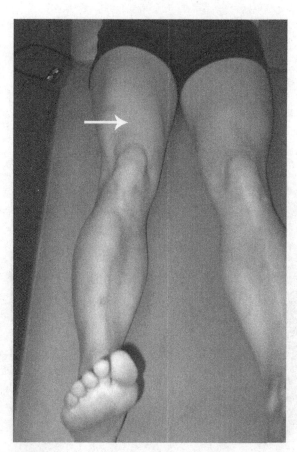

Fig. 6.35

TREATMENT OF THE PATELLA

Patellar dysfunction is typically compensatory or secondary to a problem in the foot, leg or hip. Consequently, before a patellar dysfunction can be treated successfully, somatic dysfunction in these other areas needs to be evaluated and treated. The patella can be treated in two ways, depending on the size of the patient and the physician. On a young athlete or a muscular leg the physician can facilitate the treatment by applying traction or compression to the knee.

BALANCED MEMBRANOUS TENSION TECHNIQUE

Patella

Seated Toddler/Child

Patellar dysfunction in toddlers is generally functional compensation to vara of the tibia, tibial torsion, or dysfunction in the hip and innominate. Rarely is patellar dysfunction a primary problem. Treatment of the patella should nevertheless be part of the overall management of the lower extremity.

1. The child is seated with his legs extended in front of him, similar to the position used to assess patellar motion. The physician uses one hand to contact the superior margin of the patella, stabilizing the femur. The other hand contacts the inferior margin, stabilizing the tibia (Fig. 6.36).

2. The physician will use a stacking method to find balanced tension in each plane of motion of the patella (Fig. 6.37).

3. The physician should use a direct rather than an indirect approach to engage the tissue in each restrictive barrier.

4. Once balanced tension is achieved, the physician maintains the position of the patella until there is a change in tissue texture or an improvement in the restrictive barrier.

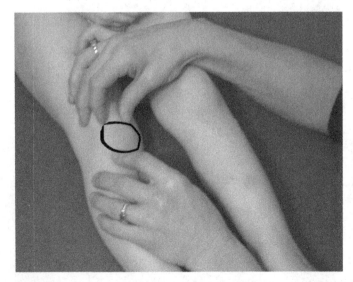

Fig. 6.36

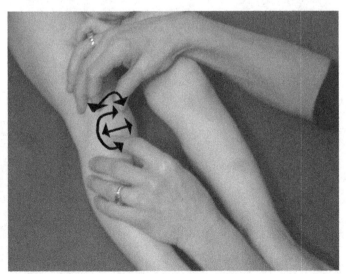

Fig. 6.37

BALANCED MEMBRANOUS TENSION TECHNIQUE

Patella

Seated Athlete

This approach is used to address tensions and stresses in the myofascial tissues influencing the patella (Fig. 6.38).

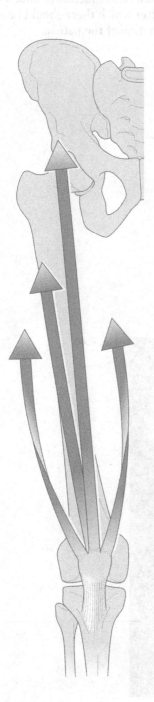

Fig. 6.38

1. The child is seated with the leg to be treated passively extended and resting on the physician's leg. The knee should have a small amount of flexion, so it is useful to have the physician sitting below the patient (Fig. 6.39).

2. The patient's leg is positioned so that the calcaneus is suspended over the lateral aspect of the physician's leg. The physician can then move her leg away from the patient to create traction on the knee.

3. The physician grasps the patella between the index fingers and thumbs of both hands.

4. As the patient's leg is tractioned away, the physician gently moves the patella through each possible plane of motion in succession, establishing balanced tension through the tissues attached to the patella. This is a stacking technique in which balanced tension is found in one plane of motion and maintained as the patella is moved through another plane of motion.

5. Balanced tension is established in each plane of motion sequentially. The point of balance is maintained until there is a change in tissue tension, after which there should be increased freedom of motion of the patella.

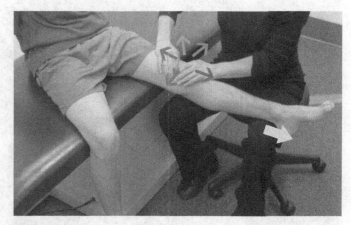

Fig. 6.39

ALTERNATIVE BALANCED LIGAMENTOUS TECHNIQUE

Patella

Supine Athlete

The patella can be treated with the leg passively extended on the table. In this case there is less knee flexion present than in the previous example, and this may not work in individuals with hyperextended knees.

1. One hand is placed under the popliteal fossa to create a small amount of flexion. The other hand grasps the patella (Fig. 6.40).

2. A stacking approach is used to achieve balanced tension. The patella is moved sequentially through each possible plane of motion, establishing balanced tension through its tissue attachments.

3. The point of balance is found and maintained until there is a change in tissue tension, after which there should be increased freedom of motion of the patella.

DIRECT MYOFASCIAL TECHNIQUE

Patella

Both of the positions of the physician and patient described above for balanced ligamentous tension may be used to apply a direct myofascial release to the patellar attachments. In direct myofascial release the patella is moved through each plane of motion to the restrictive barrier. The movements are stacked sequentially until a release of tissue tension is felt, after which there should be an improvement in the range of motion of the patella.

Fig. 6.40

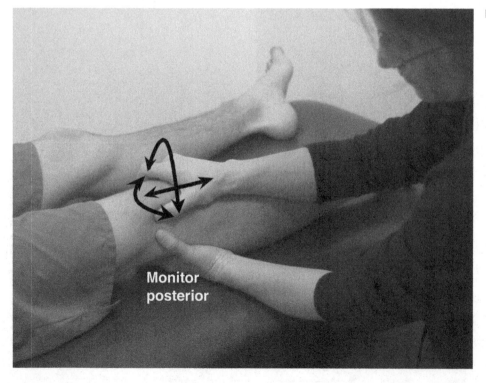

Monitor posterior

POSTERIOR TIBIAL DYSFUNCTION

Clinical Notes

A posterior tibial dysfunction is usually a traumatic injury that occurs when the foot and/or ankle is stabilized as the body weight and pelvis move forward. The momentum of the forward-moving body carries the pelvis and femur anteriorly on the stabilized tibia. In extreme cases this dysfunction may be associated with injury to the posterior cruciate ligament. This dysfunction is typically seen in sports in which the athlete wears cleated footwear, such as soccer, football and lacrosse; or sports in which the foot and ankle are fixed, such as skiing. It can also occur in equestrians during forward spills where the foot is delayed by the stirrup.

Typically the patient complains of knee pain that is worse when the knee is extended and weightbearing. Normally during extension there is some anterior glide of the tibia on the femur and a relative external rotation of the tibia and internal rotation of the femur. This is referred to as the 'screw home mechanism.' With the tibia locked posteriorly, full extension is limited, the screw home mechanism is impaired, and there is abnormal placement of the meniscus between the tibia and the femur. Consequently, with weightbearing the knee may feel unstable, although there is no true ligamentous disruption. The symptoms may be particularly exacerbated with climbing stairs, running, or hiking downhill. Full flexion may also be limited and painful.

In a posterior tibial somatic dysfunction, motion testing will reveal resistance to anterior motion of the tibia, or resistance to both anterior and posterior motion. Tenderness may or may not be present. Often there is increased tone in the quadriceps, and an anteriorly rotated innominate may be present.

Assessment of Posterior Tibia

Supine Athlete

1. The patient is supine with the hip flexed to 90°, similar to the position used to assess quadriceps tension. The physician sits beside the patient on the affected side and supports the thigh (Fig. 6.41).

2. The physician grasps the lower leg at the ankle and stabilizes the distal femur and knee with the other hand.

3. The foot is slowly brought towards the ischial tuberosity, flexing the knee. In the presence of a posteriorly displaced tibia the physician will meet a firm restrictive barrier that is associated with tenderness or 'pressure' in the knee joint. Meniscal injury should be ruled out using the Apley Compression or McMurray tests described later.

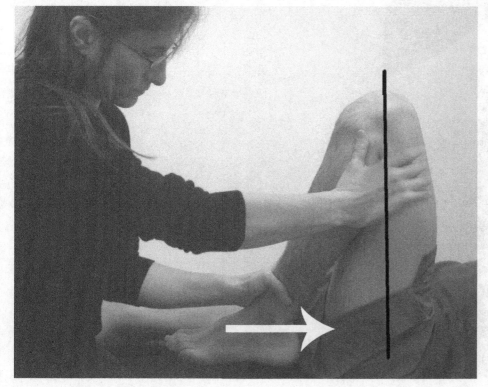

Fig. 6.41

Assessment of Hamstrings – Passive

1. The patient is supine with the hip flexed. The physician stands on the side to be tested and grasps the distal tibia just proximal to the ankle. The other hand stabilizes the distal femur (Fig. 6.42).

2. The knee is passively extended to the restrictive barrier.

3. The same maneuver is performed on the opposite leg and the findings are compared. The athlete in the figure has hamstring spasm, as evidenced by the reduced knee extension.

4. The physician's hand that is stabilizing the femur can palpate the medial and lateral hamstring groups to determine which is tighter.

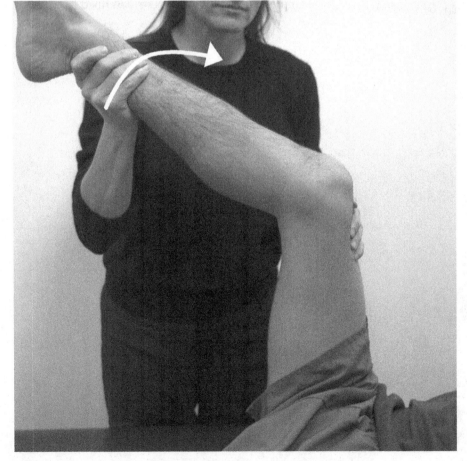

Fig. 6.42

Treatment Notes

In an acute situation a direct technique may be used as long as there is no suspicion of ligamentous disruption. If ligamentous injury is suspected, balancing techniques may be employed. Indirect techniques should be avoided in the acute phase if ligamentous injury is suspected.

In chronic situations the biceps femoris, semitendinosus and semimembranosus muscles may have shortened to compensate for the posterior tibia. It may be necessary to address the resting lengths of the quadriceps and hamstring muscles using muscle energy techniques before applying any direct technique to the tibia.

ISOMETRIC MUSCLE ENERGY TECHNIQUE

Hamstring Muscle Group

1. The patient is supine with the hip flexed. The physician stands beside the leg to be treated. The physician stabilizes the distal femur with one hand and grasps the distal tibia with the other. The hand on the femur will monitor contraction in the medial and lateral compartments of the hamstring muscle group (Fig. 6.43).

2. The knee is extended to the restrictive barrier. The patient is instructed to bend their knee (black arrow). The physician resists the motion with an equal and opposite force (white arrow). The physician adapts her counterforce to ensure that contraction is occurring in the appropriate compartment of the hamstring group.

3. This isometric contraction is maintained for 5–6 seconds. The patient is instructed to relax the contraction as the physician simultaneously relaxes her force.

4. The physician maintains this position until a change in tissue texture is noted (approximately 4–5 seconds).

5. The knee is extended to a new barrier and the sequence is repeated twice.

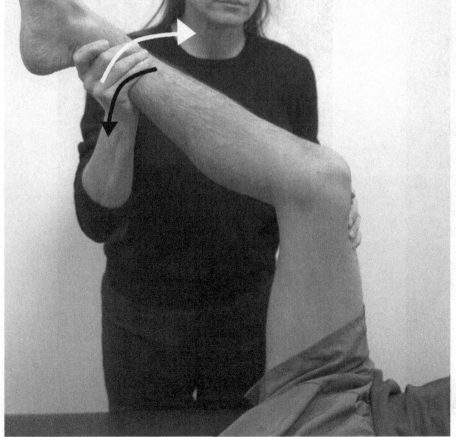

Fig. 6.43

THRUST TECHNIQUE

Posterior Tibia (Fig. 6.44)

1. The patient is supine with the hip flexed and knee flexed to the motion barrier. The foot is resting on the table.
2. The physician grasps the tibia along the proximal margin with both hands. The thumbs are placed over the tibial tubercle.
3. Gentle motion testing is performed to ascertain the rotational barrier with internal and external rotation, as well as the barrier to anterior motion.
4. Once the barriers are engaged, a short, firm thrust is applied in an anterior direction along the plane of the tibial tubercle. Motion characteristics are reassessed.

ALTERNATE THRUST TECHNIQUE

Posterior Tibia (Fig. 6.45)

1. The patient is supine and the hip is flexed.
2. The physician grasps the distal tibia above the ankle with one hand, and the other is placed posterior to the proximal tibia just below the knee.
3. The knee is flexed to the barrier.
4. The distal tibia is gently rotated internally and externally to fine-tune the barrier.
5. A short, firm thrust is used to bring the distal tibia and foot towards the ischial tuberosity as the superior hand resists the posterior motion of the tibia.

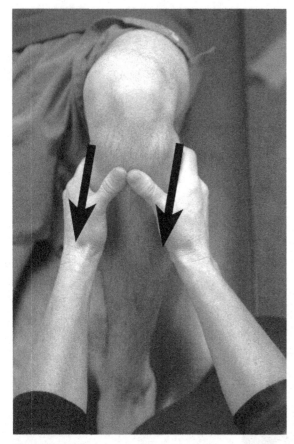

Fig. 6.44

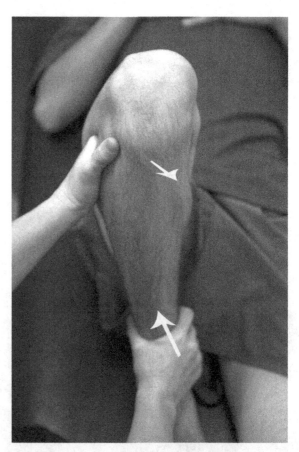

Fig. 6.45

BOWLEGS/TIBIA VARA/BLOUNT'S DISEASE (Fig. 6.46)

Clinical Notes

Bowlegs can be differentiated from genu varum by the apex of the curvature. If the apex of the curvature occurs at the knee, the child has genu varum. If the apex occurs in the shaft of the tibia, the child has a tibia vara (bowlegs). Bowing may be physiological, due to intrauterine position or mechanical strains, or it may be pathological, as occurs when the growth at the proximal tibial epiphyses is asymmetrical, as in Blount's disease. In Blount's disease there is delayed or suppressed growth of the medial epiphyseal plate due to compressive forces. As the lateral plate expands, the tibia bends around the medial epiphysis, creating the bowed appearance. Compression of the medial epiphysis may result from forces generated by myofascial strain, biomechanical dysfunction, abnormal uterine lie, obesity or trauma. Blount's disease is sometimes called tibia vara. There are three peaks in age of onset: before 3 years, between 4 and 10 years, and adolescence. The early onset is more common, usually bilateral, and associated with heavier children who are early walkers. A palpable bony prominence called a beak is present at the medial aspect of the tibial plateau. Bowlegs in infants are often associated with internal torsion of the distal tibia, and sometimes foot deformities. In ambulating toddlers there may be leg length discrepancy.

When bowlegs develop in older children or adults they are just as likely to be unilateral as bilateral. Like the infantile form, late-onset bowlegs may be associated with obesity, leg length discrepancy and internal torsion of the distal tibia. Unlike the early form, late-onset bowlegs are often coupled with a dull, achy pain. Although there are radiographic changes at the medial metaphysis, there is typically no palpable beak. Late-onset Blount's disease typically arises secondary to trauma or damage to the epiphysis of the femoral condyle.

Assessment of Bowed Legs

Infant (Fig. 6.47)

1. The infant or newborn is supine on a flat surface. Both legs are extended. If necessary, the physician may hold the legs in the extended position.

2. The forelegs are compared for alignment.

3. In Figure 6.47 the little girl has right tibia vara. There is also internal rotation of the right femur compared to the left.

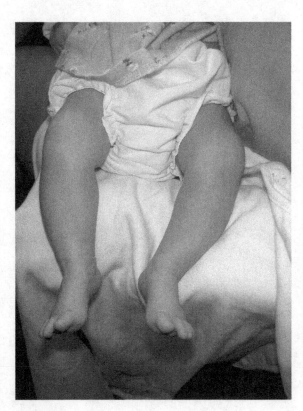

Fig. 6.46

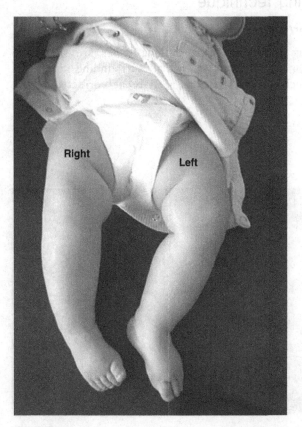

Fig. 6.47

Treatment Notes

Orthopedic consultation should be considered in children with bowlegs, especially if it is late in onset, severe, or does not respond to conservative treatment. The goal of osteopathic treatment of infantile-onset bowlegs is to correct any myofascial strains influencing the normal linear growth pattern of the leg. Marked internal rotation of the hip, tibial torsion, increased tension in the tissues of the lateral column of the femur or the medial column of the foreleg can all play a role in the bowing deformity. Difference in leg length should be evaluated using a scanogram X-ray and corrected with lift therapy in older children or athletes. With discrepancies greater than 8 or 9 mm, full-size shoe lifts are preferential to heel lifts. Lifts of this size isolated to the heel of the shoe will exacerbate shortening of the plantar flexor muscles and distort foot mechanics.

In all children with bowlegs the somatic dysfunction of the myofascial structures should be addressed to eliminate abnormal tensile forces on the bones and promote normal remodeling. As with other bony deformities, the age of the child has a direct impact on the clinical outcome. Bony remodeling occurs through growth. Older children and athletes have fewer growth opportunities available for remodeling.

Molding Technique

Todder/Child

Molding techniques used in long bones are similar to those in other bones, in that all surrounding myofascial and mechanical restrictions need to be corrected before the technique is attempted (Magoun 1951). The molding technique is best applied after there has been a significant improvement in somatic dysfunction affecting the muscles, ligaments and fasciae. Molding techniques will be most useful in young children, toddlers and infants. The basis of the molding technique is to create a counterbalance to the abnormal tensile forces acting on the bone so that the normal tensile forces may influence the bone appropriately.

1. The child is supine or held on a parent's lap. The physician contacts the proximal tibia with one hand and the distal tibia with the other (Fig. 6.48).

2. A slow, gentle compression is introduced between the two hands. The physician uses direct action to address the intraosseous strain and 'unload' the tensile forces in the tissue. For example, if there is an intraosseous torsion the physician matches and counterbalances the forces acting on it until the tissue feels more homogeneous. This is akin to the point of balanced tension.

3. Once the tissue fees homogeneous, the physician maintains that position until there is a general change in the tissue and improved inherent motion.

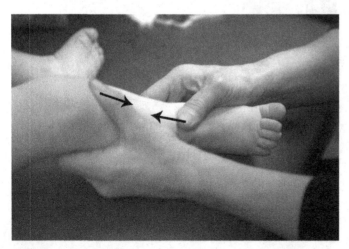

Fig. 6.48

LIGAMENTOUS STRAINS

Ligamentous strains usually develop as a result of trauma or overuse. They are not typically the result of compensatory changes unless the change is creating non-physiological forces on the ligament. Point tenderness over the medial or lateral collateral ligaments suggests ligamentous strain. Point tenderness over the midline joint space suggests strain to the articular capsule or menisci. The integrity of the capsule and ligaments can be assessed using the Apley test.

Assessment

Apley Test for Ligaments (Fig. 6.49)

1. The patient is prone with the knee passively flexed. The physician grasps the leg just proximal to the ankle.

2. The leg is lifted towards the ceiling, thereby distracting the tibia from the femur. This places traction on the ligaments and articular capsule of the knee.

3. The leg is then internally and externally rotated. Pain or excessive motion is suggestive of ligamentous injury.

Cruciate Drawer Test (Figs 6.50 and 6.51)

1. The anterior and posterior cruciate ligaments can be assessed using the anterior and posterior drawer tests. Both knees are tested, beginning with the normal knee.

2. The patient is supine with the knee bent. The physician sits at the patient's foot, stabilizing the foot with her hip or thigh. The knee is grasped at the proximal tibia.

3. The physician applies an anterior force to translate the tibia anteriorly (black arrows), noting the degree of motion, the quality of the endpoint of motion, and the presence or absence of pain or discomfort.

4. Then the physician applies a posterior force to translate the tibia posteriorly (white arrows), noting the degree of motion, the quality of the endpoint of motion, and the presence or absence of pain and discomfort.

5. The two knees are compared for symmetry of range and quality of motion.

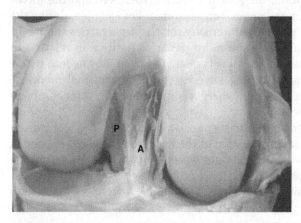

Fig. 6.50 • Anterior view of a dissection into the knee joint. The patella and superficial tissue have been removed. The knee is flexed and distracted to expose the anterior (A) and posterior (P) cruciate ligaments. The insertion of the anterior cruciate into the periosteum of the anterior tibial tubercle is clearly visible.

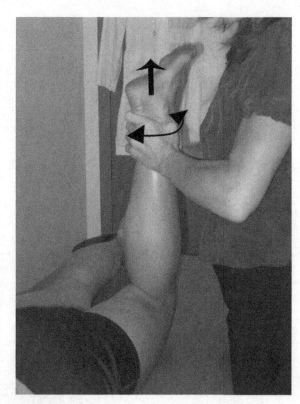

Fig. 6.49

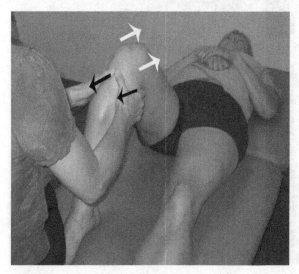

Fig. 6.51

MENISCAL INJURIES

Clinical Notes

The menisci provide lubrication, cushioning and stability to the incongruous articular surfaces of the femur and tibia. Their position between the two large weightbearing bones makes the menisci vulnerable to compressive and torsional forces. The menisci have ligamentous attachments to both the tibia and femur, and are moved by these attachments as the knee flexes and extends. During full extension with weightbearing there is enough space between the articular surfaces of the knee to accommodate the menisci, provided the correct rotational relationship between the tibia and femur is maintained. If, however, one or the other of these components is restricted from adapting its physiological position, the articular space is narrowed and the forces acting on the menisci are distorted. For example, during the flexion phase the internally rotating tibia carries the medical meniscus into a more posterior position in relation to the femur. If the tibia is restricted from moving into external rotation during knee extension, the medial meniscus remains posterior, where it is subjected to greater compressive forces.

Acute injuries to the menisci occur when the foot is fixed during rapid extension of the knee, such as might happen in sports when the athlete wears cleats. The foot, and hence the tibia, is locked into position as the running athlete's cleat hits the ground. The femur forcefully moves into internal rotation, but the tibia is prevented from externally rotating, trapping the menisci between the femoral condyle and the tibial plateau. Traumatic injuries also occur with a blow to the knee that causes either pinching of the meniscus or rapid stretching. This typically happens when the knee is slightly flexed and weightbearing, a position which allows the contacting force to drive the condyle over the meniscus.

Chronic stress due to altered knee mechanics can produce microtrauma of the menisci, resulting in edema and tears.

Assessment of Menisci

Apley Compression Test for Meniscus (Fig. 6.52)

1. The patient is prone with the knee flexed and the foot up. The physician grasps the foot with one hand and the flexed knee with the other.

2. A downward pressure is applied through the tibia to create compression at the knee.

3. The tibia is then internally and externally rotated while the compressive force is maintained. Internal rotation compresses the medial meniscus and external rotation compresses the lateral meniscus.

4. Pain, crepitus or grating during the maneuver suggests that the meniscus is injured.

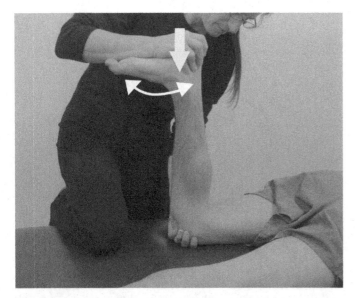

Fig. 6.52

McMurray Test for Meniscus

1. The patient is supine with the hip flexed. The lower leg is grasped at the ankle or foot and the knee is passively flexed to 90°. With the knee flexed, the lower leg is internally and externally rotated. Pain, grinding, restriction and crepitus are noted (Fig. 6.53).

2. The lower leg is then internally rotated and the knee slowly extended to test the integrity of the medial meniscus (Fig. 6.54). Pain, restriction, crepitus or a palpable click suggest medial meniscal injury.

3. The leg is returned to the starting position, hip and knee flexed at 90°. The lower leg is then externally rotated and the knee slowly extended to test the integrity of the lateral meniscus. Similarly, pain, restriction, crepitus or a palpable click suggest lateral meniscal injury.

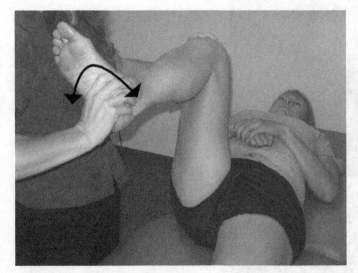

Fig. 6.53

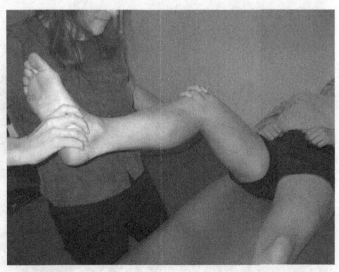

Fig. 6.54

Treatment Notes

Balanced ligamentous technique can be used as a general approach to ligamentous and connective tissue conditions of the knee. It can be particularly beneficial in treating meniscal and ligamentous injuries during the acute phase. It can also be used in post-arthroscopy patients to improve overall function from a respiratory–circulatory as well as a mechanical standpoint.

LYMPHATIC DRAINAGE TECHNIQUE

This may be applied in any situation where there is edema of the lower extremity.

1. The athlete is supine with the knee flexed and suspended from the table. The physician stands at the patient's foot on the ipsilateral side. The physician contacts the biceps femoris and the semimembranosus and semitendinosus and their fasciae at the popliteal space (Fig. 6.55).

2. The physician applies a firm but gentle traction to the soft tissue structures (white arrows) while simultaneously spreading the tissues away from the popliteal space and the hip.

3. This contact and force is maintained until the physician feels a change in tissue texture. There may also be a sensation of warmth along the back of the thigh.

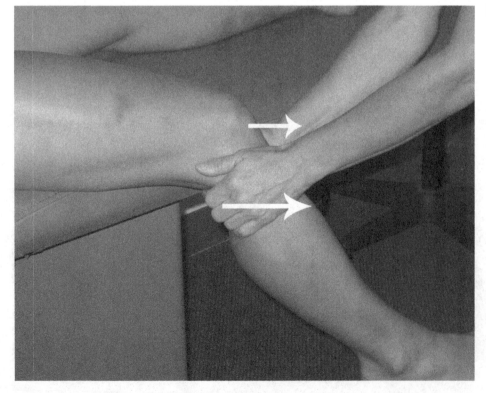

Fig. 6.55

KNEE WOBBLE TECHNIQUE

This is a general range of motion technique for the knee. It introduces motion in multiple planes. The goal of the technique is to improve joint mechanics. It may be used in cases of mild to moderately injured menisci or mildly injured ligaments. This technique is contraindicated in suspected cases of acute moderate or severe ligamentous injuries.

1. The athlete is supine with the foot and knee suspended off the table. The physician stands on the ipsilateral side. The physician contacts the proximal tibia just below the joint line and holds the athlete's foot just above her knees (Fig. 6.56).

2. The physician introduces a steady gentle translation to the knee in a figure-of-eight direction as she simultaneously allows the knee to extend.

3. The speed and distance of the translation will depend on the clinical condition of the knee. In acute injuries with significant edema the translation will be very small and the speed quite slow. In an older or more chronic condition the distance will be greater and the speed rather quick. The physician needs to adopt her force to the response of the tissue and the patient.

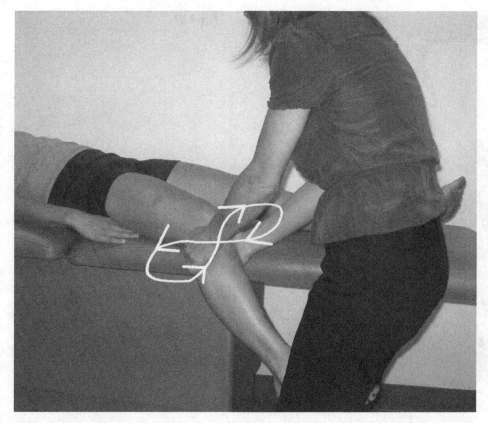

Fig. 6.56

COMPRESSIVE BALANCING TECHNIQUE

Knee Joint (Fig. 6.57)

Prone Athlete/Older Child

In cases of recurrent or chronic problems, low-grade inflammation and tissue scarring may be present. This creates a general resistance to passive motion, especially joint glide. A compressive balanced tension approach can sometimes be helpful as an initial treatment method to improve passive motion so that a more definitive biomechanical diagnosis can be made. This is more likely the case in young athletes or older children who are quite muscular.

1. The patient is prone with the knee flexed.

2. The physician stands beside the patient and places one hand under the knee and the other over the heel and plantar surface of the foot. This position allows the physician to control the degree of dorsiflexion of the foot and ankle.

3. The knee is initially flexed to 90°, although that position of flexion may change as the technique progresses.

4. A gentle but firm compressive force is placed through the tibia into the tibiofemoral articulation. The response of the associated tissues is monitored. The compression is applied to achieve slack in the periarticular tissues, not to compress the joint.

5. A stacking approach is used in which balanced tension is found in one plane of motion and maintained as the tibia is moved through another plane of motion. Using the stacking technique, the upper hand induces a combination of valgus, varus, and internal and/or external rotation to create balanced tissue tension.

6. Knee flexion may be slightly adjusted to accommodate improved balanced tension.

7. Once balanced tension is found, the position is maintained until an improvement in tissue function or a correction of the strain is noted. The physician then slowly returns the limb to the neutral position.

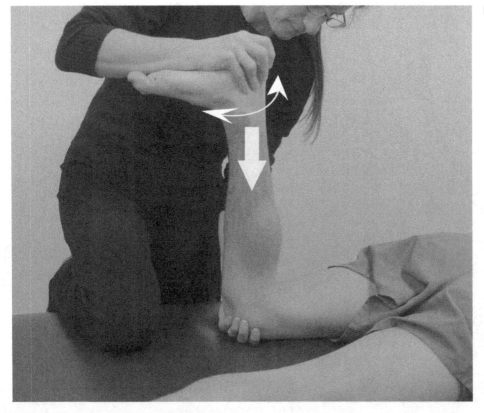

Fig. 6.57

ALTERNATIVE TECHNIQUE

Alternatively, the principles of facilitated positional release as described by Schiowitz (1990) may be used.

1. The patient and physician are in the same positions as described previously for the compressive balancing technique.

2. The tibia is moved through all planes into the direction of ease until minimum tissue tension is noted.

3. A compressive force is then placed through the tibia into the knee to facilitate the tissue release.

BALANCED MEMBRANOUS TENSION TECHNIQUE

Knee Joint

Seated Athlete/Child

The physician should direct her balancing forces through the superficial myofascial structures to the deep ligamentous and connective tissue components: the cruciate and collateral ligaments (see Fig. 6.50) and the menisci (Fig. 6.58).

1. The patient is seated with the legs flexed off the table.

2. The physician is seated facing the patient. The patient's foot and distal leg on the involved side are held between the physician's distal legs (Fig. 6.59).

3. The physician grasps the proximal tibia (Fig. 6.60) just below the mid-joint line (MJL), with the thumbs crossed over the tibial tubercle (TT) and the attachment of the patellar tendon (PT).

4. The physician monitors the tissue tension at the mid-joint line.

5. The physician attempts to bring the ligamentous articular relations into balanced tension by moving the tissues of

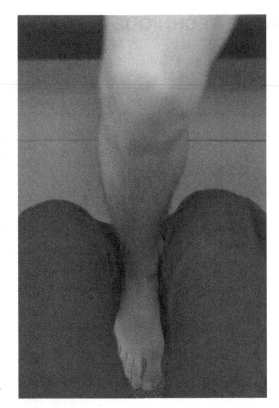

Fig. 6.59

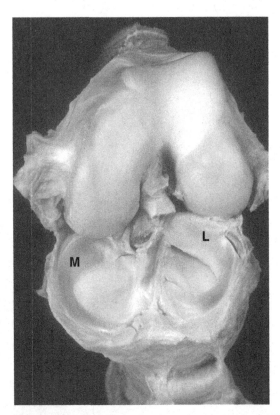

Fig. 6.58 • Anterior view of a dissection into the knee joint. The cruciate ligaments have been cut and the femur hyperflexed to reveal the medial (M) and lateral (L) menisci.

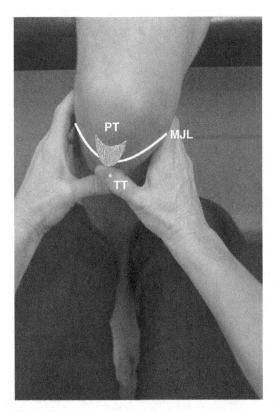

Fig. 6.60

the knee through all planes using a stacking method. The tibia is moved sequentially through each plane of motion until equal or balanced tissue tension is felt.

6. The physician begins the technique by balancing the tibia and femur in relation to the compressive or distractive forces in the knee. The physician does this by raising or lowering her heels, which places an upward or downward force into the patient's tibia. This lifts the tibia towards the femur or tractions it away, creating compression and decompression (Fig. 6.61).

7. The physician can introduce internal and external rotation of the tibia by using her hands to directly rotate the tibia, or by moving her knees in opposite directions to 'turn' the tibia. For example, in Figure 6.62 the physician externally rotates the tibia by sliding her left leg anteriorly while moving the right leg posteriorly. This turns the patient's tibia, which is clasped between the physician's lower legs.

8. Valgus and varus stresses can be introduced by tilting the physician's legs either to the left or to the right. In Figure 6.63 a varus position is created by tilting the physician's legs to the left, away from the patient.

9. A combination of these movements is used to create balanced ligamentous tension throughout the tissues

of the knee joint. Once balanced tension is achieved, the physician maintains that position until a correction in the mechanical strain or improvement in tissue function is noted.

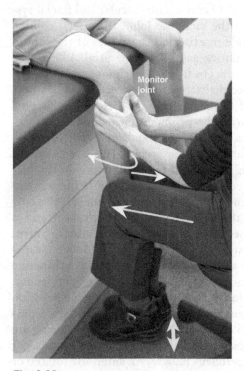

Fig. 6.62

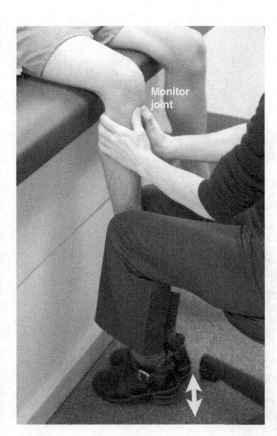

Fig. 6.61

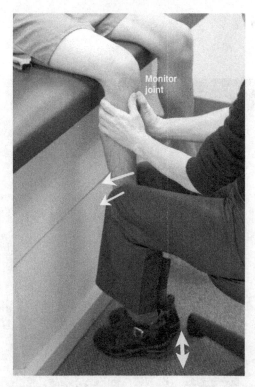

Fig. 6.63

FIBULAR DYSFUNCTIONS

Clinical Notes

The fibula is part of a continuous muscular and fascial system that stabilizes the sacroiliac joint, the lateral column of the leg, the ankle mortise and the arches of the foot as the leg is loaded during gait (Vleeming et al. 1995). The attachments of the biceps femoris reach up past the ischial tuberosity and interdigitate with the fasciae and ligamentous structures of the sacroiliac joint. Below, the bicipital insertions blend with the peroneus longus muscle, attaching along the fibula, around the cuboid and providing stability and support for the plantar arches. This lateral system is activated during weightbearing. Dysfunction in the biomechanics of any of its components disrupts the sequencing and effectiveness of the system. The fibula is the only bony structure of this bicipital peroneus mechanism, and as such it resolves the forces generated in each compartment. The fibula is also susceptible to articular dysfunction, especially through the ankle. Consequently, fibular dysfunction may have a muscular, fascial and/or articular component. Excessive supination of the foot may place undue stress on the peroneus longus muscle, pulling the fibula into a posterior position. Likewise, inversion sprains of the ankle are associated with posterior fibular dysfunction because of the strain on the peroneus muscle. An anteriorly rotated or upslipped innominate may result in an ipsilateral posterior fibular dysfunction through the stress on the biceps femoris muscle.

Posterior fibular dysfunction may present as pain in the lateral knee with weightbearing or knee flexion, paresthesias of the lateral distal leg, or pain radiating along the lateral aspect of the distal leg. The symptoms may or may not radiate into the foot and small toe. Sensory changes can be present, and in severe cases there may be weakness of the peroneus muscles and pronation of the foot.

Assessment of the Fibula

Young Adult

1. The patient is seated or supine with the leg passively extended. The fibula is grasped at each end between the thumb and finger (Fig. 6.64).

2. Inherent motion characteristics are assessed. Then the proximal end of the fibula is moved anteriorly and posteriorly to assess the passive freedom of motion.

3. To assess active motion, the patient is asked to fully dorsiflex the ankle as the physician assesses the movement at the distal and proximal ends. There should be a slight inferior and posterior motion of the fibula.

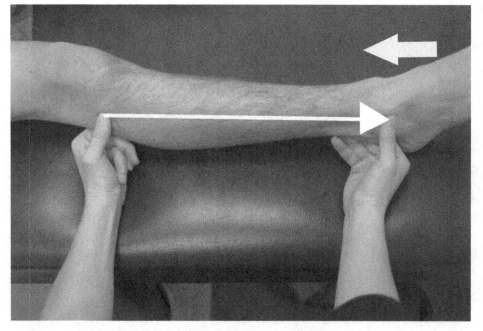

Fig. 6.64

Assessment of Proximal Fibula

Young Adult or Child

1. The patient is seated or supine with the leg passively extended. The physician grasps the head of the fibula between the thumb and finger with one hand. The tibia and knee are stabilized with the other hand (Fig. 6.65).

2. The fibular head is moved anteromedially and posterolaterally to assess freedom of motion. A firm, crisp barrier is indicative of an articular dysfunction and typically responds best to a direct technique.

3. To assess active motion, the patient is asked to flex his knee by pushing his foot into the table. This engages the biceps femoris. The response of the fibular head is noted. There should be a slight superior posterior movement of the fibula when the biceps contracts, and a return to an inferior anterior position when the biceps relaxes. Failure of the fibula to return to its initial position may be indicative of biceps femoris hypertonicity, which may respond to a muscle energy technique.

Assessment of the Fibula

Toddler and Infant (Fig. 6.66)

Neither the fibular head nor the articular fossa of the tibia is formed at birth. There is a ligamentous attachment between the fibula and the tibia. Dysfunction in this area is primarily ligamentous or muscular and usually secondary to conditions in the foot, tibia or hip. Primary problems of the fibula are rare.

1. The child is seated or supine. The fibula is contacted at the proximal and distal ends. Inherent motion characteristics are assessed.

2. The proximal end of the fibula is gently moved anteriorly and posteriorly to assess passive motion mechanics.

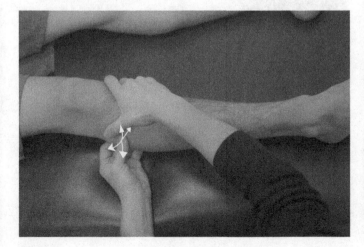

Fig. 6.65

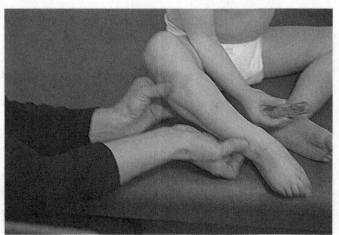

Fig. 6.66

Treatment Notes (Fig. 6.67)

The fibular head is most commonly found in a posterior position, with limited anterior and superior movement. This may be due to an articular or a myofascial dysfunction. Direct techniques are more effective in articular strains. Muscle energy and BLT techniques may be used in either type of strain.

THRUST TECHNIQUE FOR A POSTERIOR FIBULAR HEAD

(Fig. 6.68)

This technique is used for an articular dysfunction of the fibular head.

1. The patient is supine with the hip and knee flexed.

2. The physician places the metacarpophalangeal joint of the first and second fingers posteriorly to the fibular head. The other hand grasps the distal ends of the tibia and fibula.

3. The knee is flexed to the barrier while maintaining contact with the fibular head.

4. A short, firm thrust is made, simultaneously bringing the patient's foot towards the ischial tuberosity and the fibular head anteriorly.

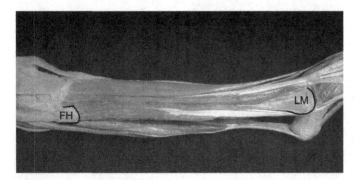

Fig. 6.67

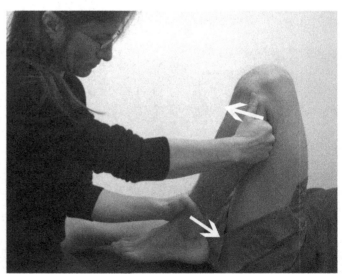

Fig. 6.68

ISOMETRIC MUSCLE ENERGY TECHNIQUE

Posterior Fibular Head/Peroneus

Supine Athlete

This technique is used on a posterior fibula where the primary problem is muscular and resulting from dysfunction in the peroneus muscles and fasciae.

1. The patient is supine with the knee bent and the foot resting on the physician's thigh in a dorsiflexed position (Fig. 6.69).

2. The fibular head is contacted and brought anterior to the restrictive barrier as the foot is repositioned to maximize dorsiflexion.

3. The patient is instructed to plantarflex his foot into the physician's thigh while the physician resists the posterior motion of the fibular head.

4. This contraction is maintained for 4–5 seconds, then the patient is told to relax. The physician maintains her contact, and after 4–5 seconds the fibular head is passively moved anteriorly as the foot is passively repositioned to increase dorsiflexion.

5. The sequence is repeated twice.

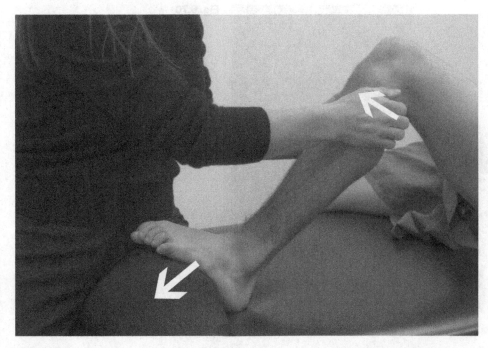

Fig. 6.69

ISOTONIC MUSCLE ENERGY TECHNIQUE

Posterior Fibular Head/Biceps Femoris

Supine Athlete

This technique is used if the dysfunction is primarily muscular and due to a biceps femoris dysfunction.

1. The patient is supine with the knee bent and the foot resting on the physician's thigh in a dorsiflexed position (Fig. 6.70).

2. The physician uses one hand to contact the fibular head and bring it anterior to the restrictive barrier. The other hand reaches behind the knee on the medial side and stabilizes the tibia.

3. The patient is instructed to 'gently try to bend his knee' (white arrow) until the physician feels the biceps femoris engage. The physician resists the knee flexion at the tibia and fibula with an equal and opposite force.

4. This contraction is maintained for 4–5 seconds, then the patient is told to relax. As the patient is relaxing, the physician increases her anterior force on the fibula, moving a small distance into the restrictive barrier (black arrow).

5. The sequence is repeated twice.

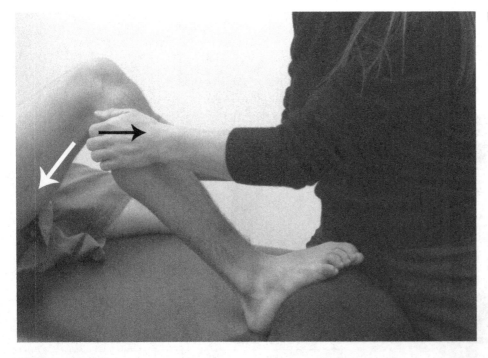

Fig. 6.70

BALANCED LIGAMENTOUS TECHNIQUE

Fibula

This may be done using either of two hand positions, depending on the level of restriction and the size of the patient.

1. The patient is supine with the leg passively extended. The proximal and distal ends of the fibula are contacted (Figs 6.71 and 6.72). A firm, constant compression is placed through the long axis of the fibula to disengage the restrictive barriers at the distal and proximal ends and unload the tensile forces.

2. If the patient has a very muscular leg or there is a significant amount of compression in the tissue, it is mechanically advantageous to position oneself medial to the leg using the thenar eminence to contact the lateral malleolus (Fig. 6.73). The other hand reaches across the leg to grasp the fibular head. This position allows the physician to lean her weight back to decompress the proximal area as she simultaneously leans inferiorly to decompress the malleolus and place a compressive force into the fibula.

3. Once the restrictive barriers at the articular ends are disengaged, the fibula is then balanced in relationship to the surrounding tissues, specifically the tibiofibular interosseous membrane. A stacking technique is applied.

4. The physician introduces flexion, extension, rotation, torsion and translation into the fibula and surrounding tissues to achieve balanced tension. In toddlers and infants, a direct rather than an indirect approach should be used to find the balanced tension. In older children and adolescents, an indirect approach can also be used.

5. Balanced tension is maintained until a change in tissue texture or a correction in the strain pattern is felt. This technique can also be applied as a molding technique.

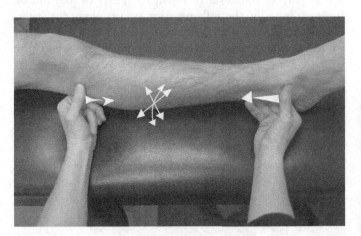

Fig. 6.71

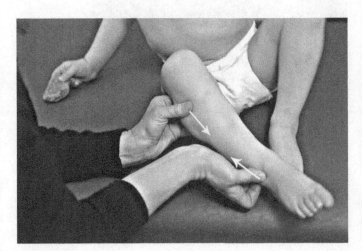

Fig. 6.72

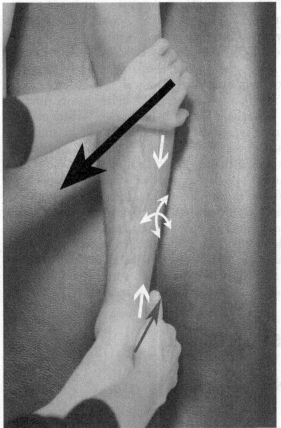

Fig. 6.73

COMPARTMENT SYNDROME

Clinical Notes

The distal lower leg is comprised of anterior and posterior compartments that are clinically significant because of the vulnerability of the structures within them. Compartment syndrome is a condition whereby the intracompartmental pressure increases to the point where it impedes microcirculation of the structures within the compartment. In extreme cases the microcirculation to the muscular structures within these compartments is compromised, resulting in ischemia and eventual tissue necrosis. Although compartment syndrome may result from direct trauma, it can also arise from repetitive strain and may be exercise induced. Compartment syndrome is a medical emergency if the ischemia does not resolve, requiring fasciotomy and debridement of necrotic muscle. Compartment syndrome usually occurs in the anterior tibial compartment and is more common in runners. Fluid pressure in the compartment rises in response to excessive activity, impeding the microcirculation to the muscles and nerves within the compartment. Larger vessels are usually not affected, so tissues distal to the compartment are also not affected. Typically, the athlete complains of a deep ache or tingling feeling with running which subsides once the activity is stopped. However, if the activity continues, the symptoms may progress to sensory changes and eventual loss of strength. This may present as tripping or clumsiness due to ischemia of the extensor hallucis longus muscle. In the early stages the symptoms of compartment syndrome will abort immediately or very soon after the exercise stops. However, in more severe cases the inflammatory products from the ischemia maintain or further exacerbate elevated compartment pressures. A cycle of ischemia, inflammation and elevated pressure is established. This is the prelude to tissue necrosis. Athletes should be instructed to stop exercising immediately, and to apply ice and elevate the leg if symptoms appear. Exercise-induced compartment syndrome is often associated with muscle hypertrophy, biomechanical dysfunction of the lower leg and altered foot mechanics. In chronic or mild cases, osteopathic evaluation and treatment of somatic dysfunction should be coupled with muscle retraining. In severe cases with suspected neurological involvement, surgical consultation is necessary.

SHIN SPLINTS

Clinical Notes

A more common – and fortunately less destructive – condition of the lower leg is shin splints. Shin splints typically occur in the posterior or anterior compartments of the lower leg. They are essentially an overuse syndrome that usually starts as an inflammation of the insertions of the anterior or posterior tibialis muscles (although they may also occur in the lateral muscle groups). Left untreated, this tendonitis may progress to a myositis and then a periostitis. Shin splints may develop as a result of poor training practices, excessive training, improper footwear, training on inappropriate surfaces, poor foot mechanics, tibial torsion, muscle imbalances, and hip or pelvic dysfunction.

ANTERIOR SHIN SPLINTS

(Figs 6.74 and 6.75)

Clinical Notes

Anterior shin splints most commonly present as pain in the lateral and anterior aspects of the mid-shaft of the lower leg. The symptoms are exacerbated with activity, especially running and repetitive pronation such as one might see in soccer players. Tenderness to palpation may or may not be present. Initially, the inflammation occurs along the insertion of the tibialis anterior muscle and probably arises from excessive dorsiflexion and plantarflexion. During gait, the

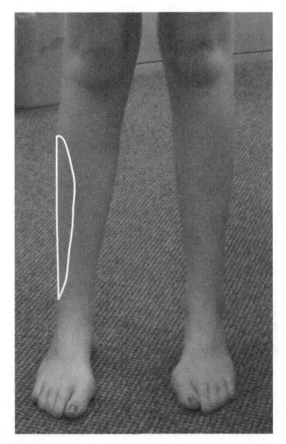

Fig. 6.74

tibialis anterior undergoes eccentric contraction as the foot moves from heel strike to stance phase. The inflammation associated with anterior shin splints inhibits the tibialis muscle so that the extensor hallucis longus and extensor digitalis are subjected to a greater workload. If the irritation to the tibialis is not addressed, these other muscles also begin to develop microtrauma. If treatment is delayed further, the inflammation and strain will progress to the muscle belly, resulting in a myositis. Athletes who continue to 'play through the pain' are at risk of developing periosteal inflammation and, in severe cases, stress fractures.

As a stabilizer of the medial longitudinal arch of the foot, the tibialis anterior is placed under excessive stress in an athlete who over-pronates during running. Likewise, runners who land with a flat or semi-flat foot, rather than a proper heel strike, place increased stress on the tibialis anterior. As the foot contacts the ground, the forces generated during the gait cycle are dissipated through the fascial tissues of the foot. When heel strike is eliminated the forces are absorbed by the tibialis anterior as it tries to control the plantarflexion of the foot. This overloads the muscle and results in microtears at its insertion.

Overloading of the tibialis anterior during concentric contraction also contributes to shin splints. There are two common culprits for this: running on graded surfaces, especially uphill or downhill, requires the tibialis anterior to contract more quickly to clear the ground; and shortening or hypertonicity of the muscles of the posterior compartment, such as occurs in soccer players and kickers, increases the preload on the tibialis anterior during dorsiflexion.

Somatic dysfunctions often associated with anterior shin splints include an internally rotated tibia, pes planus (both functional and structural), everted calcaneus, pronated talus, tight internal hip rotators, and an inflared innominate. These biomechanical dysfunctions should be corrected before muscle retraining is initiated.

POSTERIOR SHIN SPLINTS
(Figs 6.76 and 6.77)

Clinical Notes

Posterior shin splints generally involve the plantarflexor muscles of the foot and ankle, and present as pain in the

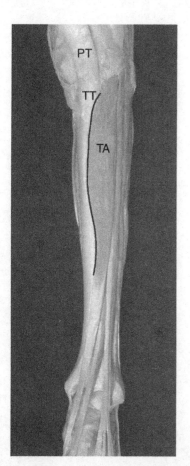

Fig. 6.75 • Anterior view of the left lower leg. The patellar tendon (PT), tibial tuberosity (TT) and tibialis anterior (TA) are identified. The dark line indicates the attachment of the tibialis anterior to the tibial shaft.

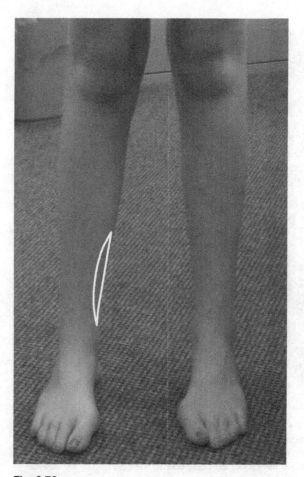

Fig. 6.76

posteromedial aspect of the lower extremity, sometimes extending as low as the medial malleolus. Like anterior shin splints they are a form of overuse syndrome, but whereas anterior shin splints generally involve the muscle insertions onto the tibia, posterior shin splints are an inflammation of the flexor tendons, particularly the tibialis posterior. Like its anterior counterpart, the tibialis posterior supports the medial longitudinal arch. The long tendon of the tibialis posterior passes under the flexor retinaculum and around the medial malleolus to insert on the navicular. This route provides several areas for potential friction upon the tendon as it passes around the ankle and under the navicular. During gait, eccentric contraction of the tibialis posterior, flexor hallucis longus, and flexor digitorum longus muscles control the foot and provide a mechanism to absorb some of the forces placed into the foot and ankle. Consequently, repetitive ankle inversion, excessive pronation and varus posture of the foot place abnormal loads on these muscles and their tendons.

Treatment Notes

Tibial torsions, altered foot mechanics and somatic dysfunction in the legs, hip and pelvis all need to be addressed when treating shin splints or compartment syndrome. Muscle retraining is an important component of rehabilitation. The child's footwear needs to be evaluated and, where necessary, changes made. In general, the use of orthotic devices should be influenced by the age of the child and the intensity of the sport training. A younger athlete who still has several years of growth ahead of him is more likely to respond to and retain manual correction of foot biomechanics than an athlete who is almost fully grown. Likewise, an athlete competing at an elite level is under greater mechanical strain and more likely to need an orthotic device to support her activity.

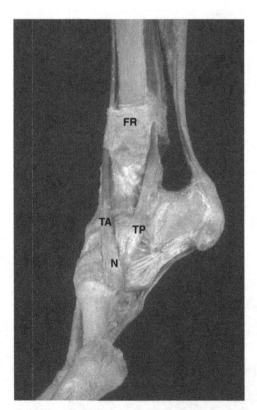

Fig. 6.77 • Medial view of the distal left leg. The superficial muscles have been removed. The tendon of tibialis posterior (TP) can be seen passing beneath the flexor retinaculum (FR) and inserting on the navicular (N) inferior and posterior to the insertion of the tibialis anterior (TA).

Isolytic Technique Anterior Compartment
(Fig. 6.78)

Isolytic techniques can be used to address myofascial contractures and improve fluid mechanics. The technique can be performed on both legs simultaneously or on one at a time.

1. The athlete is supine with the legs extended. The physician stands at the patient's feet. The physician contacts the dorsum of the patient's feet.

2. The patient is instructed to 'point your toes at your head' (black arrow), thereby contracting the tibialis anterior muscle and the dorsiflexor muscles.

3. The physician applies an equal and opposite force to induce isometric contraction of the dorsiflexor muscle group (white arrow).

4. The physician maintains this isometric contraction for 3–5 seconds and then rapidly overcomes it with a short quick impulse towards plantar flexion (Fig. 6.79, broken white arrow). The impulse should occur over a distance of 1–2 cm only. This may be repeated up to three times.

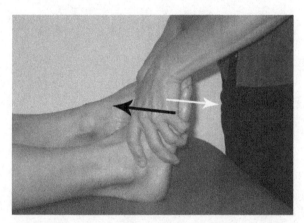

Fig. 6.78

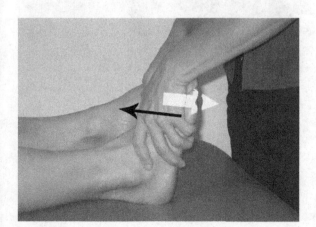

Fig. 6.79

Isolytic Technique Posterior Compartment
(Fig. 6.80)

1. The athlete is supine with the legs extended. The physician stands at the patient's feet. The physician contacts the plantar surface of the patient's feet.

2. The patient is instructed to 'point your toes at the physician' (black arrow), thereby contracting the tibialis posterior muscle and the dorsiflexor muscles.

3. The physician applies an equal and opposite force to induce isometric contraction of the plantarflexor muscle group (white arrow).

4. The physician maintains this isometric contraction for 3–5 seconds and then rapidly overcomes it with a short quick impulse towards dorsiflexion (Fig. 6.81, broken white arrow). The impulse should occur over a distance of 1–2 cm only. This may be repeated up to three times.

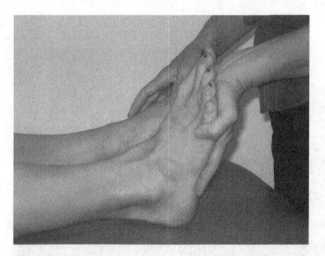

Fig. 6.80

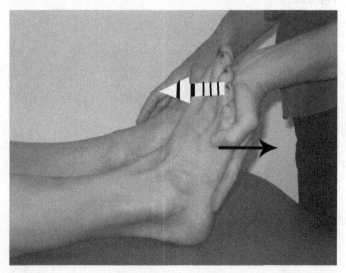

Fig. 6.81

Myofascial Milking (Figs 6.82, 6.83, 6.84)

This is a general soft tissue effleurage technique that can be employed in clinical conditions where there is edema in the distal leg, ankle or foot. The hip, knee and thorax should be treated before the distal extremity.

1. The athlete is supine. The physician stands opposite to the leg to be treated. The distal leg is visually divided into three sections, proximal, middle and distal. The physician will first treat the proximal section, then the middle, then the distal.

2. The physician contacts the myofascial tissues just distal to the knee and applies a firm but gentle kneading force

(Fig. 6.82). Her hands should move back and forth (white arrows) in opposite directions to the restrictive barriers but not through them.

3. This is continued until there is a change in tissue texture. Then the physician moves her contact to the middle third of the leg (Fig. 6.83) and repeats the kneading maneuver here until there is a change in tissue texture.

4. Finally, the physician moves her contact to the distal third of the leg (Fig. 6.84) and the procedure is repeated.

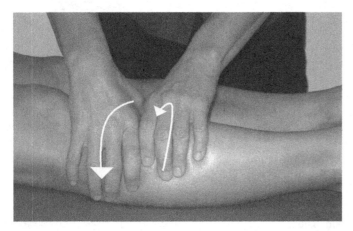

Fig. 6.82

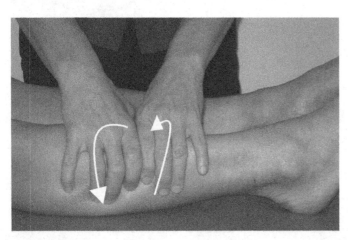

Fig. 6.83

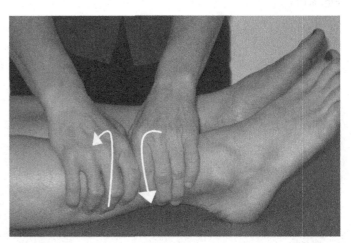

Fig. 6.84

References

Magoun HS. Osteopathy in the cranial field. Kirksville, MO: Journal Printing Company, 1951.

Schiowitz S. Facilitated positional release. J Am Osteopath Assoc 1990; 901: 145–155.

Travell JG, Simons DG. Myofascial pain and dysfunction. The trigger point manual: lower. Philadelphia: Lippincott, Williams & Wilkins, 1983.

Vleeming A, Snijders CJ, Stoeckart R, Mens JMA. A new light on low back pain: the

selflocking mechanism of the sacroiliac joints and its implication for sitting, standing, and walking. In: Vleeming A, Mooney V, Snijders CJ, Dorman T, eds. European Conference Organisers 1995; 149–168.

Chapter Seven

7

Foot and ankle

CHAPTER CONTENTS

OVERVIEW

The foot is a marvelous instrument that meets all the challenges nature has placed upon it. It is flexible but stable. It is sensitive to slight changes in surface texture and position, but insensitive to the 40-pound rucksack on your back. In utero, the feet are typically supinated and tucked against the thighs. The knees and hips are flexed, with the tibias crossed and internally rotated. This intrauterine position influences the shape of the long bones of the leg, such that congenital torsions and bowing are often present at birth. The shape of the long bones will in turn affect the morphology of the feet, especially the integrity of the arches, which are dependent upon normal functional relationships in the long restrictor muscles of the ankle and distal leg. The arch arrangement is also dependent on the bony framework of the foot and is supported by the long restrictor muscles of the distal leg: the tibialis anterior and posterior, and the peroneus longus. Bony deformities such as tibial torsions can distort the relationship of the soft tissue structures that support the platform upon which the arches are built. This influences foot mechanics.

The arches of the feet are extremely important for several reasons. The arch arrangement provides the foot with the flexibility to adapt to the various contours and textures of the surfaces it contacts. The arches help to disperse the forces of gait, thereby protecting the articular surfaces of the feet, ankles and knees. The arches are instrumental in the tensegrity system of the foot and contribute to the propulsive mechanism of gait. During gait, energy is absorbed and released through a musculofascial–ligamentous sling involving the plantar tissues of the feet, the peroneus longus, biceps femoris, gluteal muscles, contralateral latissimus dorsi and upper extremity. This system allows conservation of energy. The small short restrictor muscles of the plantar surface are heavily innervated with proprioceptive fibers that play a role in balance and posture. Biomechanical dysfunctions affecting the structural relations of the foot or its flexibility have the potential to alter the mechanics of the ankle, knee, hip, pelvis, back and even upper extremity through both mechanical and neurological mechanisms.

The ankle has its greatest range of dorsiflexion at birth. If dorsiflexion is limited, one must consider deformity, spasticity or strictures. Because the nervous system is immature, spasticity is often difficult to detect in newborns and young infants. Deep tendon reflexes are unreliable. Muscle tone is greater in flexor muscles than extensor muscles, which increases the baby's resistance to passive extension. Strictures or tightness may develop in the gastrocnemius or soleus muscles due to abnormal lie. To differentiate spasticity from strictures, one can compare ankle dorsiflexion with the knee extended and flexed. Restricted ankle motion in both positions suggests involvement of both muscles. This finding points to a neurological problem, whereas if restriction is present only in knee extension then the gastrocnemius is probably the cause, and the etiology is more likely to be mechanical and focal to that muscle. Deformity of the ankle or subtalar joint will present as abnormal positioning of the foot. Ankle dorsiflexion should be measured to rule out bony pathology. In infants and toddlers it is necessary to stabilize the subtalar joint and isolate the motion to the ankle mortise to accurately assess pure ankle motion. Active dorsiflexion of the foot typically includes ankle and mid-foot motion. In younger children, dorsiflexion of the forefoot is greater than of the hindfoot. As a result, intact forefoot dorsiflexion can mask limited talocrural motion.

As the infant matures, spasticity may present as delayed motor skills or persistence of primitive reflexes, such as the plantar or Babinski reflex. For some children, toe-walking is a normal variant in the early stages of learning to walk. However, spasticity and undiagnosed deformity need to be included in the differential diagnosis of toe-walking. In toddlers and older children the talocrural motion should be assessed from three perspectives: muscle resistance to the passive stretch required for movement, the presence of an abnormal physiological barrier due to bony abnormality, and mechanical resistance producing a restrictive barrier. Muscular resistance to passive stretch at the ankle associated with elevated deep tendon reflexes or persistence of primitive reflexes is indicative of neuropathology above the lumbar cord. Deformities of the foot can cause toe-walking and delayed motor milestones. Primitive reflexes will not persist in these children, and although resistance to joint motion is often present, the deep tendon reflexes are bilaterally symmetrical and not elevated. Neuropathology typically involves more than one muscle group, such as the knee and hip flexors on the ipsilateral side. Biomechanical dysfunction can also cause the child to toe-walk. For example, excessive pronation of the forefoot can present as limited range of motion without elevated reflexes.

GAIT

Infants typically begin walking after their first birthday. Their gait is wide based – about 70% of the width of the pelvis. Contralateral arm swing is absent, step length is short and step cadence is increased. This pattern emerges because of immature motor patterning and balance mechanisms. Early walkers lack good control of ankle dorsiflexor muscles. This affects forceful dorsiflexion at heel-strike and eccentric contraction during the stance phase. Consequently, the ankle is unable to transition smoothly from dorsiflexion to plantar flexion. This gives the appearance of a mild foot drop and results in a flatfoot strike rather than a true heel-strike. During swing and stance phases, infants tend to keep the knee more flexed because of the immature quadriceps. There is an appearance of exaggerated ankle dorsiflexion as the weight of the body is carried forward. During the second year of life, most children establish contralateral arm swing patterns, ankle dorsiflexion improves a little, the appearance of foot drop resolves, and the time spent in single-leg support during the swing phase increases. Around the age of 2 years, the child may begin to develop a heel-strike pattern. This corresponds with the ability to flex the weightbearing knee during the mid-stance phase (Burnett and Johnson 1971). Achieving knee flexion on the supporting limb requires eccentric contraction of the quadriceps and stabilization of the hip. Children with primary muscle disease or neurological conditions may not be able to sustain this position owing to weakness and/or lack of postural control mechanisms. Step length should increase and cadence decrease as the child's gait cycle matures. The step length should correspond to limb length. By 3 years of age, hip rotation improves and the base of support has narrowed to 45% of the pelvic width. Gait continues to mature, and by 7 years most children have a mature gait pattern with a narrow base of support, a true heel-strike mechanism and appropriate single-leg stance time. Although cadence is higher and velocity slower in this age group, these will improve with limb growth.

During early walking the toddler does not use the heel-strike and toe-off phases of gait. Instead, the child lands with a flat foot and the following stride is initiated by the knee and hip, rather than the propulsive mechanism of the foot. At this age the plantar arches are typically flat with weightbearing, although they are flexible with passive testing. The range of motion in the joints of the foot is greater in infants and early walkers than in older children. Limited motion between the joints or in the arches suggests bony deformation or soft tissue rigidity. Restriction in the arches will impede development of the heel-to-toe sequence, which creates the propulsion for the next stride. This sequence of movements generally does not appear until the third year. The weightbearing arches should begin to develop around the same time. Valgus and varus deformities of the forefoot can impede normal development of this sequence. Most children will not 'grow out' of deformities or misalignments at the midtarsal joint. These generally require conservative treatment, although surgical correction may be necessary in severe cases.

Gait abnormalities can be differentiated by observing the relationship of the foot to the leg and hip. Intoeing may be due to internal torsion of the tibia or femur, internal tibial rotation, clubfoot or metatarsus adductus. The alignment of the patella and foot when the leg is extended and in a neutral position or the child is standing, can determine the location of the problem. Generally, if the patella and foot are turned in the same direction, the problem is usually in the hip or femur. If the patella is in the midline and the foot is deviated, then the problem involves the tibia or the

foot itself. For example, an inturned but normal-appearing foot associated with a medially positioned patella suggests a tightness of the hip rotator muscles or a femoral torsion. A normal but inturned foot associated with a neutral or lateral patella suggests a tibial torsion, internally rotated tibia or a rotational deformity of the foot. An externally positioned patella and foot suggests external femoral torsion, slipped capital femoral epiphysis (in an older child) or biomechanical dysfunction involving the hip rotators.

An abnormal appearance of the foot with a neutral or deviated patella suggests a primary foot deformity. Clubfoot and metatarsus adductus are rotational foot deformities. Clubfoot involves positional changes of the entire foot in which the forefoot and part of the midfoot are adducted on the midtarsal joint. Metatarsus adductus is a deformity isolated to the forefoot, which is adducted on the midfoot.

CONDITIONS RESULTING IN AN INTURNED FOOT

CALCANEUS VARUS/INVERTED CALCANEUS/REARFOOT VARUS

Clinical Notes

Heel varus refers to the angle created by the calcaneus and Achilles tendon during stance. The varus angle occurs when the calcaneus is inverted and the midfoot and forefoot are positioned medially in relation to the talus. Calcaneus varus may be congenital or late onset. At birth the calcaneus is in a relative varus position that is exacerbated in appearance by the presence of primitive reflexes and the increased flexor tone in the hips and legs. As the plantar reflex is lost, the foot assumes a more neutral posture. Once the child begins standing the absence of developed plantar arches gives the foot a functional pes planus, and the calcaneus may even appear to be everted or valgus. However, by the age of 4 or 5 the calcaneus should be in a neutral position during weightbearing. Excessive inversion at birth or persistence of the inverted appearance after 4 years may be structural or functional. Abnormal positioning or morphology of the talus or calcaneus will cause a structural varus that is typically rigid. More often, however, calcaneus varus is functional and due to biomechanical strains in the hindfoot, leg or hip.

In newborns and infants with calcaneus varus the foot is inverted and supinated, but flexible. Both active and passive repositioning of the foot is possible. The Achilles tendon is palpable and deviates medially from the midline of the leg. There may be increased tension through the adductor muscle group of the femur and the somatic tissues of the medial column of the distal leg. The femur is typically externally rotated, which may be secondary to myofascial restriction or increased adductor tone. However, in some cases the position of the femur is due to an articular dysfunction and is contributing to the adductor hypertonicity. The presence of a mild genu varus or tibia varus may be due to intrauterine molding.

In older children and adolescents with calcaneus varus the medial longitudinal arch often appears functionally intact in the stance position. However, during gait the foot compensates for the inverted calcaneus by creating excessive eversion at the subtalar joint, resulting in a flattened medial arch. The resultant torque placed into the foot compromises the stability of the ankle and forefoot. This gait adaptation also increases the load on the posterior tibialis muscle and may contribute to shin splints in older children and athletes. Compensation for the varus position of the foot often includes adaptations at the knee that result in an internally rotated tibia. This further exacerbates the functional pes planus during gait and contributes to stresses in the patella and medial joint line of the knee. Older children and athletes with heel varus may complain of pain in the forefoot due to increased stress under the second and third metatarsals. Younger children may alter their stride to reduce the time spent in single-leg stance on the affected limb. Often the plantar surface of the metatarsals is callused and the shoes may show wear under the metatarsal arch.

Assessment of Calcaneus Varus (Fig. 7.1)

1. The patient is standing. The alignment of the Achilles tendon is noted. In calcaneus varus the tendon may splay medially.

2. The child is observed from behind while walking. At heel-strike the lateral aspect of the foot initially comes into contact with the ground. Then the foot rolls into pronation. It may appear that the foot slaps against the ground. (The calcaneus in this child appears almost normal; however, it is rather pronounced with walking.)

3. Shoes will be unevenly worn, with marked wear along the lateral aspect of the heel and the medial aspect of the forefoot. The first and second metatarsal heads may be callused.

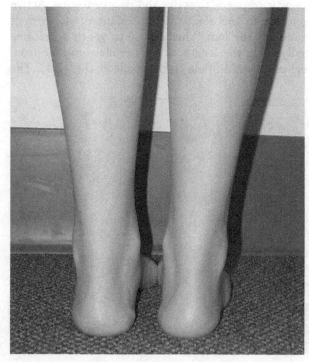

Fig. 7.1

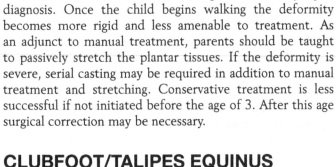

METATARSUS ADDUCTUS

Clinical Notes

Metatarsus adductus is a deformity of the foot usually noted in infancy. The metatarsal bones and toes are positioned medially (Fig. 7.2) in relation to the hindfoot. Some molding of the forefoot may be present. Severe metatarsus adductus can be confused with clubfoot in infants and newborns. However, unlike clubfoot, the adduction deformity only involves the forefoot whereas the hindfoot is quite flexible. When the condition is mild it is often missed at birth and may first present with walking. The affected child exhibits an intoed gait with a neutral patella and femur. Metatarsus adductus is most often idiopathic and probably due to intrauterine positioning. It is associated with restrictions in the transverse arch, manifesting as a resistance to passive lifting. There is tightness in the medial fasciae and adductor muscles of the forefoot, as well as torsion of the first and second metatarsal bones and inversion rotation of the first cuneiform. The calcaneus may be everted. The lateral longitudinal arch is sometimes flattened with the fibula posterior.

Initiation of treatment should begin immediately upon diagnosis. Once the child begins walking the deformity becomes more rigid and less amenable to treatment. As an adjunct to manual treatment, parents should be taught to passively stretch the plantar tissues. If the deformity is severe, serial casting may be required in addition to manual treatment and stretching. Conservative treatment is less successful if not initiated before the age of 3. After this age surgical correction may be necessary.

CLUBFOOT/TALIPES EQUINUS VARUS (Fig. 7.3)

Clinical Notes

Clubfoot is a complex deformity involving dislocation of the talonavicular joint, deformity of the neck of the talus, inversion of the calcaneus, supination of the midfoot and adduction of the forefoot. Internal torsion of the tibia is present, with external rotation of the ankle. In severe cases mild hypoplasia of the fibula, tibia and osseous components of the foot may be present, as well as mild atrophy of the gastrocnemius, soleus, peroneus and tibialis muscles. The blood vessels supplying the dorsal tissues of the foot may be narrowed or absent. Clubfoot can be described as an abnormal molding of the foot, the severity of which is determined by the degree of resistance to correction. Clubfoot is typically classified into three groups: rigid or uncorrectable, postural or partially correctable, and correctable, depending on how it responds to active and passive testing. Active testing refers to the ability of the infant to self-correct the position of the foot. This is done by gently scratching repeatedly along the length of the peroneus muscle from the level of the mid-fibula to the malleoli (Fig. 7.4). The

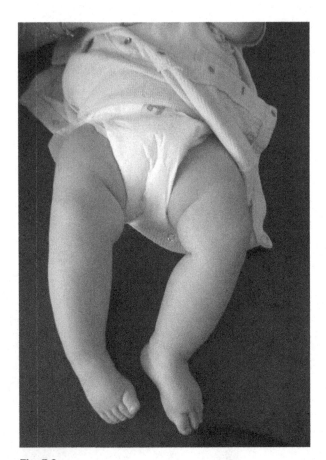

Fig. 7.2

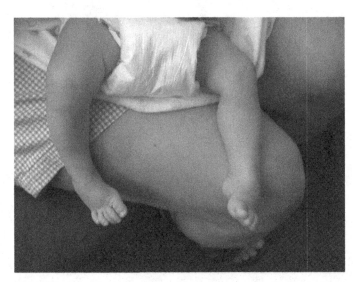

Fig. 7.3

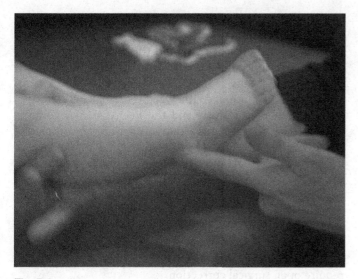

Fig. 7.4

irritation causes the peroneus longus to contract reflexively, which should evert and abduct the foot. If the child can actively reduce the deformity via this reflex, the condition should respond to conservative management.

Treatment Notes

The definitive etiology of clubfoot is unknown; however, intrauterine position, neuromuscular disorder and hereditary factors may all play a role. There have been reports of abnormalities in nerve conduction studies, monosynaptic reflexes, somatosensory fibers and the histochemical analysis of the involved muscles. In spite of this no conclusive studies have been carried out, and as a result specific treatment protocols vary. Consultation with an orthopedic surgeon should be obtained with a suspected diagnosis of clubfoot. In all but the worst cases, conservative management such as casting, taping and manual therapy are tried during the first 3–4 months of life. When conservative management fails, surgery is necessary. This usually involves correction of the talonavicular and subtalar joints and release or lengthening of the flexor tendons of the toes, the peroneus, Achilles and tibialis tendons. Serial casting, splinting and stretching are performed in the postoperative months. Most authors recommend weightbearing as soon as possible to reinforce the surgical corrections. If not corrected, the deformity will worsen as the child grows, the muscles shorten and the lateral aspect of the foot becomes longer than the medial. Some authors suggest that surgical correction should take place before the first birthday to prevent additional bone deformity secondary to growth. Other authors suggest that surgery be delayed until after the first birthday, closer to the time when the child will walk.

In the newborn, the clubfoot deformity most directly influences the structures throughout the limb, pelvis and lumbar spine. The somatic tissues of the medial column of the leg are taut, with myofascial restriction. Shortening of the tibialis anterior and posterior muscles is usually present, with compensatory lengthening of the peroneus muscles. Bowing of the tibia is also present. There is often restriction in the iliotibial band with an outflared and posterior innominate, which usually produces compression of the ipsilateral sacroiliac joint.

The foot abductor muscles need to be strengthened and their resting length shortened. In the newborn, this can be done by repeated stimulation of the peroneus muscles and passive stretching by the parents or caregivers. This is a good home assignment for parents, who can use each diaper change and feed as an opportunity to stimulate the eversion reflex and apply gentle stretching to the medial column of the leg and foot.

CONDITIONS RESULTING IN AN OUT-TURNED FOOT

TALIPES CALCANEOVALGUS/ REARFOOT VALGUS

Clinical Notes

Calcaneus valgus is a condition that occurs in the newborn due to the intrauterine position. It is typically unilateral. The forefoot is dorsiflexed and abducted and the heel is in a valgus position. There is reduced motion at the ankle. An external tibial torsion may occur as compensation for the foot position, and in some cases there is an externally rotated tibia. The fibular head may be posterior, with increased tension in the ipsilateral peroneus longus muscle and iliotibial band, as well as restricted ipsilateral sacroiliac mechanics. As with other congenital deformities, muscle deconditioning and abnormal firing patterns are often present. The plantarflexor and inversion muscles need to be rehabilitated. Parents should be taught to stimulate the foot to encourage plantar flexion and inversion. This can be done by stimulating the plantar grasp reflex or gently pressing on the medial plantar aspect of the infant's foot. The stimulus should not be irritating or the withdrawal reflex will be activated. If the child is unable to right the foot with stimulation, the valgus position may be maintained by somatic dysfunction of the peroneal muscles, and in some cases muscle contractures may even be present.

The differential diagnosis for calcaneus valgus in newborns includes vertical talus. Differentiation can be made on physical examination. Whereas in calcaneus valgus there is normal positioning of the bones of the hindfoot, in congenital vertical talus there is true displacement of the talus and the foot is rigid. Congenital calcaneus valgus typically resolves with conservative treatment such as manipulation and stimulation. As with many other congenital molding deformities, growth plays a role in resolution of the problem. However, if muscle imbalances and dysfunction are not addressed, the deformity may actually worsen with growth. When treating young children, it is prudent to remember the old adage: 'as the twig is bent, so grows the tree.'

Calcaneus valgus may also present in older ambulating children or young athletes. It is then referred to as rearfoot valgus. If it is congenital, there is typically a history of delayed walking. However, more often it is late onset and due to postural factors rather than an undiagnosed congenital condition. Adolescents and young athletes with rearfoot valgus typically present with complaints of ankle or knee pain. Rearfoot valgus is usually associated with increased adductor and internal hip rotator tone and weak gluteus and abdominal muscles. This combination allows the pelvis to tilt anteriorly and the femurs to internally rotate, which loads the medial leg and foot, encouraging further eversion of the calcaneus and pronation of the midfoot. In older children and young athletes the rearfoot valgus is associated with flattening of the medial longitudinal arch with weightbearing. However, the medial arch is flexible and is usually present in non-weightbearing positions. The pes planus is a functional adaptation to the abnormal loading placed on the mid and forefoot by the calcaneal misalignment. The rearfoot mechanics must be addressed before any change in the arch can be sustained. The valgus position of the calcaneus undermines the support system for the anterior talus. Consequently, the talus tends to be in a more plantarflexed position when the foot is loaded in weightbearing. This restricts talocrural motion and places increased stress on the ankle mortise and the medial aspect of the knee. The plantar talus allows the navicular to drop and the integrity of both the medial longitudinal and transverse arches is compromised.

ROCKER-BOTTOM FOOT/ VERTICAL TALUS

Clinical Notes

A rocker-bottom foot is a rare deformity that is often associated with other malformations or part of a congenital syndrome. There are, however, instances where uterine lie or improper casting may produce a rocker-bottom type foot. This occurs when the forefoot is cast in a more dorsiflexed position than the hindfoot. Although the foot appears deformed, it will be quite flexible, unlike a true rocker-bottom foot. In a true rocker-bottom or vertical talus, the talus is displaced inferiorly and medially, towards the plantar surface of the foot. The calcaneus lies lateral to the talus,

the forefoot is dorsiflexed and the talonavicular joint is dislocated. The plantar surface has a convex appearance. The subtalar joint is stiff or rigid, and the level of flexibility in the forefoot depends on the severity of the deformity. The displaced talus fails to articulate correctly with the tibia, limiting ankle motion. With weightbearing the calcaneus moves further posteriorly and the heel does not come in contact with the ground. Contractures of the muscles of the lower leg often develop, contributing to the overall rigidity of the foot and restriction in ankle dorsiflexion. Orthopedic consultation should be sought for all children with suspected vertical talus. In most cases orthotics can be introduced as the child grows, to assist with gait mechanics and improve function. A trial of manipulation and casting is often employed as the initial treatment. In moderate and mild cases this may be enough. However, some children require open surgical correction.

PES PLANUS

Clinical Notes

Pes planus describes a pronated foot with flattening of the medial longitudinal arch. The foot may be flexible or rigid. Rigid pes planus is rare and may be due to peroneal spasm, fusion of the tarsal bones or rigid deformity, such as vertical talus. Flexible pes planus can be either structural or functional.

In toddlers, the plantar arch system is not well formed, giving a flat foot appearance. This is due in part to the immaturity of the osseous structures, particularly the navicular, which does not begin its ossification process until the child is 2 or 3 years old. The ligamentous structures supporting the arches are also immature, and there is a certain amount of physiological ligamentous laxity, which peaks by 3 years and then diminishes. These factors, combined with neuromotor immaturity and the normal varus position of birth, encourage foot pronation. By the age of 4 or 5 the arch system should be established and maintained in the weightbearing position.

Structural pes planus is caused by foot deformities such as calcaneus valgus, accessory navicular and vertical talus. Depending on the severity of the deformity, there is reduced flexibility to passive motion testing of the medial and transverse arches. Structural pes planus is typically present early in life and is often first noted in 3–5-year-olds as the foot thins out and the appearance of the talus becomes more prominent with weightbearing. Structural pes planus may arise as compensation for minor congenital deformities in the forefoot, leg and hips. In early walkers, excessive genu or tibia varum results in compensatory over-pronation at the subtalar and midtarsal joints. If the deformity of the leg does not correct, the foot develops with a pronated stance. There will be tightness and restriction in the somatic tissues of the medial column of the leg, but the peroneus muscle will be tight as well. In children with a varus forefoot, the foot compensates by everting the calcaneus and pronating the midfoot to maintain contact with the ground. The everted calcaneus produces shortening in the tissues of the lateral column. Excessive external rotation at the hip also promotes pronation by abducting the foot. Although at birth external rotation is greater than internal rotation, this discrepancy should improve by the age of 4. Persistent shortening or restriction in the external hip rotators will maintain the pronated posture in the foot. Weakness of the tibialis muscles due to immaturity or neurological paresis will also result in a pes planus.

In most cases flexible pes planus is functional (i.e. postural) and develops later, in early childhood. It usually arises as a postural compensation in the foot to a mechanical or motor dysfunction in the leg, hip or hindfoot. In these children the calcaneus is everted, the talus is in a position of plantar flexion and may be prominent, and the navicular is abducted and dorsiflexed. The key finding is flexibility. Passive dorsiflexion may produce some change at the medial arch, but active engagement of the arch usually fails in these children. Often the concave appearance of the foot diminishes when non-weightbearing is compared to weightbearing. Persistence of the convex appearance in non-weightbearing is typically said to be indicative of a rigid pes planus. However, the author has found that in older children and athletes who have a history of untreated functional pes planus, the convex appearance of the foot may not change in the non-weightbearing position. Children with this problem typically have articular and myofascial dysfunction in the foot which has resulted in shortening of the plantar tissues. Similarly, children who have been wearing rigid orthotics and have not received manipulative treatment of the articular dysfunction or appropriate muscle rehabilitation may also present with persistent pes planus in the non-weightbearing position. In these cases, passive and active testing should be performed to ascertain the functional capabilities and rehabilitation potential of the foot.

Finally, functional pes planus may be caused by poor footwear, deconditioning of muscles and lazy gait mechanics. Biomechanical dysfunctions associated with functional pes planus include internal rotation of the tibia, internal torsion of the tibia or femur, genu valgus, eversion of the calcaneus, and anteriorly tipped pelvis. With chronic pronation the peroneus and Achilles tendons shorten and the tibialis tendons stretch, reinforcing the abnormal posture. During rapid growth phases the appearance of the pes planus may worsen due to the postural influences on the developing bones. The influences of the foot extend beyond the ankle. Poor foot mechanics increase the load on the joints and muscles of the feet, knees and hips. As these areas become strained, the child will compensate by altering gait mechanics, which may further exacerbate the mechanical dysfunctions. As a result, pes planus can be a contributing factor in Osgood–Schlatter syndrome, patellofemoral issues, recurrent ankle sprains, midline joint pain in the knee, shin splints and mechanical hip pain.

In terms of assessment, three components need to be considered in functional pes planus: the change in the arch from non-weightbearing to weightbearing posture; the degree of pronation present with gait; and the flexibility of the arch. If the arch resists active correction but changes with passive correction, manipulative treatment and retraining will be effective. If the arch resists passive correction and the talus is displaced, then treatment will be more protracted and it may be necessary to augment manipulation with a supportive orthotic. Over-pronation during gait needs to be addressed before any correction in the arch can occur. Often simply treating an everted calcaneus will correct the medial arch deformity, but in many patients dysfunctions of the limb and pelvis contribute to the hindfoot dysfunction. Over-pronation not only affects the medial arch, it will also cause loss of the anterior and lateral longitudinal arches and, if excessive, the transverse arch can become rigid and somewhat flattened.

Assessment of Medial Arch

Passive Testing Arch (Figs 7.5 and 7.6)

The child is standing with his weight evenly distributed on both feet. The great toe of one foot is passively dorsiflexed (Fig. 7.6). This maneuver puts tension through the plantar fascia and compresses the first ray of the foot, elevating the medial arch. If the arch does not elevate, one must consider congenital joint fusion, contractures of the plantar tissues, primary muscle disease, rheumatoid arthropathy and spasticity. If the arch can be stimulated this suggests functional pes planus even if the pes planus persists in the non-weightbearing position. Older children should then be assessed for active engagement of the arch.

Non-weightbearing and Weightbearing

The distance from the floor to the base of the navicular can be measured both in weightbearing and non-weightbearing. The difference should be less than 3 mm.

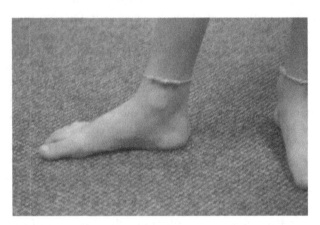

Fig. 7.5

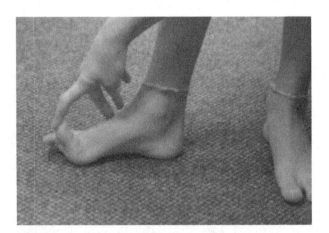

Fig. 7.6

Active Testing Arch

In an older child, functional pes planus can be differentiated from a neurological pes planus by asking the child to grip the ground with his toes (Figs 7.7 and 7.8). This should cause the arch to elevate to some degree. The change in arch height should be compared with that which was achieved with the passive testing (Fig. 7.9). A common reason that the arch does not elevate is muscle weakness, particularly the tibialis muscles. The weakness may be due to neuropathology, myopathy or deconditioning. Strictures of the plantar tissues may also prevent the child from actively engaging the arch.

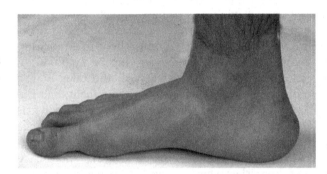

Fig. 7.7

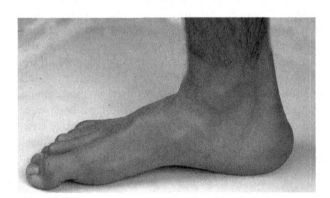

Fig. 7.8

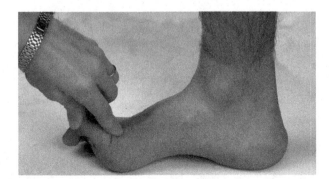

Fig. 7.9

Active Testing of the Calcaneus (Fig. 7.10)

Asking the child to stand on his toes will cause the everted calcaneus to move to a neutral or inverted position. If the foot is truly rigid, the calcaneus will remain everted. This is also a useful test in children with hypotonia or deconditioning of the plantar flexors to assess the level of dysfunction.

Treatment

Retraining Dorsal and Plantar Flexor Muscles

The child can be taught to do repetitive toe raises and heel walking to stimulate recruitment of the muscles supporting the arches (Figs 7.10 and 7.11). Asking the child to slowly rise up on his toes and then to slowly drop down requires eccentric contraction of the gastrocnemius, peroneus longus and flexor hallucis. Asking the child to walk on his heels recruits the tibialis anterior and posterior muscles.

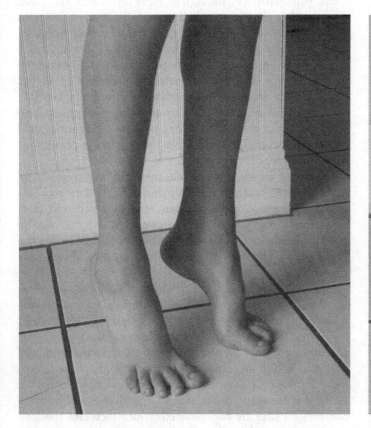

Fig. 7.10

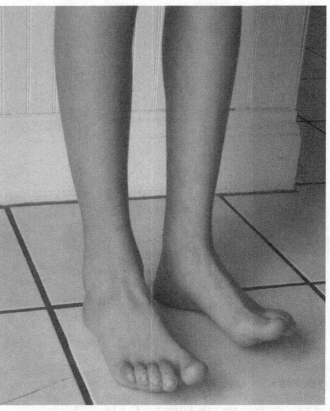

Fig. 7.11

DROPPED LATERAL ARCH

Clinical Notes

Flattening of the lateral arch may be a concurrent finding with pes planus, or it may be secondary to calcaneus varus or peroneus muscle imbalance. Flattening of the lateral arch is often associated with a posterior fibula and may develop after an ipsilateral inversion ankle sprain. The child may complain of discomfort on the lateral aspect of the foot, heel or lateral malleoli. Calluses or blisters may develop on the small toe, which tends to be curled and supinated. In addition to a primary foot problem, flattening of the lateral arch may be secondary to somatic dysfunctions of the fibula, pelvis and sacrum, as well as the peroneus muscle or the hamstring group. The lateral arch is part of the myofascial lateral column system, which supports the sacroiliac joint. This column extends from the inferior sacroiliac ligaments that insert onto the ischial tuberosity. It is contiguous with the tendon of biceps femoris muscle, through the adjacent tendon of the peroneus longus muscle along the fibula and across the lateral arch to the plantar surface of the foot (Fig. 7.12).

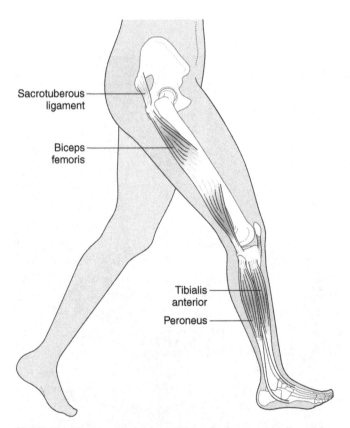

Sacrotuberous ligament

Biceps femoris

Tibialis anterior

Peroneus

Fig. 7.12 • The lateral column stabilizing the lower extremity, pelvis and sacrum during gait. (Adapted from Vleeming A. Movement, stability and low back pain. Edinburgh: Elsevier, 1997, with permission.)

This tensegrity system supports the pelvis, torso and limb in weightbearing and contributes to the propulsion mechanism of gait. Dysfunction of any of the components of the system affects the other components and undermines the integrity of the entire system. This leads to altered gait mechanics, increased load across articular cartilage, overuse syndrome in muscles and increased oxygen consumption.

The lateral column tensegrity system is dependent on proper conditioning of the muscular components. In addition to organic pathology, muscular imbalances can develop as a result of improper training, a sedentary lifestyle and improper footwear. Once this system is disrupted by one dysfunction, the other components develop compensatory adaptations that themselves often represent mechanical dysfunctions. This is particularly important in children with spasticity and hypotonia, where the workload of ambulation is already increased.

PES CAVUS

Clinical Notes

Pes cavus refers to a markedly high medial longitudinal arch. It is not present at birth, but develops in mid to late childhood. It is often uncomfortable, and may present with frank pain with weightbearing. In severe cases the child may develop claw toes or hallucis valgus. It can be seen in demyelinating neuropathies, spina bifida, cerebral palsy, muscular dystrophies and cerebellar disease. In many cases the cause is an imbalance between agonist and antagonist muscle groups. Common imbalances contributing to pes cavus include weak gastrocnemius and strong plantar flexors, weak tibialis anterior and strong hallucis extensors, and weak peroneus brevis and strong peroneus longus. In mild cases orthotics and stretching may help with symptoms, but surgical release may be necessary in severe cases.

When the arch is exaggerated, the child may compensate by turning the forefoot medially during weightbearing. This creates a forefoot varus position. The navicular and talus resist this varus position, so the calcaneus compensates by everting or moving into a valgus position. This increases the pronation of the entire foot, further stressing the plantar tissues.

Some families have hereditary high arches. These children should use footwear that will support their arch, especially when engaged in running or activities requiring sudden stops and starts. In general, children with high medial arches are at risk for injuries and overuse syndrome owing to the rigidity of the arch. A high arch tends to be more tightly packed, with less interosseous movement to accommodate sudden changes in the surface shape or weight. The transverse arch is often compressed laterally and elevated, which increases the load on the metatarsal heads and plantar fasciae. Consequently, young athletes are at risk for developing stress fractures, and children with pes cavus are at risk for developing plantar fasciitis in adulthood.

PEDAL COMPENSATION IN LEG LENGTH DISCREPANCIES

Foot mechanics are affected by differences in leg length. When the child has a short leg, the foot on the ipsilateral side is under greater compressive force from the weight load and may assume a more pronated position. The foot may then compensate by over-supinating at the subtalar joint and by carrying the weight on the lateral aspect of the heel and foot. The contralateral foot will assume a more pronated position with internal rotation of the tibia and femur (see Chapter 5, Femur, Hip, Pelvis for a discussion of evaluation of leg length differences).

PLANTAR FASCIITIS

Clinical Notes

Although commonly thought of as a condition of aging, plantar fasciitis can develop in young athletes through a combination of improper training, poor footwear and/or abnormal foot mechanics. Plantar fasciitis is an overuse syndrome that develops when excessive tensile loads are placed on the plantar fascia, causing repetitive microtrauma. Typically it is common in running sports and sports with sudden stops and starts. However, in the author's experience, plantar fasciitis can also occur in situations where ankle dorsiflexion is limited but forward propulsion is still used, such as roller blades with rigid bottoms, and alpine skiers who spend significant time walking in their boots. Dancers who train *en pointe* place significant stress on the plantar fascia and are at risk for developing plantar fasciitis, especially in the early stages of training or during periods of intense training.

The plantar fasciae can be subjected to excessive tensile loads through several mechanisms. Under normal conditions the plantar fascia lengthens as the foot contacts the ground from the heel-strike to the stance phase of gait, and then shortens as the foot moves into toe-off. This action is a component of the forward propulsion mechanism of the foot. Limited ankle dorsiflexion during stance forces the forefoot to compensate with dorsiflexion and pronation, which increases the stretch on the plantar fascia. Calcaneus varus or a posterior calcaneus shifts the origin and insertion of the fasciae away from each other, increasing the tensile force. Children with pes cavus have naturally shortened and tight plantar fasciae, which are more susceptible to trauma from stretch.

The forces generated during gait are normally absorbed by the plantar arch system. If the arch system is dysfunctional, greater forces are transferred into the fasciae and plantar ligaments, causing microtrauma and inflammation. Overpronation of the subtalar joint stretches the plantar fascia with weightbearing. This can occur because the calcaneus is everted or the tibia is internally rotated. The plantar fascia is an extension of the Achilles tendon; consequently, tight calf muscles or tibial dysfunction may play a role in the development of fasciitis. Tightness of the gastrocnemius and soleus affects the tensile forces in the plantar fasciae by lifting the calcaneus. Hamstring tightness that prevents full knee extension can also be a contributing factor. Consequently, children with spasticity are at risk for developing fasciitis. Children with subtle leg length discrepancy often compensate by limiting heel-strike on the affected side. This places increased stress on the plantar fascia and may progress to fasciitis.

Most plantar foot pain is due to plantar fasciitis. However, when symptoms do not improve with appropriate management one must consider other causes, such as rheumatological disease, tarsal tunnel syndrome with or without thyroid disease, calcaneal apophysitis, myositis of the abductor hallucis or Achilles tendon, and rheumatoid arthritis. In most cases the etiology is mechanical. Leg length discrepancy should be ruled out with leg length tomography. A standing postural study only evaluates standing sacral base unleveling and femoral head heights. Both may be altered by pelvic rotation. In addition, total leg length may be equal, with discrepancies between the lengths of the femurs and tibias. This will significantly affect gait mechanics and alter plantar forces.

SEVER DISEASE (CALCANEAL APOPHYSITIS)

Calcaneal apophysitis is a condition where the apophysis at the insertion of the Achilles tendon becomes inflamed secondary to repetitive microtrauma from either elevated tensile forces or repetitive compression. It tends to be more common in boys than girls, and in children who participate in activities that require repetitive running and stopping, such as soccer, track and basketball. It typically presents between 8 and 16 years, when the two ossification centers of the calcaneus begin to fuse. There are two proposed mechanisms for the condition. Both involve microtrauma and microtears to either the Sharpey's fibers inserting onto the apophysis or the apophysis itself. The patient complains of pain with weightbearing. A highly indicative sign is focal pain when the lateral and medial aspects of the calcaneus are squeezed together. Increased tone or tension in the gastrocnemius and soleus will exacerbate the condition. The goal of treatment is to reduce the tensile load on the tissues. Techniques to stretch the dorsiflexor muscles and fasciae, and to correct mechanical dysfunction in the hind and midfoot should be employed. Heel lifts may be used to shift the center of gravity forward and reduce the tensile load on the calcaneus. In severe conditions casting may be necessary. In general, recovery is slow and may take up to a year.

TREATMENT OF THE FOOT AND ANKLE

Treatment Notes

In the vast majority of chronic foot deformities, gait disturbances and developmental conditions in all age groups, it is necessary to treat all the structures of the foot to correct the problem. In children, the flexibility of the structural relationships allows for significant adaptive and compensatory changes to develop. The interrelatedness of the structures is so profound that it is extremely rare for any condition to localize to any one structure without creating compensatory changes throughout the entire unit. This is especially true in developmental and chronic problems, but may also be appropriately suitable in non-acute traumatic injuries and athletes. Obviously, specific approaches are more effective in certain conditions, but an overall rebalancing of foot biomechanics should be carried out in addition to the specific manipulation.

As a general rule, balanced ligamentous techniques are used in the treatment of congenital and chronic problems in all age groups, even in younger children. Articulatory and thrust techniques may be useful in the treatment of acute injuries in athletes and older children. As a rule, treatment of the hindfoot and ankle mortise should precede treatment of the forefoot. The hindfoot and ankle need to be treated as a functional unit. Typically, this area is addressed first because it is subjected to most of the compressive force entering the foot. The medial arch is treated next because its keystone, the navicular bone, influences both the medial and the transverse arches. This is followed by the transverse and lateral arches. The position of the metatarsals and phalanges is dependent on the arches, so they are addressed once the arches are treated. The plantar fasciae are typically left for last because the tensile forces on these tissues are determined by the functional relations of the aforementioned structures.

BALANCED LIGAMENTOUS TECHNIQUE

Calcaneus

Child

Depending on the size of the child, one of two hand positions can be used (see Alternate technique).

1. The patient is seated or supine with the knee extended.

2. The calcaneus is held in the palm of the physician's hand with the fingers around it posterior and inferior to the malleoli. The other hand stabilizes the talus and the ankle mortise (Fig. 7.13).

3. A firm but gentle traction is placed on the calcaneus to decompress it from the talus and establish balanced ligamentous tension. Initially the traction is in a posterior inferior direction and then the vector is changed to anterior and superior, following the path described in Figure 7.14. Valgus, varus, eversion, inversion, supination, and pronation vectors are introduced to establish balanced ligamentous tension in the talocalcaneal, tibiocalcaneal, and calcaneofibular tissues.

4. Once balanced tension is established, the position is maintained until there is a change in tissue texture, a correction of the mechanical strain or an improvement in tissue function.

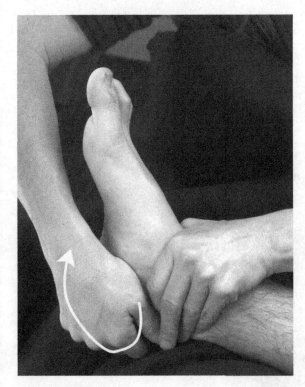

Fig. 7.13

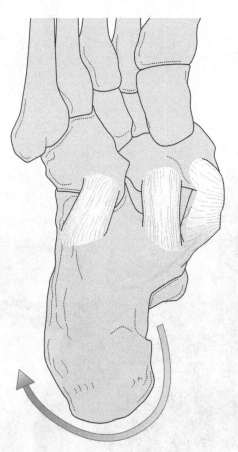

Fig. 7.14

Alternate Hand Position

Athletes and Adolescents

1. The athlete or adolescent is seated or supine with the knee extended and the foot suspended off the table.

2. In athletes and adolescents the physician grasps the calcaneus inferior to the malleoli with the thenar eminences of both hands, interlacing the fingers around the posterior aspect of the heel (Fig. 7.15).

3. A firm but gentle traction is placed on the calcaneus to decompress it from the talus and establish balanced ligamentous tension. Initially the traction is in a posterior inferior direction, and then the vector is changed to anterior and superior following the path described in Figure 7.14. Valgus, varus, eversion, inversion, supination and pronation vectors are introduced to establish balanced ligamentous tension in the talocalcaneal, tibioalcaneal, and calcaneofibular tissues.

4. Once balanced tension is established, the position is maintained until there is a change in tissue texture, a correction of the mechanical strain or an improvement in tissue function.

Fig. 7.15

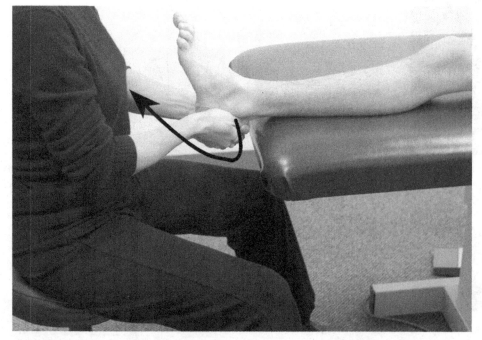

DECOMPRESSION BALANCED LIGAMENTOUS TECHNIQUE

Ankle Mortise and Talus (Talocrural Joint)

Supine Athlete

1. The patient is seated or supine with the knee extended. In an athlete or adolescent, the foot is suspended off the edge of the table.

2. The physician grasps the malleoli bilaterally, either between the index finger and thumb of each hand, or by hooking the knuckle of each index finger posterior to the malleoli (Fig. 7.16).

3. The physician places a firm but gentle traction on the malleoli in an anterior direction allowing the heel and foot to be suspended (Fig. 7.17) (gray arrow). The weight of the suspended foot places a natural posterior traction on the talus and calcaneus (stippled arrow). This counterbalances the anterior lift applied by the physician. A slight lateral vector is introduced into the malleoli through the posterior contact, which distracts the malleoli away from each other (black arrow).

4. This position is fine-tuned to achieve balanced ligamentous tension between the talus, tibia and fibula. Once balanced tension is established the position is maintained until there is a change in tissue texture, a correction of the mechanical strain or an improvement in tissue function.

5. Fibular dysfunction may need to be treated prior to the ankle mortise, especially in traumatic injuries such as inversion sprains.

6. There are instances when more decompression needs to occur at the talocrural articulation than can be generated by the suspended foot. To augment the decompression created by the weight of the foot, the physician can contact the sides of the calcaneus with the knuckles of the middle and ring fingers and provide an inferior traction by spreading the fingers that are contacting the calcaneus away from the thumbs, which are contacting the malleoli.

7. In infants and younger children, the physician may be tempted to grasp both malleoli with the thumb and fingers of one hand and the calcaneus with the other, similar to the position used for treatment of the calcaneus. However, this hand position creates compression across the distal tibiofibular articulation and interferes with the decompression used in this approach.

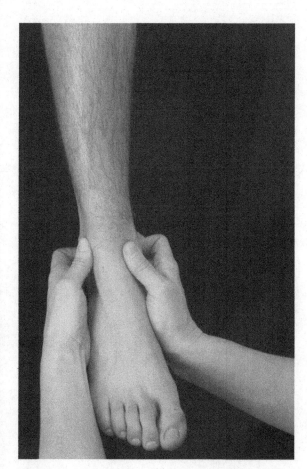

Fig. 7.16

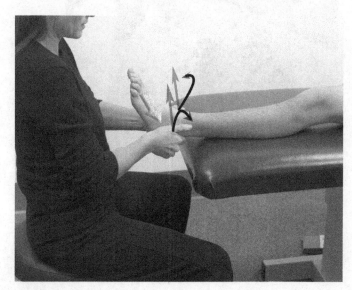

Fig. 7.17

COMPRESSION BALANCED LIGAMENTOUS TECHNIQUE

Talocrural Joint

In traumatic injuries and in larger children and athletes there may be significant compression in the ankle mortise. Often these patients will not respond to decompression but need to be treated with compression.

1. The patient is prone with the knee flexed and the foot up. The physician stands beside the patient (Fig. 7.18).

2. The hand distal to the patient is placed over the plantar surface of the foot, grasping the calcaneus. The other hand wraps around the ankle so that contact is made with the distal end of the tibia.

3. With the foot in a neutral position the hand contacting the calcaneus introduces a firm but gentle compression towards the knee to engage the talus. At the same time the tibia is gently taken posteriorly.

4. Dorsiflexion, plantar flexion, inversion and eversion of the calcaneus and talus are introduced as the tibia is gently taken into internal and external rotation to achieve balanced ligamentous tension.

5. Once balanced tension is established, the position is maintained until there is a change in tissue texture, a correction of the mechanical strain or an improvement in tissue function.

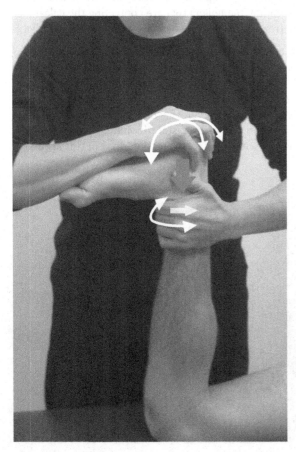

Fig. 7.18

BALANCED LIGAMENTOUS TECHNIQUE

Talocalcaneonavicular Joint

1. The patient is seated or supine with the knee extended and the calcaneus resting on the table or on the physician's leg in a slightly dorsiflexed position. This stabilizes the calcaneus.

2. The physician reaches across the ankle mortise and contacts each malleolus and the tibia (Fig. 7.19). This creates a compressive force across the ankle mortise and stabilizes the talocrural joint. With the other hand, the physician reaches over the dorsum of the foot and wraps her fingers around the medial longitudinal arch, contacting the navicular and talus (Fig. 7.20).

3. With the lateral three fingers grasping the navicular, cuneiform and metatarsals, a gentle anterior traction is used to disengage the subtalar joint (gray arrow). The index finger and thumb of the two hands apply anterior, posterior, dorsiflexion, plantar flexion, inversion and eversion movements to the talus and navicular to achieve balanced tension in the talocalcaneonavicular joint (white arrows).

4. Once balanced tension is established, the position is maintained until there is a change in tissue texture, a correction of the mechanical strain or an improvement in tissue function.

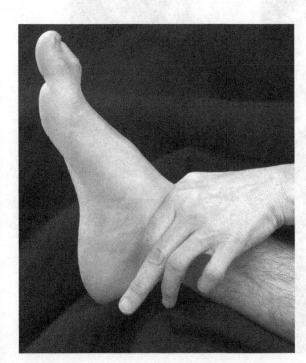

Fig. 7.19

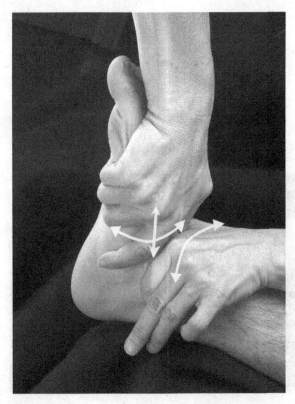

Fig. 7.20

SPRINGING/ARTICULATORY TECHNIQUE

Navicular and Medial Longitudinal Arch

1. The patient is seated or supine with the knee extended. The foot is resting on the table or off the table's edge.

2. The physician sits alongside the patient's leg. The hand that is nearest to the patient's knee is positioned so that the forearm lies on top of the tibia. The talus and ankle are stabilized by the hypothenar eminence and the weight of the arm. The index finger is wrapped around the navicular (Fig. 7.21)

3. The other hand is placed across the dorsum of the foot with the index finger wrapped around the first cuneiform. The index finger contacting the navicular acts as a fulcrum. The cuneiform and forefoot are taken into pronation as the navicular is taken into supination until the restrictive barrier is engaged.

4. A short quick thrust is applied simultaneously with both hands in opposite directions, taking the navicular into supination and the cuneiform and forefoot into pronation (Fig. 7.22). This buckles the arch and allows the navicular to spring back into position.

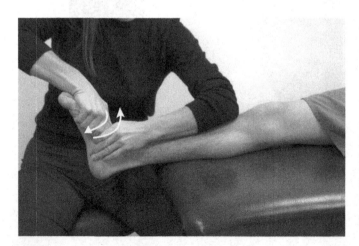

Fig. 7.21

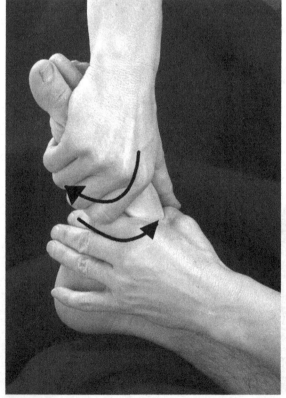

Fig. 7.22

BALANCED LIGAMENTOUS TECHNIQUE

Navicular and Medial Longitudinal Arch

1. The patient is seated or supine with the knee extended and the foot resting on or suspended from the table. The physician sits beside the leg to be treated. The hand that is closest to the patient's knee is positioned so that the arm rests on top of the distal leg, stabilizing the tibia and the ankle. The index finger grasps the talus (Fig. 7.23).

2. The other hand is placed across the dorsum of the foot, with the index finger grasping the navicular and the other fingers grasping the first cuneiform and metatarsal.

3. The cuneiform and metatarsal are tractioned anteriorly away from the navicular (gray arrow). Using opposing motions, the talus and navicular are alternately brought into supination, pronation, plantar and dorsiflexion, compression and decompression to achieve balanced ligamentous tension between the talus and navicular.

4. Once balanced tension is established, the position is maintained until there is a change in tissue texture, a correction of the mechanical strain or an improvement in tissue function.

Fig. 7.23

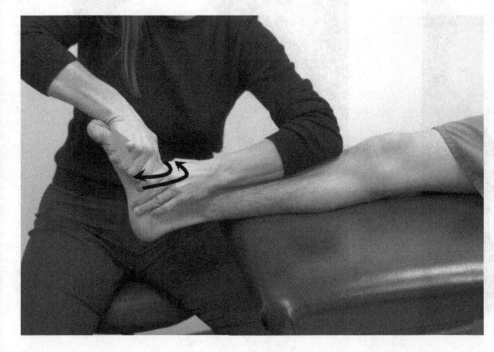

BALANCED LIGAMENTOUS TECHNIQUE

Cuboid and Lateral Longitudinal Arch

In most patients the lateral arch is dysfunctional or flattened. In children it is generally the last arch to develop.

1. The patient is supine or seated with the knee extended and the foot resting on the table or the physician's leg. The physician is positioned opposite to the side of the foot that needs to be treated. The hand proximal to the patient reaches across the leg and grasps the cuboid between the thumb and the index finger (Fig. 7.24).

2. The other hand reaches over the dorsum of the forefoot to grasp the fourth and fifth metatarsals along their entire lengths (Figs 7.25 and 7.26).

3. The metatarsals are gently tractioned away from the cuboid (gray arrow) until a slight freedom of motion is perceived at the cuboid. Then the metatarsals are taken into adduction and supination as the cuboid is lifted superiorly (dorsally) and taken into pronation or supination to establish balanced tension (black arrows).

4. Once balanced tension is established, the position is maintained until there is a change in tissue texture, a correction of the mechanical strain or an improvement in tissue function.

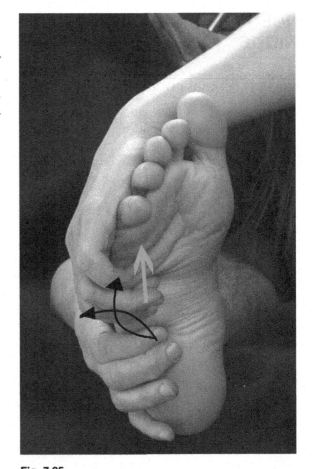

Fig. 7.25

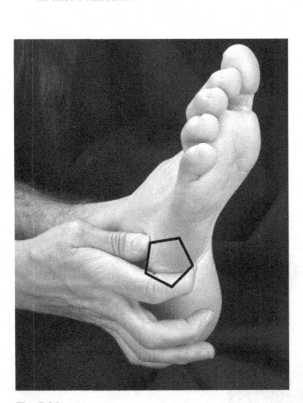

Fig. 7.24

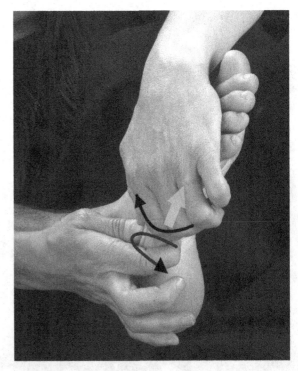

Fig. 7.26

DECOMPRESSION

Transverse Arch and Second Cuneiform

The transverse arch usually becomes compressed and rigid as a result of poor foot mechanics or ankle trauma. Typically the middle cuneiform is wedged between the first and third cuneiforms. This packs the arch tightly, so that it loses what little flexibility it has. As a result, the forces entering the foot are transferred to the metatarsal heads. This can create pain at the ball of the foot or between the metatarsal bones. The second and third metatarsals are most often affected.

1. The patient is supine with the knee extended and the foot resting on the table. The physician sits facing the foot. The thumbs are placed on the plantar surface (Fig. 7.27) under the middle (second) cuneiform, with the fingers over the dorsum of the foot.

2. The thumbs lift the cuneiform as the fingers spread the transverse arch. This position is maintained until there is a tissue release. In older children positional cooperation can be employed and the child is asked to curl his toes down, thereby exaggerating the lift on the cuneiforms.

Fig. 7.27

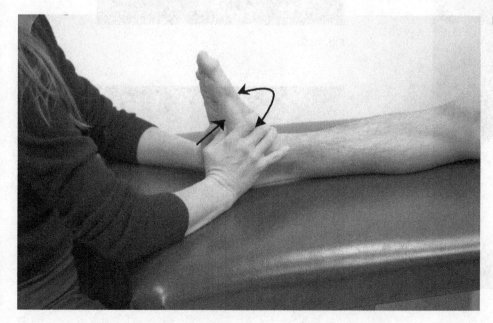

BALANCED LIGAMENTOUS TECHNIQUE

Metatarsal–Cuneiform Articulation

Both the position and the function of the metatarsals are directly influenced by the transverse arch. Compression or dropping of the transverse arch produces flattening at the anterior arch and splaying of the metatarsal heads. With weightbearing, there is increased pressure on the plantar surfaces of the proximal part of the metatarsals. The splaying causes curling of the toes. The line of gravity is shifted laterally in the foot, increasing pressure between the second and third metatarsals, and often causing pain in the lumbrical muscles.

Elevation of the transverse arch can result from wearing rigid orthotics or from trauma to the plantar surface of the foot. When the arch is elevated, the second cuneiform is compressed between the first and third cuneiforms. The medial and lateral arches may appear to be intact, but they are inflexible. There is increased pressure on the heads of the metatarsals, especially the first, with weightbearing, which may result in a flexor hallucis longus tendonitis.

1. The patient is supine or seated with the knee extended. The physician grasps the proximal metatarsal between the thumb and index finger of one hand and its articulating cuneiform with the other (Figs 7.28, 7.29 and 7.30). For the fourth and fifth metatarsals, the cuboid is contacted.

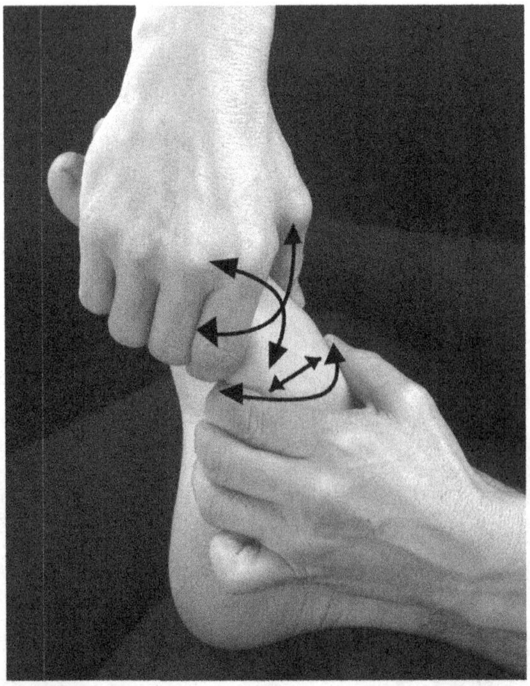

2. Balanced ligamentous tension is established at the articulation by simultaneously introducing vectors of motion into the metatarsal and the articulating bone. Figure 7.26 demonstrates treatment of the first metatarsal. The metatarsal is gently taken into supination, pronation, abduction, adduction, plantarflexion and dorsiflexion as the cuneiform is rotated and translated.

3. Once balanced tension is established, the position is maintained until there is a change in tissue texture, a correction of the mechanical strain or an improvement in tissue function.

4. In older children this same handhold can be used to apply an articulatory force into the joint to establish correction.

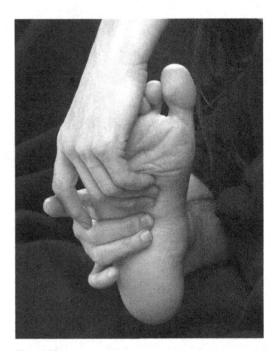

Fig. 7.29

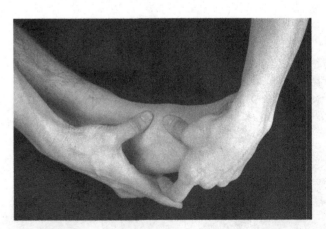

Fig. 7.30

Fig. 7.28

THE USE OF FOOT ORTHOTICS

Clinical Notes

Orthotic devices can be very useful to support the foot in a physiological position and in reinforcing proper mechanics. In general, for ambulating children the author prefers orthotics with some flexibility. Whereas the foot seems to mold passively to a rigid orthotic, orthotics made of polypropylene or some other flexible material encourage some degree of movement between the structures of the foot. It is normal for a few degrees of pronation to occur when one moves from heel-strike to midstance position and there is a minimal amount of pronation in the forefoot which occurs at terminal stance. Rigid orthotics often prevent this natural change to the medial arch and forefoot. Many rigid orthotics are cast with the subtalar joint in a neutral position. In recent years some controversy has arisen around this positioning. The subtalar neutral position is only present for a fraction of the gait cycle, and in single stance most people are slightly dorsiflexed. Although subtalar neutral is an anatomically correct position it is an artificial one from a functional perspective. Furthermore, in the context of the respiratory–circulatory model of osteopathic treatment, passive motion of the plantar tissues plays a role in the arterial, venous and lymphatic circulation in the foot. Rigid orthotics are more likely to limit the involuntary natural movements of plantar tissues than are flexible orthotics.

Although orthotics are typically considered for over-pronation of the medial arch, all three arches should be addressed by any orthotic placed in the shoe. In children, orthotics should be used as an adjunct to manipulation and rehabilitation in all but the most extreme cases. All too often orthotics turn into a crutch that allow the child's foot and leg to become deconditioned and lose any functional capacity it once had. The younger the child, the better the chances are for optimizing functional capacity. This is an important consideration in children with spasticity who are placed in ankle foot orthotics with locked ankle position. The combination of a locked ankle position and a rigid foot orthotic forces the child to adapt to postural perturbations at the knee, hip and pelvis. This produces greater sway and torque, leading to instability.

The hindfoot also needs to be taken into account when using orthotics. A well-structured heel cup that stabilizes the calcaneus in a neutral position is important to encourage a neutral heel when the child has a calcaneal displacement, tibial torsion or genu deformity. Owing to the flexibility of the pedal structures, younger children will often accommodate dysfunction in the tibia, knee or hip by altering the placement of the foot. For example, toddlers with untreated internal tibial torsions or genu valgus may compensate by shifting their weight medially and creating a rearfoot valgus. If these developmental deformities are not addressed, the child will 'grow into' the pattern through training of muscle firing patterns, resting muscle lengths and bone growth adaptations. The foot adaptation reinforces the dysfunction of the leg and hip and a cycle of adaptation is created. This cycle can often be interrupted by an orthotic that supports the correct rearfoot position until the dysfunctions of the leg and hip are resolved.

Good foot orthotics will affect more than the feet: changes will occur throughout the legs, pelvis and spine. The characteristics of the orthotics are determined by appropriate foot measurements and gait assessment. However, the clinician will still need to evaluate the effect of the orthotics on the child's posture and balance to determine whether or not they are appropriate. Proper fit can be assessed by viewing the child while he is standing in the orthotics. The Achilles tendon should lie in the midline of the leg without valgus or varus deviation. The tibias should be in a slightly externally rotation position, the femurs slightly internally rotated but not anteverted, and the pelvis neutral. Standing leg lengths, iliac crest heights, PSIS and ASIS landmarks should be symmetrical and equal, assuming there is no leg length difference. There should be no innominate rotation, and the standing flexion test should be negative. On forward bending evaluation there should be a decrease in a rib asymmetry. In some children, the functional component of a scoliosis can be corrected with proper foot orthotics. On lateral view there should be a direct line between the ear, shoulder, hip and ankle. On anterior view, the line of gravity from the hip should pass through the center of the leg and ankle, lying between the first and second metatarsals. Postural stress testing should demonstrate good balance and symmetry.

Obviously, regardless of the thickness of the orthotic, it is imperative that any patient requiring an orthotic wears one in both shoes. Even the thinnest orthotic will create innominate rotation, pelvic imbalance and sacral unleveling unless an orthotic of identical thickness is worn in the contralateral shoe.

TRAUMATIC INJURIES

ANTERIOR TIBIA ON TALUS

Clinical Notes

This injury typically occurs in athletes wearing cleated shoes. The athlete suddenly stops while running, the foot is locked into position by the cleat, but the momentum of the body carries the athlete forward. This mechanism can also result in a posterior tibia on the femur, and if the force is strong enough, can cause injury to the posterior cruciate ligament. If the primary problem is the anterior tibia on the talus, then the athlete will complain of discomfort in the anterior aspect of the ankle and foot with dorsiflexion. The pain typically presents with running, climbing stairs, and at the end of the stance phase of gait. Compared to the contralateral ankle, passive and active range of dorsiflexion will be reduced and movement in other planes will be restricted when the ankle is dorsiflexed. There is often tenderness over the anterior aspect to the talus and tender points in the gastrocnemius and soleus muscles.

TREATMENT

Thrust Technique

Talocrural Joint

1. The patient is prone with the knee flexed and the foot up. The physician stands beside the leg and grasps the tibia with the hand closest to the patient's hip (Fig. 7.31).

2. The other hand grasps the calcaneus. The physician's wrist and forearm are placed along the plantar surface of the foot. The physician uses her forearm to dorsiflex the ankle to the restrictive barrier.

3. A firm but gentle thrust is employed with both hands simultaneously. The plantar hand takes the foot in an arc towards dorsiflexion, and the hand on the tibia brings the distal tibia posteriorly. There should be an improvement in dorsiflexion and resolution of the tenderness.

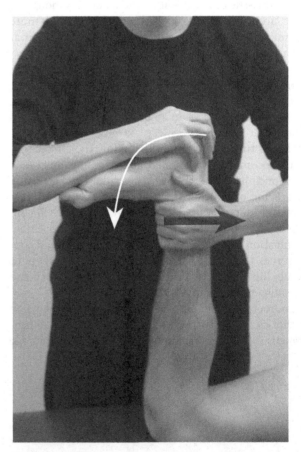

Fig. 7.31

Thrust Technique

Talocrural Joint

1. The patient is supine with the knee extended. The physician stands beside the leg to be treated. The proximal hand is placed over the ankle mortise as close to the talus as possible (Fig. 7.32).

2. The distal hand is placed under the heel. This hand cups the calcaneus while the wrist and forearm lie alongside the plantar surface of the foot.

3. A gentle pressure is used to push the tibia towards the table, as the foot is dorsiflexed to the restrictive barrier. A short firm impulse is employed to dorsiflex the ankle through the restrictive barrier as the tibia is simultaneously taken posteriorly (into the table).

BALANCED LIGAMENTOUS TECHNIQUE

Talocrural Joint

This technique (similar to one described previously) may be used to treat both talocrural and subtalar dysfunction in traumatic injuries. The forces are first directed at the talocrural and then at the subtalar joints.

1. The patient is prone with the knee flexed and the foot elevated. The physician stands alongside the involved ankle. Similar to the articulatory technique, the proximal hand grasps the tibia and the distal hand grasps the heel with the wrist and forearm along the plantar surface (see Fig. 7.16).

2. A firm but gentle compression is placed into the subtalar joint until a slight increase in freedom of motion is perceived. If too much compression is used the joint will lock. The compression should create slack in the surrounding tissues, not engage the joint.

3. The tissues of the talocrural and subtalar joints are brought into balanced tension through the movements of the tibia and the foot. The tibia is internally and externally rotated and translated anteriorly and posteriorly. Abduction, adduction, inversion, eversion, plantar and dorsiflexion are introduced simultaneously into the subtalar and talocrural joints.

4. Once balanced tension is established, the position is held until there is a change in tissue texture, an improvement in tissue function or correction of the strain occurs.

Fig. 7.32

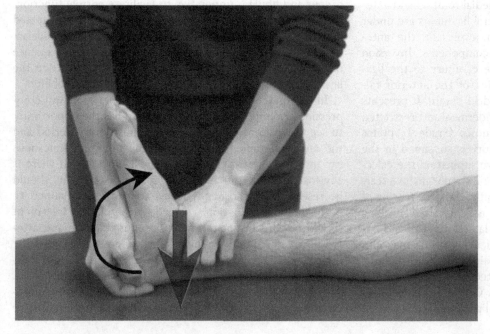

INVERSION ANKLE SPRAIN

Clinical Notes

Inversion sprains are the most common form of ankle injury and involve injury to the lateral collateral ligaments. In severe injuries, the ligaments may rupture and the talus maybe displaced anteriorly on the tibia. Athletes with inversion sprains are at risk for recurrent injury. Almost a third of patients with ankle sprains will develop mechanical instability, and up to 30% continue to have problems months after the acute injury. One of the key points of concern in ankle injuries is the function of the talus. The weight of the body is transmitted through the tibia to the dome of the talus and then into the foot. The talus forms three important joints: one with the ankle, one with the calcaneus and one with the navicular. Consequently, normal function of the foot and ankle is dependent on the talus. The movement of the talus at the ankle mortise involves dorsiflexion with lateral rotation and plantar flexion with medial rotation. The talocrural joint is more stable in dorsiflexion owing to the posterior wedged shape of the talus and the long fibula, which limit posterior motion and lateral rotation, respectively. In plantar flexion the joint is vulnerable. The wider anterior surface of the dome allows for anterior glide of the talus on the tibia when the joint is open, and the short medial malleoli allow for medial rotation. Furthermore, in plantar flexion only the posterior aspect of the talus dome comes in contact with the tibia, and stability depends more on the surrounding ligaments than the bony mechanics.

In an inversion sprain the talus is plantar flexed and supinated as the weight descends onto the foot. This is the most vulnerable position for the talus. Its articulation with the ankle mortise is open, allowing for medial rotation and anterior displacement. The lateral collateral ligaments are under the greatest strain in this position, especially the anterior talofibular and calcaneofibular components. Inversion sprains can be graded by the degree of injury to the ligamentous structures. Minimum tearing of the anterior talofibular ligament is considered a grade 1 sprain. It presents as mild localized swelling, point tenderness and restricted motion. There is usually no ecchymosis. Grade 1 sprains usually occur when most of the injury is sustained in the plantarflexed position. With excessive supination the calcaneofibular ligament is stressed. Grade 2 sprains involve tearing or rupture of the anterior ligament and partial tearing of the calcaneofibular ligament. There is generalized swelling ecchymosis and tenderness over the lateral malleoli and lateral aspect of the hindfoot. The articular capsule may also be injured. The patient will have pain with weightbearing and be unable to stand on the affected foot. There may be some instability with passive testing. Grade 3 sprains occur when both the anterior and lateral ligaments are ruptured

as well as the capsule. The patient is unable to bear weight. The lateral foot and ankle are diffusely swollen, ecchymotic and tender. There is obvious instability with passive testing. Anterior drawer sign will be positive if the anterior talofibular ligament has been ruptured. If it has been strained, the patient will complain of pain and there may be guarding. The talar tilt test evaluates calcaneal inversion. The foot is slightly plantarflexed and the heel inverted. The motion is compared with the contralateral leg. In grade 3 sprains the talar tilt and anterior drawer test will be positive. In grade 2 sprains the talar tilt test will result in pain but no instability if the ligament is still intact. Fractures need to be ruled out in younger children because of the vulnerability of the epiphyseal plate. The two most common fractures in inversion ankle sprains are Salter–Harris and avulsion type. The child with a fracture will have exquisite point tenderness over the site.

Inversion sprains create primary dysfunction at the subtalar and talocrural joints and secondary dysfunction in other areas. With an inversion sprain, the talus is drawn anteriorly and rotated medially, the calcaneus inverts and the transverse arch is bowed. The fibula is brought posteriorly by the stretch on the peroneus longus, and the tibia may rotate laterally. The displacement of the talus affects the subtalar joint and drops the medial longitudinal arch. The momentum of the forward-moving body collapsing the foot often creates a fascial strain extending into the pelvis, thoracolumbar fascia and contralateral rib cage (Blood 1980).

Treatment Notes

The treatment sequence will depend on the chronicity and severity of the injury. However, correction of the talus, calcaneus and fibula is imperative to facilitate normal function.

In general, the displaced or strained talus can be treated immediately after injury by a trained and qualified clinician. Once the inflammatory phase begins, the treatment sequence often changes because the presence of the edema restricts the ligamentous tissues and can significantly limit joint mobility.

In the first 24 hours after the injury, elevation and compression are important. If the physician has the opportunity to see the patient in the immediate post-injury period and the ankle is stable, correction of the talus and calcaneus can improve the patient's condition significantly. If there is any instability of the ankle, correction of the talus should be reserved for those physicians trained and qualified to perform joint reduction. Instead, manipulative treatment should be directed at improving venous drainage and arterial flow to facilitate wound healing. Venous and lymphatic drainage may be improved by addressing the junctional areas of the torso, the pelvic diaphragm and the popliteal fossa. The use of anti-inflammatory medication for pain management is somewhat controversial because of its suppressive effects on connective tissue healing. Assisted weightbearing with a crutch or cane is prudent, even in grade 1 sprains, because the distorted proprioceptive input from the area can lead to temporary balance issues.

In patients with grade 1 and 2 injuries management will depend on the severity of the injury at presentation. The sequence of treatment of the primary and secondary strains is based on the level of discomfort. Commonly, once the initial inflammatory response has occurred, pain and swelling often make it difficult to mechanically address the primary sprain in the subtalar and talocrural joints. In these cases, initial treatment goals should include lymphatic drainage, relieving muscle spasm and correcting secondary strains. This can be done by treating the junctional areas of the spine, the rib cage, the pelvis, popliteal fossa, peroneus and fibula. Gentle passive techniques such as BLT, passive range of motion and FPR can be introduced after the first 24–36 hours. Venous and lymphatic drainage techniques, elevation and compression should continue to be employed. As the edema improves, it becomes easier to address the foot mechanics. In general, patients should begin non-weightbearing range of motion exercises on the day after the injury. A very comfortable manner in which to begin this process is to have the patient soak the foot and ankle in a cool bath while slowly moving them through the full range of motions. Such motions should include abduction, adduction, flexion, extension, inversion and eversion, as well as more subtle movements to stimulate proprioception, such as outlining the letters of the alphabet with her foot. This should be done without a wrap or compression, and it should be painless. Pain should not be ignored. The patient should rehabilitate the ankle within the confines of painless activities only. In young adolescents, persistent pain with non-weightbearing may be indicative of occult fracture. As soon as possible the patient should progress to exercises against controlled resistance, such as riding a stationary bicycle. Again, this should be painless. Depending on the extent of tissue damage, sometime between the first and third weeks after the injury, the patient should begin weightbearing exercises such as side-stepping, climbing stairs, stepping backwards, rising on toes, rising on heels. Complaints of stiffness are typical, but the exercises should be modified if there is pain.

In patients with grade 3 injuries, casting or rigid bracing is usually necessary. Initial osteopathic management should focus on facilitating arterial, venous and lymphatic flow to support tissue healing and treating other areas of the body affected by the abnormal gait and use of crutches. The thoracolumbar and lumbosacral junctions, the rib cage, thoracic spine, shoulders, and thoracic inlet are common areas of dysfunction due to the walking cast or crutches. Strains involving the fibular head, tibia, peroneus, biceps femoris and innominate are usually secondary to the injury and should be treated using gentle techniques. From an osteopathic perspective, removing the secondary strains facilitates the body's natural healing ability and assists repair at the site of injury. The patient should be re-examined at least weekly to maintain function in these areas. Towards the end of the second week, the mechanics of the foot may be gently addressed. Again, begin away from the talus, freeing and rebalancing the structures surrounding it. Articulatory, thrust and muscle energy techniques are contraindicated in unstable ankles, with one exception: a trained and qualified clinician may perform manipulative adjustment for specific reduction of a displaced or dislocated structure. Gentle balancing, unwinding or myofascial techniques can be used to treat the calcaneus, the distal fibula, the navicular and distal tibia. Once there is some freedom in the structures surrounding the subtalar and talocrural joints, treatment can be directed at the mechanical strain or displacement of the talus. The specific technique chosen will depend on the feel of the tissue, the age of the patient, patient comorbidities and practitioner preference. It may take the unstable ankle 3 or more weeks to achieve sufficient ligamentous integrity to perform non-weightbearing range of motion exercises, which should begin as soon as is appropriate. Use of a water bath provides some passive resistance. The same types of motions should be employed as described for milder sprains. Muscle atrophy is a problem in the cast leg, and patients benefit from both isometric exercises and visualized movements while still in the cast.

In patients with chronic or recurrent ankle problems after an ankle sprain the problem is often related to non-reduction of the talus dysfunction coupled with compensatory adaptations in the midfoot and calcaneus. In these patients, the talus may still have some component of plantar flexion, medial rotation or supination remaining after the sprain has healed. The calcaneus and navicular have to adapt to the subsequent shift in the placement of weight. Typically the calcaneus was inverted by the injury, so contact on heel-strike is displaced laterally. The patient compensates by over-pronating the forefoot. The medial longitudinal arch may be flat with standing, but sometimes the pronation is only present with ambulation. The calcaneus often shifts posteriorly, placing more stress on the plantar tissues. Myofascial restriction extending through the peroneus–biceps femoris mechanism may further complicate the biomechanical picture with lumbar, pelvic and sacral dysfunctions. In addition to normalizing foot mechanics, these other areas need to be addressed with a combination of manipulation, proprioceptive retraining and rebalancing and strengthening exercises.

Myofascial Milking Technique

Athlete

A general rule in all fluid, lymphatic and fascial milking techniques is to treat the most proximal areas first, then move distally. In all cases, the junctional areas of the spine should be treated before the extremity. This technique was also described in the treatment of compartment syndrome and shin splints; whereas in those conditions the palpatory focus is the compartment and the pressure is very light, in the case of foot and ankle edema the palpatory focus is more superficial but the pressure applied is increased.

1. The patient is supine. The physician stands contralateral to the leg to be treated. The lower leg (inferior to the knee) is visually divided into thirds. Beginning at the most distal end of the most proximal third, the physician contacts the tissues with both hands.

2. Using both hands, the physician employs a gentle kneading motion moving in a distal to proximal direction within that proximal third of the lower leg (Fig. 7.33). This is repeated twice.

3. Then the physician moves her hands to the distal end of the middle third of the leg (Fig. 7.34). Working in a distal to proximal direction the physician employs a gentle kneading motion with both hands noting any change in tissue texture. This is repeated twice.

4. The physician then moves her hands to the distal end of the distal third of the lower leg (Fig. 7.35). Working in a distal to proximal direction, the physician employs a gentle kneading motion with both hands, noting any change in tissue texture. This is repeated twice.

5. The entire sequence may be repeated two to three times until a change in tissue texture or an improvement in tissue function is noted.

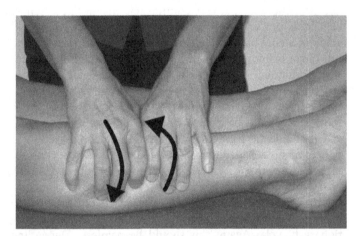

Fig. 7.34

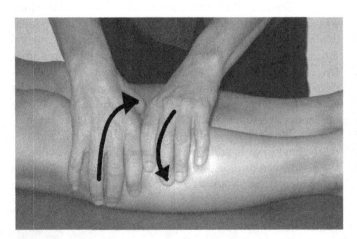

Fig. 7.33

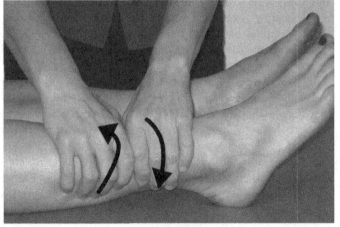

Fig. 7.35

HIGH-VELOCITY LOW-AMPLITUDE TALOTIBIAL/INVERSION SPRAIN

The patient often complains of pain with dorsiflexion and loading, there is tenderness at the anterior aspect of the talotibial junction, and dorsiflexion is limited on active and passive testing.

1. The patient is supine with the hips and knees extended. The physician sits at the patient's feet. The physician's hands are clasped over the dorsum of the foot with the thumbs on the plantar surface (Fig. 7.36).

2. The physician dorsiflexes and everts the foot to engage the restrictive barrier.

3. A short, quick impulse introducing traction, dorsiflexion and eversion is applied to the foot to reseat the talus in the ankle mortise.

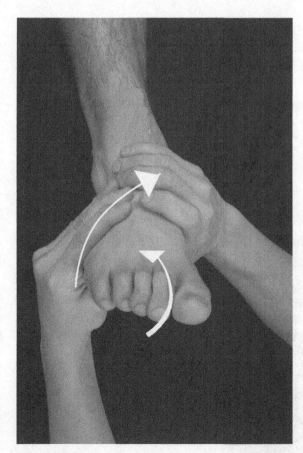

Fig. 7.36

THRUST TECHNIQUE FOR A POSTERIOR FIBULAR HEAD

This technique is also described in Chapter 6, on the Lower Leg. It is repeated here because it should be done following the reseating of the talus in patients with inversion ankle sprains. This is especially true if there is tenderness at the posterior margin of the fibular head or restricted motion of the fibula with ankle dorsiflexion and plantar flexion.

1. The patient is supine with the hip and knee flexed.

2. The physician places the metacarpophalangeal joint of the first and second fingers posterior to the fibular head. The other hand grasps the distal end of the tibia and fibula (Fig. 7.37).

3. The knee is flexed to the barrier while maintaining contact with the fibular head.

4. Simultaneously the physician employs two short, firm thrusts. One brings the patient's foot towards the ischial tuberosity (white arrow) and the other (black arrow) moves the fibular head anteriorly.

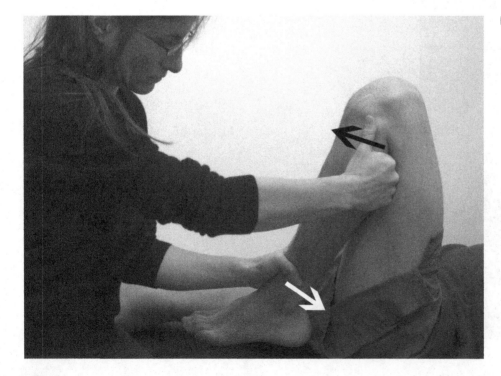

Fig. 7.37

References

Blood SD. Treatment of the sprained ankle. J Am Osteopath Assoc 1980; 79: 680–692.

Burnett C, Johnson E. Development of gait in childhood II. Dev Med Child Neurol 1971; 13: 207–215.

Printed in the United States
By Bookmasters